This book should be returned by the last date stamped
above. You may renew the loan for a further period
if the book is not required by another reader.

Practical Hemostasis and Thrombosis

Practical Hemostasis and Thrombosis

EDITED BY

Denise O'Shaughnessy

Director of Laboratory Haematology, Consultant Haematologist (Haemostasis and Transfusion), Southampton University Hospitals, Southampton, UK

Michael Makris

Director, Sheffield Haemophilia and Thrombosis Centre, Royal Hallamshire Hospital, Sheffield, UK

David Lillicrap

Professor, Department of Pathology and Molecular Medicine, Richardson Laboratories, Queen's University, Kingston, Ontario, Canada

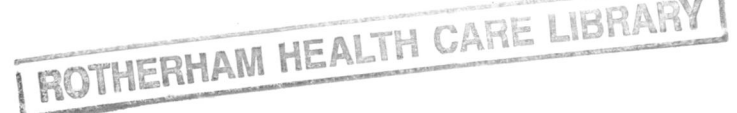
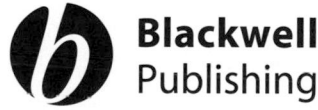
Blackwell Publishing

Blackwell Publishing, Inc., 350 Main Street, Malden, Massachusetts 02148-5020, USA
Blackwell Publishing Ltd, 9600 Garsington Road, Oxford OX4 2DQ, UK
Blackwell Publishing Asia Pty Ltd, 550 Swanston Street, Carlton, Victoria 3053, Australia

First published 2005

Library of Congress Cataloging-in-Publication Data
Practical hemostasis and thrombosis / edited by Denise O'Shaughnessy, Michael Makris, David Lillicrap.
    p. ; cm.
  ISBN-13: 978-1-4051-3030-1 (alk. paper)
  ISBN-10: 1-4051-3030-X (alk. paper)
1. Blood coagulation disorders. 2. Thrombosis. 3. Hemostasis.
  [DNLM: 1. Hemostasis—physiology. 2. Blood Coagulation Disorders. 3. Hemorrhagic Disorders. 4. Thromboembolism. 5. Thrombosis. WH 310 P895 2005] I. O'Shaughnessy, Denise. II. Makris, Michael. III. Lillicrap, David. IV. Title.

  RC647.C55P734 2004
  616.1'57—dc22

                                                    2004028924

ISBN-13: 978-1-4051-3030-1
ISBN-10: 1-4051-3030-X

A catalogue record for this title is available from the British Library

Set in 9.5/12pt Sabon by Graphicraft Limited, Hong Kong
Printed and bound in India by Replika Press Pvt. Ltd

Commissioning Editor: Maria Khan
Development Editor: Claire Bonnett
Production Controller: Kate Charman

For further information on Blackwell Publishing, visit our website:
http://www.blackwellpublishing.com

The publisher's policy is to use permanent paper from mills that operate a sustainable forestry policy, and which has been manufactured from pulp processed using acid-free and elementary chlorine-free practices. Furthermore, the publisher ensures that the text paper and cover board used have met acceptable environmental accreditation standards.

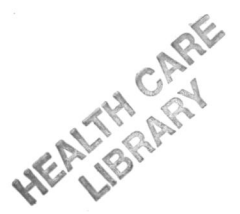

Contents

List of Contributors

Roopen Arya
MA, PhD, MRCPath, FRCP
Consultant Hematologist
Department of Hematological Medicine
King's College Hospital
London
UK

Mary Bauman
RN, BA
Advanced Practice Nurse Intern
Pediatric Thrombosis Program
Stollery Children's Hospital
University of Alberta
Edmonton
Alberta
Canada

Victor S. Blanchette
MD, FRCPC, FRCP
Professor
Department of Pediatrics
University of Toronto
Toronto
Ontario
Canada
and
Hospital For Sick Children
Toronto
Ontario
Canada

Paula Bolton-Maggs
FRCP, FRCPath, FRCPCH
Consultant Hematologist
Manchester Royal Infirmary
Manchester
UK

Giancarlo Castaman
Department of Hematology and
Hemophilia and Thrombosis Center
San Bortolo Hospital
Italy

Marco Cattaneo
MD
Professor
Unit of Hematology and Thrombosis
Ospedale San Paolo

Department of Medicine, Surgery and
Dentistry
University of Milan
Milan
Italy

Adrian Copplestone
MB BS, FRCP, FRCPath, ILMT
Consultant Hematologist
Derriford Hospital
Plymouth
UK

Benilde Cosmi
MD, PhD
Lecturer
Department of Angiology and Blood
Coagulation
University Hospital S. Orsola–Malpighi
Bologna
Italy

Anna Falanga
MD
Associate Professor, Research Associate
Hematology–Oncology Department
Ospedali Riuniti Bergamo
Bergamo
Italy

Paul Harrison
BSc, PhD, MRCPath
Clinical Scientist
Oxford Hemophilia Centre and
Thrombosis Unit
Churchill Hospital
Oxford
UK

Beverley J. Hunt
MD, FRCP, FRCPath
Consultant
Department of Hematology and
Rheumatology
Guy's & St Thomas' Trust
London
UK

Paula James
MD, FRCPC
Assistant Professor

Department of Pathology and Molecular
Medicine
Department of Medicine
Queen's University
Kingston
Ontario
Canada

Walter H.A. Kahr
MD, FRCPC
Assistant Professor
Division of Hematology/Oncology
Hospital for Sick Children
Toronto
Canada

Raj S. Kasthuri
MD
Fellow in Hematology and Oncology
Department of Medicine
Division of Hematology and Oncology and
Transplantation
University of Minnesota Medical School
Minneapolis
USA

Clive Kearon
MB, PhD
Professor
McMaster Medical Unit
Henderson General Hospital
Hamilton
Ontario
Canada

Nigel S. Key
MB ChB, FRCP
Professor of Medicine
MMC 480 Mayo Building
Minneapolis
USA

Steve Kitchen
BSc, PhD
Principal Clinical Scientist
Sheffield Hemophilia and Thrombosis
Centre
Royal Hallamshire Hospital
Sheffield
UK

David Lillicrap
MD, FRCPC
Professor
Department of Pathology and Molecular
Medicine
Richardson Laboratories
Queen's University
Kingston
Ontario
Canada

Lori-Ann Linkins
MD
McMaster Medical Unit
Henderson General Hospital
Hamilton
Ontario
Canada

Gordon D.O. Lowe
MD, FRCP, FFPH
Professor of Vascular Medicine
University of Glasgow
Glasgow Royal Infirmary
Glasgow
UK

Rhona M. Maclean
MRCP, MRCPath
Consultant Hematologist
Sheffield Hemophilia and Thrombosis
Centre
Royal Hallamshire Hospital
Sheffield
UK

Michael Makris
MA, MD, FRCP, FRCPath
Director
Sheffield Haemophilia and Thrombosis
Centre
Royal Hallamshire Hospital
Sheffield
UK

Marina Marchetti
BioSC
Research Associate
Hematology–Oncology Department
Ospedail Riunti Bergamo
Bergamo
Italy

Patricia Massicotte
MSc, MD, FRCPC
Peter Olley Chair
Pediatric Thrombosis Program
Stollery Children's Hospital
University Of Alberta
Edmonton
Alberta
Canada

Niamh M. O'Connell
MB, MRCPI, MRCPath
Consultant Hematologist
The Adelaide and Meath Hospital and
Trinity College
Dublin
Ireland

Denise O'Shaughnessy
DPhil, FRCP, FRCPath, MBA
Director of Laboratory Haematology
Consultant Haematologist (Haemostasis
and Transfusion)
Southampton University Hospitals
Southampton
UK

Raj K. Patel
MRCP, MRCPath
Consultant Hematologist
Department of Hematological Medicine
King's College Hospital
London
UK

Gualtiero Palareti
MD
Professor
Department of Angiology and Blood
Coagulation
University Hospital S. Orsola–Malpighi
Bologna
Italy

Francesco Rodeghiero
Department of Hematology and
Hemophilia and Thrombosis Center
San Bortolo Hospital
Vicenza
Italy

Sara E. Stuart-Smith
MRCP
Research Associate
Departments of Hematology and
Rheumatology
Guy's & St Thomas' Trust
London
UK

R. Campbell Tait
BSc, MB ChB, FRCP, FRCPath
Consultant Hematologist
Glasgow Royal Infirmary
Glasgow
UK

Alberto Tosetto
Department of Hematology and
Hemophilia and Thrombosis Center
San Bortolo Hospital
Vicenza
Italy

Steven von Kier
DA, MBSc, FCIBM
Divisional Programme Manager
Integrated Blood Management Programme
Oxford Radcliffe Hospital NHS Trust
UK

Isobel D. Walker
MD, FRCP, FRCPath
Professor of Hematology
Glasgow Royal Infirmary
Scotland
UK

Henry G. Watson
MD, FRCP, FRCPath
Consultant Hematologist
Department of Hematology
Aberdeen Royal Infirmary
Aberdeen
Scotland
UK

Jonathan Wilde
MD, FRCP, FRCPath
Consultant Hematologist
Manchester Royal Infirmary
Manchester
UK

Part 1

The laboratory interface

Chapter 1

Basic principles underlying the coagulation system

Niamh M. O'Connell

Introduction

The coagulation system, incorporating pro- and anticoagulant proteins, the fibrinolytic system, platelets and the vascular endothelium, is a critical system in homeostasis. An efficient system to repair defects in the vessel wall is clearly beneficial but thrombosis in critical sites can also be detrimental to normal physiology, hence the highly developed anticoagulant and fibrinolytic systems. The importance of elements of the system is indicated by the presence of homologous proteins in primitive organisms and studies suggest that these proteins evolved at least 450 million years ago.

Coagulation factors also have a role in normal embryonic growth and development, and complete deficiencies in tissue factor (TF), factor VII (FVII), tissue factor pathway inhibitor (TFPI), factor X (FX), factor V (FV), prothrombin (PT) or protein C (PC) result in embryonic lethality in transgenic mice.

In recent years, the interplay between coagulation and inflammation/sepsis has been increasingly recognized with a number of anticoagulant proteins associated with pronounced anti-inflammatory effects. PC and antithrombin (AT) have both been used effectively in the treatment of sepsis and improvements in mortality rates are seen with infusions of activated PC which are independent of pretreatment levels.

The current model of coagulation

Formation of a fibrin clot is the final result of a complex series of proteolytic events.

Previous models of coagulation suggested that the intrinsic and extrinsic coagulation cascades functioned independently. It is now understood that there are two phases of coagulation, which are intimately linked:
1 initiation, and
2 propagation.

Thrombin plays a central part:
1 in the activation of factors and cofactors that promote further thrombin generation;
2 in the activation of anticoagulant factors that extinguish thrombin generation; and
3 in determining the balance of fibrinolysis.

The role of platelets in both primary hemostasis (generation of the platelet plug) and secondary hemostasis (formation of a fibrin clot) is also recognized.

Platelets

Platelets are central to primary hemostasis. They are responsible for the initial closure of the defect in the vessel wall through the formation of the platelet plug. Important pro- and anticoagulant factors are stored within platelet granules and these are released into the microenvironment around vessel injury. In secondary hemostasis, platelets provide the membrane surface to which the activated clotting factors bind, leading to increased enzyme efficiency and increased thrombin generation.

Platelets are produced from megakaryocytes in the bone marrow and are released into the circulation. The platelet count is in the range $150-400 \times 10^3/L$ in normal individuals and the circulating half-life is approximately 10 days.

The platelet structure has a number of specialized features:

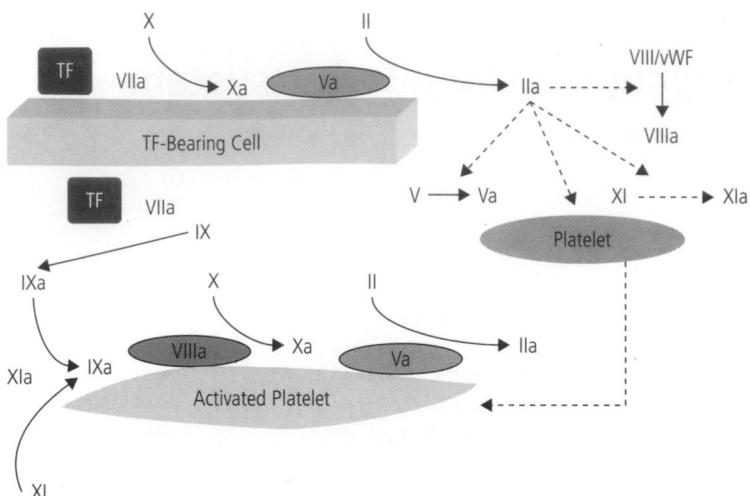

Figure 1.1 Initiation and propagation of coagulation.

• Surface glycoproteins (Gp) are present on the platelet membrane, which enable binding to collagen and von Willebrand factor (VWF) on the subendothelial surface (Gp Ia-IIa, Gp Ib/IX/V), to fibrinogen (Gp IIb-IIIa) and to other platelets via thrombospondin (Gp IV).

• The membrane surface is invaginated, increasing the surface area for release of the contents of intracellular granules.

• Within the platelet, alpha granules contain a variety of hemostatic proteins including FV, VWF, fibrinogen and fibrinolytic proteins. Dense granules contain adenosine diphosphate and triphosphate as well as serotonin.

• The dense tubular system mediates calcium flux.

• Peripheral microtubules and cytoplasmic filaments are present, which control platelet shape change.

On vessel injury and exposure of the subendothelium, circulating platelets bind via the surface glycoproteins, Gp Ia-IIa and Gp Ib/IX/V. The platelets then undergo shape change, becoming spherical and extending pseudopods.

The intracellular granules are moved towards the surface and release of their contents into the microenvironment is mediated by the mobilization of calcium. Two metabolic pathways govern both the mobilization of calcium and the activation of platelets.

Activation of platelets results in exposure of Gp IIb-IIIa and binding to fibrinogen.

Platelet aggregation leads to a "flip" in the platelet membrane with exposure of the procoagulant phosphatidylserine which provides the surface for binding of the coagulation factors and secondary hemostasis.

Coagulation

Step 1: Initiation

In the current model of coagulation, initiation of clotting occurs when TF binds to activated factor VII (FVIIa) (Figure 1.1).

TF is constitutively expressed on cells such as smooth muscle cells and fibroblasts but not on resting endothelium. TF is exposed to the circulating blood by disruption of the endothelium or by activation of endothelial cells or monocytes.

Approximately 1–2% of circulating FVII exists in the active form, FVIIa, but this serine protease is not catalytically active until it binds to TF.

The FVIIa–TF complex activates both FIX and FX although FX is a more efficient substrate for the complex.

Activated FX (FXa) binds to the platelet membrane and cleaves prothrombin to thrombin. The small amount of thrombin initially formed activates a number of factors that are critical for the second phase of coagulation, propagation; namely factors V, VIII and XI.

Another crucial role is the activation of platelets

Table 1.1 Procoagulant clotting factors.

Current nomenclature	Name	Function	Half-life (h)
Factor I	Fibrinogen	Precursor of fibrin	90
Factor II	Prothrombin	Serine protease in prothrombinase complex	65
(Factor III)	Calcium	Cofactor	
(Factor IV)	Tissue factor	Initiation of coagulation	
Factor V	Proaccelerin	Cofactor in prothrombinase complex	15
Factor VII	Proconvertin	Initiation of coagulation	5
Factor VIII	Antihemophilic factor	Cofactor in tenase complex	12
Factor IX	Christmas factor	Serine protease in tenase complex	24
Factor X	Stuart–Prower factor	Serine protease in prothrombinase complex	40
Factor XI	Plasma thromboplastin antecedent	Amplification of coagulation	45
Factor XII	Hageman factor	Contact factor	50
Factor XIII	Fibrin stabilizing factor	Cross-linkage of fibrin	200
Prekallikrein	Fletcher factor	Contact factor	35
High molecular weight kininogen	Fitzgerald factor	Contact factor	150

that provide the surface on which the propagation phase of coagulation occurs.

Step 2: Propagation of coagulation

Propagation of coagulation depends on the presence of sufficient concentrations of activated serine proteases, cofactors and platelets from the initiation phase (Table 1.1).

Whereas initiation of coagulation depended on the TF–FVIIa complex, propagation depends on two complexes:
1 the intrinsic factor tenase; and
2 the prothrombinase complexes.

These complexes have unique specificity but many common features. All consist of a vitamin K-dependent serine protease with an accessory cofactor bound to a membrane. The proteins are structurally similar and the assembly of the complexes increases enzymatic efficiency over the efficiency of the serine protease alone.

The intrinsic tenase complex

In the intrinsic tenase complex, membrane-bound FIXa forms a complex with its cofactor FVIIIa and calcium. This complex is the major activator of FX and is 50 times more active than the FVIIa–TF complex. In comparison to the FIX serine protease alone, the catalytic efficiency of the intrinsic tenase complex is increased by 5–6 orders of magnitude. More than 90% of the FXa produced in the coagulation cascade is produced by the intrinsic tenase complex. Additional FIX is generated by activated FXI to further augment FXa and thrombin generation.

The prothrombinase complex

The prothrombinase complex is formed when FXa binds to the membrane surface by its Gla domain and complexes with its cofactor FVa and calcium. The prothrombinase complex is 300,000-fold more active than FXa alone in catalyzing the conversion of prothrombin to thrombin. The rate-limiting component of the propagation phase is the concentration of FXa. The consequence of the interplay of the activated factors and cofactors in the propagation phase of coagulation is that 96% of the total thrombin generated is produced in this phase.

Natural anticoagulants

The natural anticoagulants (Table 1.2) play a critical part in controlling thrombin generation:

Table 1.2 Natural anticoagulants.

Protein	Function
Antithrombin	Inhibits thrombin, FXa, IXa, XIa
Protein C	Inhibits FVIIIa and FVa
Protein S	Cofactor for protein C
TFPI	Inhibits TF/FVIIa
Thrombomodulin	Activates protein C and TAFI in a complex with thrombin
Heparin cofactor 2	Inhibits thrombin
α_2-Macroglobulin	Inhibits thrombin and FXa
α_1-Antitrypsin	Inhibits FXIa and other serine proteases
Protease nexin 2	Inhibits FXIa

TFPI, tissue factor pathway inhibitor.

- TFPI is an efficient inhibitor of the FVIIa–TF complex by formation of a quaternary complex with FVIIa/TF/FX, leading to rapid extinction of the initiation phase.
- AT effectively neutralizes all procoagulant serine proteases and is present at twice the concentration of its substrates. Antithrombin is a potent inhibitor of thrombin, FIXa, FXa and FXIa.
- Both AT and TFPI are stoichiometric inhibitors.

There is also a dynamic inhibitory system in the thrombomodulin–PC system. The larger amount of thrombin generated in the propagation phase (96%) binds to thrombomodulin and this complex activates PC to activated PC (aPC).

- aPC with its cofactor protein S (PS) inhibits FVa and FVIIIa, thus switching off thrombin generation by the intrinsic tenase and prothrombinase complexes.
- α_2-Macroglobulin inhibits serine proteases by steric hindrance rather than by inactivation of the active site. It is responsible for approximately 20% of the inhibition of thrombin and 10% of the inhibition of FXa. It is an acute phase reactant and may be a significant inhibitor of coagulation when levels are elevated. This is particularly important in children where the level of α_2-macroglobulin is higher.
- Protease nexin 2 and α_1-antitrypsin, inhibitors of FXIa and the serine proteases, respectively.
- Heparin cofactor II, a specific inhibitor of thrombin.

The fibrinolytic system

The role of the fibrinolytic system is to ensure that the formation of the fibrin clot is localized to the site of vessel injury and that the clot is efficiently removed once wound healing has occurred (Figure 1.2). As the fibrin clot is formed, pro- and anti-fibrinolytic proteins are incorporated into the clot by binding to fibrin (Table 1.3). Plasminogen, plasmin and tissue plasminogen activator (tPA) bind to lysine residues on fibrin while α_2-antiplasmin is cross-linked to fibrin by FXIII.

Two forms of plasmin(ogen) occur:
1 Glu-plasmin(ogen) has a glutamate residue at position 1 of the protein and is less active than
2 Lys-plasmin(ogen), which has lysine as the first amino acid after removal of the first 76 amino acids by catalytic degradation.

Plasminogen is cleaved to form plasmin by:
- tPA, which is released by endothelial cells; and
- urokinase (uPA), which is primarily found in urine.

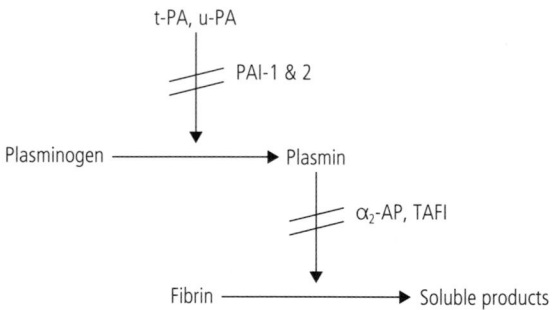

Figure 1.2 The fibrinolytic system.

Table 1.3 Fibrinolytic proteins.

Antifibrinolytic proteins	Profibrinolytic proteins
α_2-Antiplasmin	Plasminogen
PAI-1	Plasmin
PAI-2	tPA
TAFI	uPA

PAI, plasminogen activator inhibitor; TAFI, thrombin activatable fibrinolysis inhibitor; tPA, tissue plasminogen activator; uPA, urokinase.

The half-life of tPA in plasma is short because of rapid inactivation by its specific inhibitor plasminogen activator inhibitor type 1 (PAI-1) and clearance by the liver. However, the activity of fibrin bound tPA for fibrin-bound plasminogen is markedly enhanced and is protected from inhibition.

Both fibrin and fibrinogen are substrates for plasmin, which hydrolyzes arginine and lysine bonds at multiple sites resulting in cleavage products known as fibrin(ogen) degradation products (FDPs). However, only FDPs that are derived from cross-linked fibrin are detectable as D-dimers. D-dimers therefore are specific for clot-bound fibrin.

Major inhibitors of fibrinolysis

These are PAI-1 and plasminogen activator inhibitor type 2 (PAI-2), α_2-antiplasmin, α_2-macroglobulin and thrombin activatable fibrinolysis inhibitor (TAFI):
• PAI-1 and PAI-2 are found in platelets and endothelial cells.
• PAI-2 is produced in increasing amounts by the placenta during pregnancy but is also present in monocytes.
• Synthesis of α_2-antiplasmin and TAFI occurs in the liver.

Circulating plasmin is rapidly inhibited by α_2-antiplasmin, augmented by α_2-macroglobulin. Plasmin bound to fibrin is relatively protected from inhibition but the process of plasmin binding to fibrin can be inhibited by α_2-antiplasmin, especially if it is cross-linked to fibrin by FXIII. TAFI is activated by the thrombin–thrombomodulin complex and it removes lysine residues from fibrin, thus protecting it from degradation by plasmin.

Further reading

Bernard GR, Vincent JL, Laterre PF, LaRosa SP, Dhainaut JF, Lopez-Rodriguez A *et al.* Efficacy and safety of recombinant human activated protein C for severe sepsis. *N Engl J Med* 2001;**344**:699–709.

Booth NA. Fibrinolysis and thrombosis. *Baillieres Best Pract Res Clin Haematol* 1999;**12**:423–33.

Booth NA. TAFI meets the sticky ends. *Thromb Haemost* 2001;**85**:1–2.

Bouma BN, Meijers JC. Thrombin-activatable fibrinolysis inhibitor (TAFI, plasma procarboxypeptidase B, procarboxypeptidase R, procarboxypeptidase U). *J Thromb Haemost* 2003;**1**:1566–74.

Brummel KE, Paradis SG, Butenas S, Mann KG. Thrombin functions during tissue factor-induced blood coagulation. *Blood* 2002;**100**:148–52.

Butenas S, Mann KG. Blood coagulation. *Biochemistry (Mosc)* 2002;**67**:3–12.

Davidson CJ, Tuddenham EG, McVey JH. 450 million years of hemostasis. *J Thromb Haemost* 2003;**1**:1487–94.

Esmon CT. Inflammation and thrombosis. *J Thromb Haemost* 2003;**1**:1343–8.

Esmon CT. The protein C pathway. *Chest* 2003;**124**(Suppl 3):26–32.

Hotchkiss RS, Karl IE. The pathophysiology and treatment of sepsis. *N Engl J Med* 2003;**348**:138–50.

Mann KG. Thrombin formation. *Chest* 2003;**124**(Suppl 3):4–10.

Monroe DM, Hoffman M, Roberts HR. Platelets and thrombin generation. *Arterioscler Thromb Vasc Biol* 2002;**22**:1381–9.

Chapter 2
Laboratory tests of hemostasis

Steve Kitchen and Michael Makris

Introduction

In the laboratory investigation of hemostasis, the results of clotting tests can be affected by the collection and processing of blood samples and by the selection, design, quality control and interpretation of screening tests and specific assays. Such effects can have important diagnostic and therapeutic implications.

Sample collection and processing

Collection

For normal screening tests, venous blood should be collected gently but rapidly using a syringe or an evacuated collection system when possible from veins in the elbow. Application of a tourniquet to facilitate collection does not normally affect the results of most tests for bleeding disorders, although prolonged application must be avoided and the tourniquet should be applied just before sample collection.

Tests of fibrinolysis

Minimal stasis should be used because venous stasis causes local release of fibrinolytic components into the vein. The needle should not be more than 21 gauge (for infants a 22 or 23 gauge needle may be necessary).

Venous catheters

Collection through peripheral venous catheters or non-heparinized central venous catheters can be successful for prothrombin time (PT) and activated partial thromboplastin time (APTT) testing, but is best avoided; if used, sufficient blood must be discarded to prevent contamination or dilution by fluids from the line (typically 5–10 mL of blood from adults).

Mixing with anticoagulant

If there is any delay between collection and mixing with anticoagulant, or delay in filling of the collection system, the blood must be discarded because of possible activation of coagulation. Once blood and anticoagulant are mixed the container should be sealed and mixed by gentle inversion five times, even for evacuated collection systems, but vigorous shaking should be avoided.

Any difficulty in venepuncture can affect the results obtained, particularly for tests of platelet function. Prior to analysis the sample should be visually inspected and discarded if there is evidence of clotting or hemolysis. Partially clotted blood is typically associated with a dramatic false shortening of the APTT together with the loss of fibrinogen.

Anticoagulant and sample filling

The recommended anticoagulant for collection of blood for investigations of blood clotting is normally trisodium citrate. Different strengths of trisodium citrate have been employed but:
• A strength of 0.105–0.109 mol/L has been recommended for blood used for coagulation testing in general, including factor assays. One volume of anticoagulant is mixed with nine volumes of blood, and the fill volume must be at least 90% of the target volume for some test systems to give accurate results.

Table 2.1 The volume of anticoagulant required for a 5-mL sample.

Haematocrit (%)	Volume of anticoagulant (mL)	Volume of blood (mL)
25–55	0.5	4.5
20	0.7	4.3
60	0.4	4.6
70	0.25	4.75
80	0.2	4.8

- Although 0.129 mol/L trisodium citrate has been considered acceptable in the past, this is not currently recommended. Samples collected into 0.129 mol/L may be more affected by underfilling than samples collected into the 0.109 mol/L strength.
- If the patient has a hematocrit greater than 55%, results of PT and APTT can be affected and the volume of anticoagulant should be adjusted to take account of the altered plasma volume. Table 2.1 is a guide to the volume of anticoagulant required for a 5-mL sample.

Alternatively, the anticoagulant volume of 0.5 mL can be kept constant and the volume of added blood varied accordingly to the hematocrit. The volume of blood to be added (to 0.5 mL of 0.109 mol/L citrate) is calculated from the formula:

$$\frac{60}{100 - \text{hematocrit}} \times 4.5$$

Container

The inner surface of the sample container employed for blood sample collection can influence the results obtained, particularly for screening tests and should not induce contact activation (non-siliconized glass is inappropriate). For factor assays there is evidence that results on samples collected in a number of different sample types are essentially interchangeable.

Processing and storage of samples prior to analysis

Centrifugation

For preparation of platelet-rich plasma (PRP) to investigate platelet function, samples should be centrifuged at room temperature (18–25°C) at 150–200 g for 15 min, and analyzed within 2 h of sample collection.

For most other tests related to bleeding disorders, samples should be centrifuged at a speed and time that produces samples with residual platelet counts well below 10×10^9/L; for example, using 2000 g for at least 10 min.

Centrifugation at a temperature of 18–25°C is acceptable for most clotting tests. Exceptions include labile parameters such as many tests of fibrinolytic activity. After centrifugation, prolonged storage at 4–8°C should be avoided as this can cause cold activation, increasing FVII activity and shortening of the PT or APTT.

Stability

Samples for APTT should be analyzed within 4 h of collection. The results of some other clotting tests such as the D-dimer and the PT of samples from warfarinized subjects are stable for 24 h or longer. Unless a laboratory has data on the stability of testing plasmas at room temperature for a specific test, the plasmas should be deep frozen within 4 h of collection for future analysis.

Some clotting factor test results are stable for samples stored at −24°C or lower for up to 3 months and for samples stored at −74°C for up to 18 months (results within 10% of baseline defined as stable). Storage in domestic grade −20°C freezers is normally unacceptable.

If frozen samples are shipped to another laboratory for testing on dry ice, care must be taken to avoid exposure of the plasma to carbon dioxide which may affect the pH and the results of screening tests.

Prior to analysis, frozen samples must be thawed rapidly at 37°C for 3–5 min. Thawing at lower temperatures is not acceptable because some cryoprecipitation is possible.

Use of coagulation screening tests

Laboratories usually offer a set of tests (the coagulation screen) that aims to identify most clinically important hemostatic defects. Invariably this includes the PT, the APTT, fibrinogen and usually thrombin time. It is important to perform a full blood count to quantify the platelet count, but assessment of platelet function is not usually offered or performed in the initial tests. The pattern of abnormalities of the coagulation screen as shown in Table 2.2, suggests possible diagnoses and allows further tests to be performed to define the abnormality.

Prothrombin time

Tissue factor (in the form of thromboplastin) and calcium are added to plasma that has been anticoagulated with citrate during collection. Tissue factor reacts with FVIIa to activate the "extrinsic" pathway and thus form a clot.

Use of the prothrombin time test

The PT is sensitive to and thus prolonged in patients with deficiencies of factors VII, X, V, II and

Table 2.2 Interpretation of abnormalities of coagulation screening tests.

Prothrombin time	APTT	Thrombin time	Fibrinogen	Possible conditions
Prolonged	Normal	Normal	Normal	Factor VII deficiency
Normal	Prolonged	Normal	Normal	Deficiency of FVIII, FIX, FXI, FXII or contact factor
				Lupus anticoagulant
Prolonged	Prolonged	Normal	Normal	Deficiency of FII, FV or FX
				Oral anticoagulant therapy
				Vitamin K deficiency
				Combined deficiency of FV + FVIII
				Combined deficiency of FII, FVII, FIX, FX
				Liver disease
Prolonged	Prolonged	Prolonged	Normal or low	Hypo- or dysfibrinogenemia
				Liver disease
				Massive transfusion
				DIC

APTT, activated partial prothrombin time; DIC, disseminated intravascular coagulopathy.

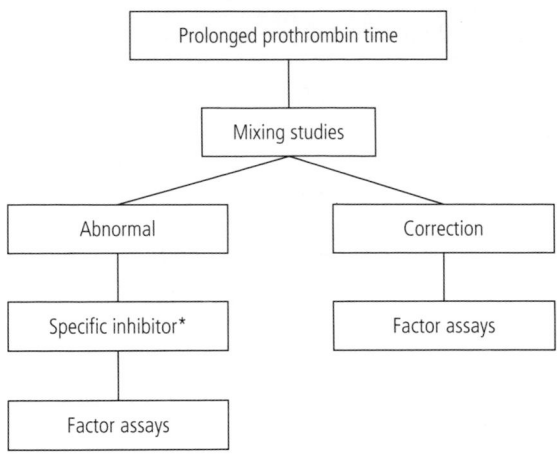

* Rarely the lupus anticoagulant can prolong the PT, but almost always the APTT will also be prolonged and appropriate tests should be carried out as in table 2.2

Figure 2.1 Investigation of a prolonged prothrombin time.

fibrinogen. It is particularly useful in monitoring anticoagulation in patients on warfarin.

Figure 2.1 suggests a pathway for investigation of a patient with a prolonged PT.

Activated partial thromboplastin time

Phospholipid (lacking tissue factor, hence the term "partial" thromboplastin) and particulate matter (such as kaolin) are added to plasma to generate a clot. Abnormalities in the "intrinsic" and "common" pathway will result in prolongation of the APTT.

Use of the APTT

This test is abnormal in patients:
• with deficiencies of factors XII, XI, X, IX, VIII, V, II and fibrinogen;
• on heparin therapy; or
• who have the lupus anticoagulant.
Figure 2.2 suggests a pathway for investigation of patients with prolonged APTT. Prolongation of the APTT, sometimes to a dramatic degree, can be seen in patients without a bleeding diathesis (Table 2.3).

Mixing studies

These are central in the investigation of a prolonged APTT. The principle is that the test is repeated, with 50% of the test plasma being replaced by normal plasma (which assumes that this contains normal amounts of all the clotting factors). The result of the mixing study is that the test will have all the clotting factors to a minimum of 50% and thus should result in:
• a normal APTT if the cause of the abnormality was a deficiency of a clotting factor;
• a prolonged APTT if an inhibitor (either to a specific factor or a lupus anticoagulant) is present.

Thrombin time

The thrombin time measures the rate of conversion of fibrinogen to polymerized fibrin after the addition of thrombin to plasma. It is sensitive to and thus prolonged in:
• hypo- and dysfibrinogenemia;
• heparin therapy (or heparin contamination of the sample);
• the presence of fibrin(ogen) degradation products and factors that influence the fibrin polymerization (e.g. the presence of a paraprotein in myeloma).

Figure 2.3 suggests a pathway for investigation of a prolonged thrombin time. Heparin contamination in a sample can also be confirmed by correction of a prolonged thrombin time after treatment of a sample with heparinase, hepzyme, reptilase or mixing with protamine, an agent that antagonizes heparin.

Fibrinogen

A number of methods are available for measurement of fibrinogen concentration. Most automated coagulation analyzers now provide a measure of fibrinogen concentration, calculated from the degree of change of light scatter or optical density during measurement of the prothrombin time (PT-derived fibrinogen). Although this is simple and cheap, it is inaccurate in some patients such as those with disseminated intravascular coagulopathy (DIC), liver disease, renal disease, dysfibrinogenemia, following thrombolytic therapy and in

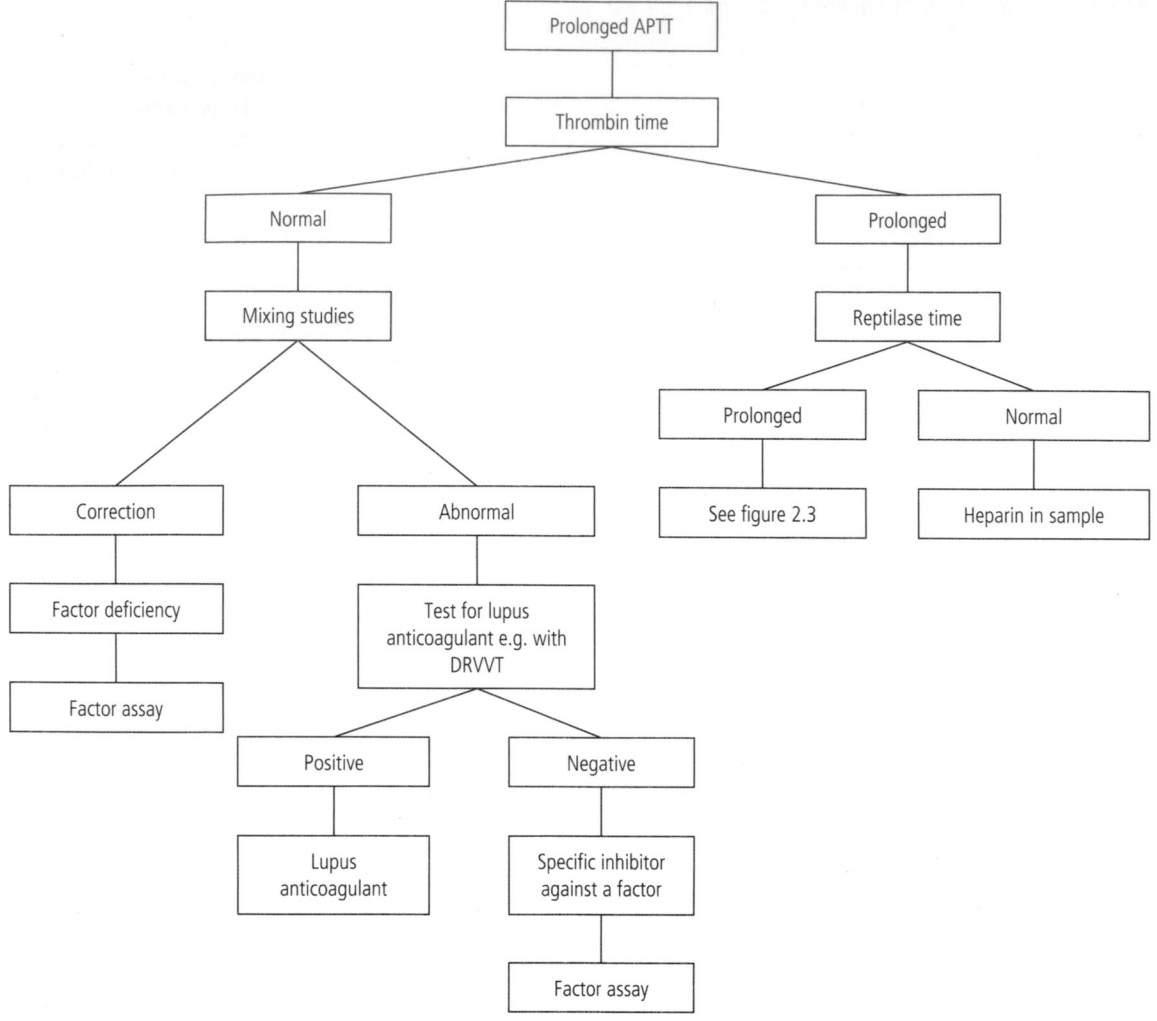

Figure 2.2 Investigation of a prolonged APTT.

those with markedly raised or reduced fibrinogen concentrations. The recommended method for measuring fibrinogen concentration as originally described by Clauss is based on the thrombin time and uses a high concentration of thrombin solution.

Screening tests – assay issues

The sensitivity of PT and APTT to the presence of clotting factor deficiencies is dependent on the test system employed. The degree of prolongation in the presence of a clotting factor deficiency can vary dramatically between reagents. There is no clear consensus on what level of clotting factor deficiency is clinically relevant and therefore the level that should be detected as an abnormal screening test result has not been defined. In relation to the APTT, one important application is the detection of deficiencies associated with bleeding, in particular factors VIII, IX and XI.

A number of APTT methods are available for which abnormal results are normally present when the level of clotting factor is below 30 u/dL and only methods for which this is the case should be used to screen for possible bleeding disorders. In the case of FVIII it has been recommended in the

Table 2.3 Conditions associated with a prolonged APTT but without a bleeding diathesis.

Deficiency of:
    factor XII
    high molecular weight kininogen
    prekallekrein
Lupus anticoagulant
Excess citrate anticoagulant

past that the APTT technique selected should have a normal reference range that closely corresponds to a FVIII reference range of 50–200 u/dL. However, it should be noted that for most methods normal APTT results will be obtained in at least some patients with FVIII in the range 30–50 u/dL, and few, if any, reagents will be associated with prolonged results in every patient of this type.

For most techniques, the APTT is less sensitive to the reduction of FIX levels than for FVIII, and most if not all currently available techniques will be associated with normal APTT results in at least some cases with FIX in the range 25–50 u/dL.

Data from published studies and from external quality assessment programs suggest that most widely used current APTT reagents will have:
• prolonged APTT results in samples from patients with FIX or FXI below 20–25 u/dL;
• a more mixed pattern of normal and abnormal results when FIX or FXI is in the region 25–60 u/dL.

Lower limit of normal range
The lower limit for FXI activity is probably between 60 and 70 u/dL. The lower limit of normal for FVIII or FIX is approximately 50 u/dL. A normal APTT does not always exclude the presence of

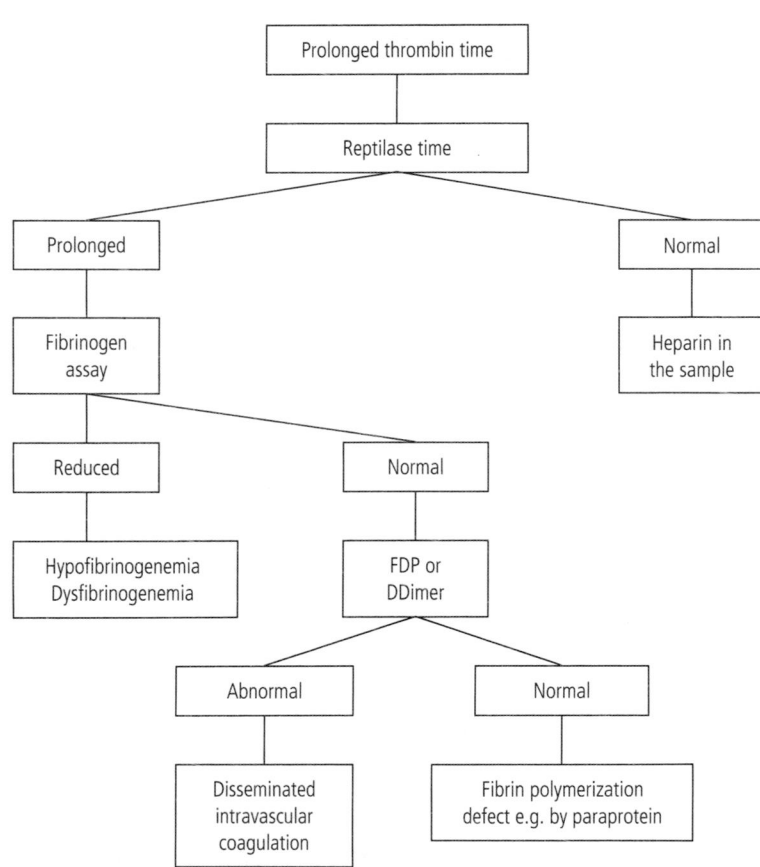

Figure 2.3 Investigation of a prolonged thrombin time.

a mild deficiency. In plasma from subjects with FIX or FXI deficiency, marked elevation of FVIII, if present, may normalize the APTT.

Variation with reagents

There is marked variation between results:
• With different APTT reagents, partly because of the use of different *activators* in APTT as well as the *phospholipid profile*. For these reasons, locally determined reference ranges are essential.
• With different PT *thromboplastins* used in the assays of factor VII or X. Sensitive PT techniques will show prolongation of PT above the upper limit of normal when there is an isolated deficiency of FVII, FX or FV with a level below 30–40 u/dL. In general, the level of factor II (prothrombin) associated with prolongation of PT is lower than for the other factors.

In the case of both the PT and APTT, it is useful to repeat borderline results on a fresh sample. It should be noted that the within subject variation of PT and APTT over time may be 6–12%.

For both the PT and APTT, the degree of prolongation may be small in the presence of mild deficiency and therefore there is a need for adequate quality control procedures and for carefully established accurate normal or reference ranges. In view of the limitations of screening tests, it is important that results are interpreted in conjunction with all relevant personal and family history details when screening for bleeding disorders. *Normal screening tests do not always exclude the presence of mild deficiency states.*

Recommendations and summary: screening tests

• PT and APTT methods vary in sensitivity to factor deficiency.
• Mild deficiency may be associated with normal PT or APTT.
• For bleeding disorders select a method for which APTT is normally prolonged when FVIII, FIX or FXI is 30 IU/dL or less.
• Elevated FVIII may normalize APTT in mild FIX or FXI deficiency.
• Assessments of APTT sensitivity should employ samples from patients.

Clotting factor assay design

One-stage assays

For many years the most commonly performed assays for clotting factors have been one-stage clotting assays based on:
• the APTT in the case of factors VIII, IX or XI;
• the PT in the case of factors II, V, VII or X.

There are a number of general features of the design of one-stage clotting assays that are necessary to ensure accurate, reliable and valid results. In factor assays, the principle depends upon the ability of a sample containing the factor under investigation to correct or shorten the delayed clotting of a plasma completely deficient in that factor. Such deficient plasmas must contain less than 1 u/dL of the clotting factor under investigation and normal levels of all other relevant clotting factors.

It is important that the clotting time measured by the APTT or PT depends directly on the amount of factor present in the mixture of deficient and reference or test plasma. For example, in a FVIII assay the level of FVIII must be rate-limiting in relation to the clotting time obtained.

This requires dilution of a reference or standard plasma of known concentration. Preparation of several different dilutions of the reference plasma allows construction of a calibration curve in which the clotting time response depends on the dose (concentration) of factor present. At lower plasma dilutions or higher factor concentrations the factor under investigation may not be rate limiting and the assay is no longer specific and therefore invalid. It may be necessary to extend the calibration curve by testing additional dilutions when analyzing test plasmas with concentrations below 10 u/dL. At very low concentrations of an individual factor (< 1–2 u/dL), the clotting time of the deficient plasma may not be even partially corrected by addition of the test plasma dilution. Dilutions are selected so that there is a linear relationship between concentration (logarithmic scale) and the response in clotting time (logarithmic or linear scale). The reference curve should be prepared using at least three different dilutions and a calibration curve should be included each time the assay is performed unless there is clear evidence that the responses are so reproducible that a calibration curve can be stored for use on other occasions. The reference plasma should be calibrated by a route traceable back to WHO international standards where these are available. Test plasmas should be analyzed using three dilutions so that it is possible to confirm that the dose–response curve of the test plasma is linear and parallel to the dose–response curve of the reference plasma. It is not acceptable to test a single test dilution because this reduces the accuracy substantially and may lead to major underestimation of the true concentration when inhibitors are present. If a dose–response curve of a test plasma is not parallel to the reference curve, and the presence of an inhibitor such as an antiphospholipid antibody is confirmed or suspected, then the estimate of activity obtained from the highest test plasma dilution is likely to be closest to the real concentration, but it should be noted that the criteria for a valid assay cannot be met and results must be interpreted with caution. In the case of one-stage APTT-based assays, the interference by antiphospholipid antibodies is frequently dependent on the APTT reagent used and its phospholipid content. Some APTT reagents such as Actin FS contain a high phospholipid concentration and this type of reagent is much less affected by these antibodies and is particularly suitable for use in factor assays in such cases.

Recommendations and summary: factor assays

• Assays should be calibrated with reference plasmas traceable back to WHO standards where available.
• Deficient plasmas must have < 1 u/dL of the clotting factor being assayed and normal levels of other relevant factors.
• Not less than three dilutions of test plasmas should be tested.
• A valid assay requires test and calibration lines to be parallel.
• Interference by antiphospholipid antibodies can be minimized by use of an APTT reagent with a high phospholipid content.

Thrombophilia testing

This section addresses some laboratory aspects of testing for heritable thrombophilia – protein C (PC), protein S (PS), antithrombin (AT), activated protein C resistance (APC-R), FV Leiden (FVL) and the prothrombin 20210A allele.

Sample collection, processing and assay

For thrombophilia testing as for other coagulation tests:
• A citrate concentration of 0.105–0.109 mol/L should be used for sample collection, because citrate strength may affect results, at least for APC-R testing.
• Centrifugation should be as for other coagulation tests described above.
• Residual platelets in plasma following centrifugation can also affect results of APC-R tests and plasmas should be centrifuged as described above, separated and recentrifuged a second time to ensure maximum removal of platelets. (Such a procedure is not necessary for AT, PC or PS testing but can used for convenience without adverse effects if the same plasma is to be used for these investigations in addition to APC-R.)
• Such double centrifuged plasma can then be stored deep frozen prior to analysis for at least 6 months for clotting PS activity and at least 18 months for PC and AT.
• In general, activity assays are preferable to antigen assays because antigen assays will be normal in some patients with type 2 defects where a normal concentration of a defective protein is present.

In the case of PS, this is complicated by the problems associated with interference by FVL in many different activity assays and can lead to important underestimation of the true level, with misdiagnosis a possibility. At present, the standardization of PS activity assays is poor in that results of different assays may differ substantially even in normal subjects. For these reasons PS activity assays must be used with caution.

FVL can also cause underestimation of the true PC level in clotting assays. A chromogenic PC assay may be used to avoid this problem or alternatively the PC clotting assay can be modified to include predilution of test sample 1 in 4 in PC-deficient plasma to restore specificity. A similar procedure can be employed to improve performance of clotting PS assays in the presence of FVL.

Clotting assays of PC and PS may also be influenced adversely by elevated FVIII causing underestimation. The presence of the lupus anticoagulant may be associated with falsely high results, with the possibility of a false normal result in the presence of deficiency.

When assaying PC, PS and AT, calibration curves should include a minimum of three dilutions and, in general, the most precise test results will be obtained if a calibration curve is prepared with each group of patient samples. As for other tests of hemostasis, it is important to use a reference plasma traceable back to WHO standards which are available for AT, PC and PS.

Testing for APC-R is largely based on APTT in the presence and absence of APC, and therefore many of the variables that affect the APTT will in turn influence APC-R test results. These include the presence of heparin or lupus anticoagulant by prolonging clotting times, or elevated FVIII, which shortens clotting times and manifest as acquired APC-R. The original APC-R test also requires normal levels of clotting factors including FII and FX which are reduced by warfarin therapy. Valid APC-R testing as originally used requires a normal PT and APTT.

There is evidence that standardization of results obtained by the original assay can be improved by calculation of the normalized APC-R ratio (test APC ratio divided by APC ratio of a pooled normal plasma tested in the same batch of tests). The test can be significantly improved by predilution of test plasma in FV-deficient plasma, making the test 100% sensitive to the presence of FVL. This modification also makes the test specific for FVL, and will be associated with normal results where APC resistance in the classic assay is not a consequence of FVL. This must be borne in mind when interpreting results. In some versions of the test there is clear separation between results obtained in heterozygotes and homozygotes, but even for such assays confirmation by genetic testing may be necessary because it is important to identify homozygotes with certainty.

When genetic testing for the FVL or prothrombin alleles is undertaken, there are fewer relevant preanalytical variables than for phenotypic tests on plasma. Whole blood samples are stable for several weeks, at least for some of the genotyping methods.

Because of the many differences between results of apparently similar assays in thrombophilia testing, it is particularly important to establish locally a reference or normal range as discussed in Appendix 1.

Recommendations and summary: thrombophilia tests

- Double centrifugation is required for APC-R testing.
- Presence of FVL may cause significant underestimation of clotting PC or PS activity.
- Results of PS activity assays are highly dependent on reagents used.
- Elevated FVIII or lupus anticoagulant can interfere with PC or PS clotting assays.
- Results of AT assays may depend on the enzyme used in the assay.
- APC-R with FV-deficient plasma dilution is the most sensitive and specific for FVL.
- Genetic testing for FVL or prothrombin allele may not be error free.

Quality assurance

All laboratory tests of blood coagulation require careful application of quality assurance procedures to ensure reliability of results. Quality assurance is used to describe all the measures that are taken to ensure the reliability of laboratory testing and reporting. This includes the choice of test, the collection of a valid sample from the patient, analysis of the specimen and the recording of results in a timely and accurate manner, through to interpretation of the results, where appropriate, and communication of these results to the referring clinicians.

Internal quality control (IQC) and external quality assessment (EQA) are complementary components of a laboratory quality assurance programme. Quality assurance is required to check that the results of laboratory investigations are reliable enough to be released to assist clinical decision making, monitoring of therapy and diagnosis of hemostatic abnormalities.

Internal quality control

IQC is used to establish whether a series of techniques and procedures are performing consistently over a period of time (precision). It is therefore deployed to ensure day-to-day laboratory consistency. It is important to recognize that a precise technique is not necessarily accurate, accuracy being a measure of the closeness of an estimated value to the true value.

IQC procedures should be applied in a way that ensures immediate and constant control of result generation. Within a laboratory setting, the quality of results obtained is influenced by maintenance of an up-to-date manual of standard operational procedures; use of reliable reagents and reference materials; selection of automation and adequate maintenance; adequate records and reporting system for results; an appropriate complement of suitably trained personnel.

For screening tests it is important to include regular and frequent testing of quality control material, which should include a normal material and at least one level of abnormal sample. For batch analysis, a quality control sample can be included with each batch. For continuous processing systems, the frequency of quality control testing must be tailored to the work pattern and should be adjusted until the frequency of repeat patient testing resulting from the limits of the quality control studies is at a minimum. For many random access coagulometers, performing screening tests, this could typically be every 2 h of continuous work or every 30–40 samples. For factor assays and parameters typically tested in batches, a quality control sample should be included with each group of tests. Patient results should only be released if quality control

results remain within acceptable target limits. It is frequently useful to include IQC material at different critical levels of abnormality.

External quality assessment

EQA is used to identify the degree of agreement between one laboratory's results and those obtained by other centers which can be used as a measure of accuracy. The main function of EQA is proficiency testing of individual laboratory testing, but larger programs provide information concerning the relative performance of analytical procedures, including the method principle, reagents and instruments. As a general principle, all centers undertaking investigations of hemostasis should participate in an accredited EQA program for all tests where available.

Recommendations and summary: quality control

- Quality control samples should be analyzed regularly and frequently for screening tests, and with each group of factor assays.
- Centers should participate in accredited external quality assessment programs for all tests where available.

Further reading

Jennings I, Cooper P. Screening for thrombophilia: a laboratory perspective. *Br J Biomed Sci* 2003.**60**;39–51.

Koepke JA. Partial thromboplastin time test: proposed performance guidelines. ICSH Panel on the PTT. *Thromb Haemost* 1986;**55**:143–4.

Lawrie AS, Kitchen S, Purdy G, Mackie IJ, Preston FE, Machin SJ. Assessment of actin FS and actin FSL sensitivity to specific clotting factor deficiencies. *Clin Lab Haematol* 1998;**20**:179–86.

Walker ID, Greaves M, Preston FE. Investigation and management of heritable thrombophilia. *Br J Haematol* 2001:**114**:512–18.

Chapter 3
Molecular diagnostic approaches to hemostasis

Paula James and David Lillicrap

Introduction

The first coagulation factor gene, factor IX, was cloned and characterized in 1982 and since that time remarkable progress has been made in the use of molecular genetic strategies to assist in the diagnosis of coagulation disorders. This chapter summarizes the current state of molecular diagnostics for the more common hemostatic conditions, with a discussion of both hemorrhagic and thrombotic problems for which genetic tests are now available.

It is important to emphasize that for most hemostatic conditions encountered in clinical practice, the initial diagnostic test of choice will still be one that is performed in a routine hemostasis laboratory. For example, the diagnosis of hemophilia A will still, in the vast majority of cases, be made using a factor VIII clotting assay. The role of molecular genetic testing for this condition will be to assist in genetic counseling and to provide predictive information relating to certain aspects of clinical management. To date, the number of conditions for which the initial diagnostic strategy demands a genetic test is small. One such example is the test for the prothrombin 20210 thrombophilic variant.

A second, general issue that merits brief discussion concerns the appropriate venue for molecular genetic testing for hemostatic disorders. The successful implementation of a molecular diagnostic service for hemostatic conditions requires access to appropriate expertise, and these tests cannot readily be added to the repertoire of a routine clinical coagulation laboratory. However, genetic testing for hemostatic problems can easily be incorporated into a general molecular diagnostic facility, although the involvement of personnel with an additional interest in the phenotypic aspects of clotting is undoubtedly beneficial for optimizing testing strategies and test interpretation.

Molecular diagnostics of bleeding disorders

Molecular genetic testing for the hemophilias have been available since the cloning of the factor VIII and IX genes, in 1984 and 1982 respectively.

Hemophilia A

To date, all inherited cases of isolated factor VIII deficiency have been linked to mutations of the factor VIII locus, which is located at the telomeric end of the long arm of the X chromosome (Xq28) and encompasses 186 kilobases (kb) of genomic DNA (Fig. 3.1). The large size of the gene, which contains 26 exons, has been a challenge for the

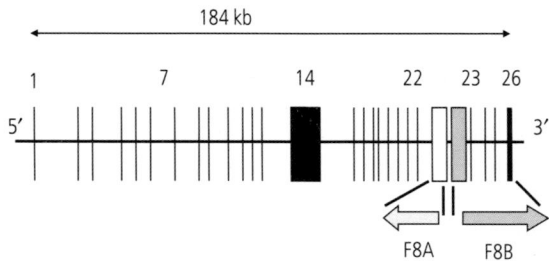

Figure 3.1 Structure of the factor VIII gene. The gene spans 184 kb of genomic DNA at the tip of the long arm of the human X chromosome. There are 26 coding exons. In addition, two further open reading frames are present in intron 22 of the gene: F8A, a product that is transcribed in the opposite direction to factor VIII; and F8B, a transcript that comprises intron 22 sequence spliced onto the final four exons of factor VIII.

development of molecular diagnostic testing. Two diagnostic strategies can be used to investigate this condition.

Polymorphism linkage analysis in hemophilia A

Where there is a family history of hemophilia, and informative intragenic polymorphisms are identified, polymorphism linkage testing can still be a useful strategy for effecting carrier diagnosis and prenatal testing. However, linkage analysis is limited in its utility by a number of factors, the most frequently encountered of which are:

• an isolated case of hemophilia (lack of prior family history);

• the absence of informative polymorphic markers; and

• the problem of non-participating family members.

In an isolated case of hemophilia, linkage data can still be used to exclude further transmission of the mutant allele by the propositus. However, because the time at which the mutation arose within the pedigree is unclear, predictions about previous transmission of the mutant allele to others within the family are not possible. There are simple sequence repeat polymorphisms in introns 13 and 22 and a *Bcl* I dimorphism in intron 18. These polymorphic markers are informative in approximately 90% of families tested, regardless of ethnic background. These studies can produce results for reporting within a few days from the receipt of the test material, an interval that is acceptable for most prenatal testing situations.

If the assays for these markers are uninformative, further analysis of less frequent polymorphisms in introns 22 (*XbaI*) and 7 (G/A dimorphism) may also be helpful. The number of instances in which a linked extragenic polymorphism has to be used, with the accompanying risk of recombination, is now fortunately very low.

Direct mutation testing for hemophilia A

Advances in molecular genetic technology over the past decade have made the direct detection of hemophilic mutations a feasible testing option in diagnostic laboratories. The current Internet-accessible Hemophilia A Mutation Database (http://europium.csc.mrc.ac.uk) lists more than 700 different factor VIII mutations. The majority of these changes represent point mutations that have now been reported in all 26 exons of the gene. The database also lists many small (less than 200 nucleotides [nt]) and large deletions and a number of factor VIII gene insertions.

Rationale for direct mutation testing in hemophilia A

In a diagnostic setting, the most frequent group of subjects for whom direct mutation testing would be beneficial are those in whom an isolated report of severe hemophilia precludes the use of linkage analysis to track the mutant factor VIII gene. These individuals require direct mutation analysis to identify the carrier state and for accurate prenatal identification of affected offspring. Direct detection of the hemophilic mutation will also eliminate the uncertainties posed by potential germline mosaicism in the setting of a newly acquired mutation.

The second reason for pursuing the causative mutation in hemophilia A is the recent documentation that specific factor VIII genotypes are more predictive for the risk of acquiring a factor VIII inhibitor. Patients with null genotypes (large deletions, nonsense mutations and the factor VIII inversion mutations) have significantly higher risks for developing an inhibitor (between 25% [inversion mutations] and 70% [large, multidomain deletions]) than those whose hemophilia is caused by missense mutations, small deletions and gene insertions for whom the risk of inhibitor development is less than 10%. Although these associations have yet to be rigorously evaluated in a prospective fashion, given the clinical consequences of inhibitor development and the potential benefit of various forms of immune tolerance protocols, one can reasonably make the case for mutation testing in all new severe cases of hemophilia A. Furthermore, there is also preliminary evidence that the outcome of immune tolerance protocols is also influenced significantly by the hemophilic genotype.

Strategies for direct mutation detection in hemophilia A

Two basic approaches can be taken to identifying the causative mutation in hemophilia A (Fig. 3.2):

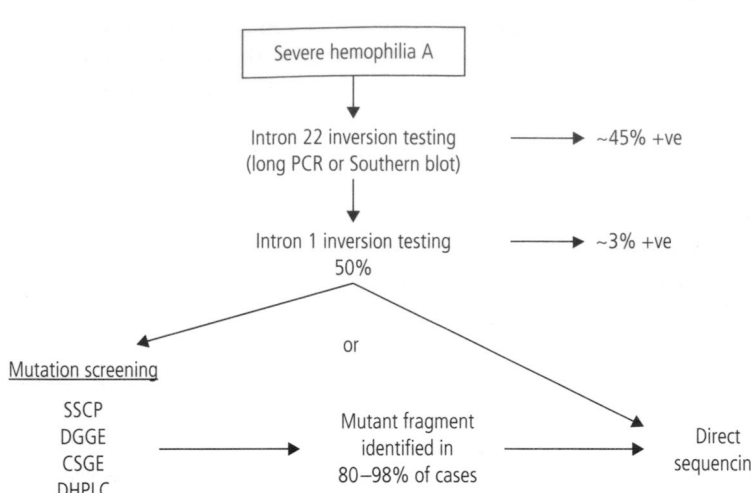

Figure 3.2 Molecular diagnostic algorithm for severe hemophilia A. The intron 22 inversion mutation will be present in ~45% of cases and another ~3% of cases are caused by the intron 1 inversion. In the remaining 50% of cases, single nucleotide substitutions comprise the majority of mutations. These can be tested through the analysis of PCR-amplified exon fragments using either a mutation screening strategy or direct sequence analysis of the amplified factor VIII exons. CSGE, conformation-sensitive gel electrophoresis; DGGE, denaturing gradient gel electrophoresis; DHPLC, denaturing high-performance liquid chromatography; SSCP, single-strand conformation polymorphism analysis.

1 A mutation screening strategy followed by sequencing of the abnormal region of the gene.
2 Direct sequencing of the factor VIII coding region.

A variety of screening techniques have now been developed for the detection of subtle mutations, including:
• single-strand conformation polymorphism (SSCP) analysis;
• denaturing gradient gel electrophoresis (DGGE);
• chemical mismatch cleavage (CMC);
• conformation-sensitive gel electrophoresis (CSGE); and
• denaturing high-performance liquid chromatography (DHPLC).

In laboratories using any one of these methods on a regular basis, the sensitivity for detecting point mutations is likely to be between 85% and 95%, with recent studies suggesting that DHPLC may have a detection rate approaching 100%.

Following the identification of an abnormality in one region of the gene, the abnormal fragment can be sequenced (see Plate 1, facing p. 24). With the rapid development of automated sequencing technology, the cost and efficiency of direct sequence analysis has now improved to the point where this strategy can be realistically considered for studying genes as large and complex as factor VIII.

Factor VIII inversion mutations

There are two significant exceptions to the mutational heterogeneity of hemophilia A:
1 The intron 22 factor VIII inversion mutation, found in approximately 45% of patients with a severe phenotype. This inversion involves exons 1–22 of the gene and is caused by an intrachromosomal recombination event between a copy of the F8A gene within intron 22 of factor VIII and additional F8A copies approximately 400 kb 5′ (telomeric) of factor VIII. The inversion is only found in patients with a severe phenotype. In the molecular diagnostic laboratory, testing for the inversion mutation should be the first step in the analysis of any kindred affected by severe hemophilia A. The inversion can be detected with either a Southern blot (Fig. 3.3) or a long-range (> 10 kb) PCR-based approach. In approximately 83% of cases, the recombination event will have been with the distal extragenic copy of F8A (type 1 inversions), in approximately 16% with the proximal F8A copy (type 2), and in approximately 1% of inversions, rare rearrangement patterns are seen.
2 A second recurring factor VIII mutation is seen in ~3% of severe hemophilia A cases and involves an inversion event with sequences in intron 1. This mutation can readily be detected with a PCR-based approach.

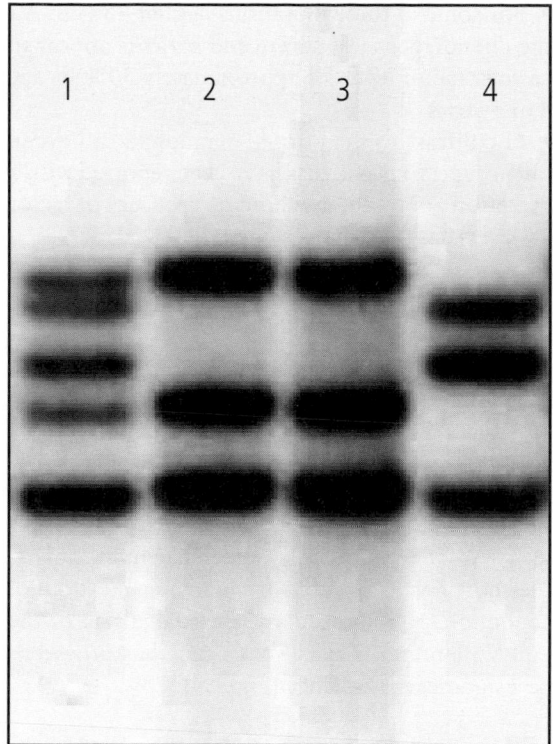

Factor VIII Intron 22 Inversion Mutation Test

Figure 3.3 Autoradiograph of the factor VIII intron 22 inversion mutation. The genomic DNA has been digested with the restriction enzyme Bcl II and, following Southern transfer, the blot has been probed with a DNA fragment derived from intron 22 of the factor VIII gene. Lanes 2 and 3 show the normal hybridization pattern. Lane 4 shows the hybridization pattern with the common form of the intron 22 inversion mutation and lane 1 shows the hybridization pattern in a heterozygous female carrier for this mutation.

Hemophilia B

All reported cases of hemophilia B have been linked to defects in the factor IX gene, which is centromeric to the factor VIII gene on the X chromosome (Xq27). As with hemophilia A, the inherited deficiency of factor IX demonstrates both phenotypic and mutational heterogeneity. The molecular diagnostic strategies employed for hemophilia B testing are similar to those discussed for hemophilia A, with the exception that in hemophilia B there is no single predominant mutation equivalent to the factor VIII inversions in hemophilia A.

Polymorphism linkage analysis in hemophilia B

The factor IX gene contains a number of polymorphisms that can be used for linkage analysis in known hemophilia B kindreds. There are no multi-allelic repeat elements in the factor IX gene and the ethnic variability of several of the factor IX polymorphisms is extreme. For instance, in Oriental populations, analysis of the intragenic markers is invariably uninformative.

Direct mutation testing for hemophilia B

In contrast to hemophilia A, where the large size of the gene has limited direct mutational analysis, many laboratories now employ direct mutation analysis for the smaller and less complex factor IX gene (186 kb/26 exons vs. 34 kb/8 exons). A worldwide Hemophilia B Mutation Database has been in existence since 1990, and the current Internet-accessible registry (http://www.kcl.ac.uk/ip/peter-green/haemBdatabase.html) lists information on more than 800 different mutations in over 2500 patients, making hemophilia B one of the most extensively investigated diseases at the molecular genetic level. As with hemophilia A, most of the mutations resulting in this phenotype are single-nucleotide variations located throughout the gene from the promoter to the end of the coding region.

Hemophilia B mutations of particular clinical significance

Many of the factor IX missense mutations have provided knowledge of the basic structure and function correlates of the factor IX protein. However, several clinically important mutation types are worth highlighting from a molecular diagnostic standpoint.

The first group of mutations of note are a variety of gross factor IX gene deletions and rearrangements which result in severe hemophilia B. These can be complicated by the development of inhibitors and anaphylactic reactions to replacement therapy. This constellation of findings has now been reported in more than 30 patients worldwide, and has further emphasized the proposal that all new cases of severe hemophilia B should be screened for gross factor IX deletions or rearrangements by both polymerase chain reaction (PCR) and Southern blotting with a cDNA probe.

The second, recently described type of factor IX mutation with important clinical consequences involves missense mutations in the propeptide-encoding sequence, resulting in a markedly reduced affinity of the mutant protein for the vitamin K-dependent carboxylase. Two different missense mutations have been described at amino acid residue-10 and these patients have normal baseline factor IX levels but show marked sensitivity to treatment with vitamin K antagonists, leading to a significantly increased risk of bleeding on oral anticoagulant therapy.

The final group of factor IX mutations that merit recognition are:
• Those in the factor IX promoter (18 different point mutations have now been described in the approximately 40 nucleotides adjacent to the transcription start site).
• These mutations are associated with the hemophilia B Leyden phenotype, where factor IX deficiency undergoes at least a partial spontaneous phenotypic resolution following puberty, as a result of androgen-dependent gene expression.

• For some of these mutations (e.g. nt −6 G to A), the phenotype is less severe and patients appear to recover factor levels of approximately 30% by age 4 or 5 years.
• In contrast to the normal hemophilia B Leyden phenotype, four patients have been reported with a mutation at nt −26, in whom no recovery of factor IX levels has been documented.

von Willebrand disease

Von Willebrand disease (VWD) is the most common inherited bleeding disorder known in humans, and there has been much interest in the genetic pathology over the past decade. The mutations resulting in this phenotype are only beginning to be understood, and the role of molecular diagnostics in VWD is consequently somewhat limited. Furthermore, with 52 exons encompassing 170 kb of genomic DNA, molecular genetic analysis of the von Willebrand factor (VWF) gene has proved to be a significant challenge (Fig. 3.4).

Type 3 VWD

Although this disorder is rare (prevalence of ~1 per

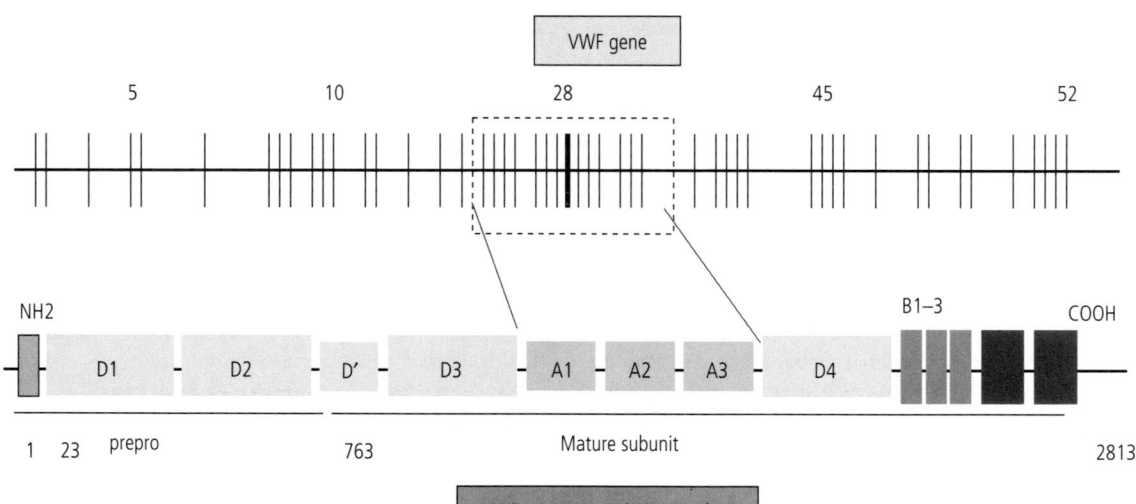

Figure 3.4 The VWF gene and primary translation product. The gene comprises 52 exons, of which exons 21–34 (outlined in the interrupted box) are duplicated, with minor variations, in a chromosome 22 pseudogene sequence. The primary translation product comprises a 22 amino acid signal peptide, a 741 residue propeptide and a mature, secreted subunit of 2050 residues.

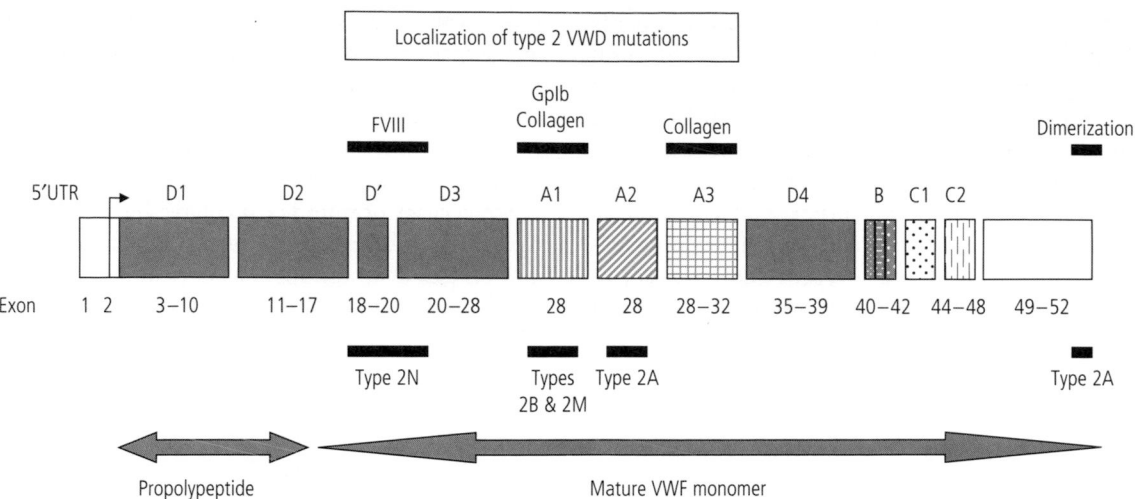

Figure 3.5 The von Willebrand factor protein comprising the large N-terminal propolypeptide (VWF: Ag II) and the mature subunit. Repeated protein domains are designated A–D and the binding sites for factor VIII, platelet Gp Ib and collagen are shown. The area critical for subunit dimerization is also shown. Sites for common mutations resulting in type 2 VWD are shown.

million population), molecular studies of families with type 3 VWD represent one instance in which molecular diagnostics can be beneficial, as parents with children diagnosed with type 3 VWD may choose prenatal testing in future pregnancies.

Highly informative repeat sequence polymorphisms are available for linkage analysis, both within the VWF gene and in the 5′ flanking region of the gene. As with the hemophilias, an Internet-accessible mutation database is also maintained for VWD (http://www.shef.ac.uk/vwf/index.html).

A review of this database indicates that some cases of type 3 VWD are the result of complete or partial deletions of the VWF gene. Type 3 patients with deletion mutations also appear to be predisposed to developing allo-antibodies to their replacement therapy. Thus, screening of type 3 patients with a VWF cDNA Southern blot might be helpful, both for direct mutation detection and also to evaluate the risk of inhibitor development.

Type 2 VWD

Type 2 variants of VWD comprise approximately 15% of these patients in most surveys. Although initial investigation of these cases must rely on the use of standard coagulation tests to evaluate the VWF–factor VIII complex, molecular genetic analysis can be used to confirm or refute first diagnostic impressions (Fig. 3.5).

Type 2A VWD

Type 2A VWD involves loss of high molecular weight (HMW) VWF multimers and a resultant decrease in platelet-mediated VWF function.

Two molecular mechanisms have been described for type 2A disease:
1 in group 1, HMW multimers are processed ineffectively by the cell;
2 in group 2, HMW multimers secreted into the plasma are more susceptible to proteolysis.
Both forms of the disorder are the result of heterozygous missense mutations affecting the A2 (rarely A1) protein domain of VWF, which are localized to exon 28 of the VWF gene and can be readily evaluated by direct sequencing of a PCR product obtained from genomic DNA.

Frameshift and missense mutations have also been described in exon 52, causing defects in dimerization. A less common recessive form of the disorder results from mutations in the propeptide sequence.

Type 2B VWD

Type 2B VWD involves dominant gain-of-function changes enhancing the affinity of mutant VWF for its platelet receptor, glycoprotein (Gp) Ib. These missense mutations are consistently clustered in the region of the gene encoding the A1 protein domain (rarely A2). Direct sequencing of exon 28 sequences can provide molecular genetic confirmation of the type 2B phenotype. Ninety percent of cases are caused by R1308C, R1306C, V1316M and R1341Q.

Type 2M VWD

The type 2M variant has reduced platelet-mediated VWF function with normal VWF multimers, with missense mutations localized to the same region of exon 28 as the type 2B mutations. They can be detected with the same sequencing strategy.

Type 2N VWD

Type 2N VWD is a recessive disorder and a condition easily confused with mild hemophilia A. The most efficient molecular genetic approach to achieve this distinction is to sequence the PCR products amplified from exons 18–20, and exon 24 of the VWF gene. In patients with type 2N VWD, this analysis will show either homozygous or compound heterozygous missense mutations affecting the factor VIII binding domain of the protein, R854Q being the most frequent mutation. Coinheritance of a type 2N allele with a severe type 1 or type 3 null allele will also result in this phenotype.

Type 1 VWD

Despite being the most prevalent form of the disorder, representing approximately 75% of all VWD cases, the molecular pathogenesis of type 1 VWD remains the least well understood. Diagnosis can often be difficult and is influenced by a variety of factors, including the temporal variability of VWF levels and the ABO blood group of patients, accounting for approximately 30% of the variability in VWF levels, with blood group O having the lowest levels. Another significant complicating factor in attempting to address the genetic basis for type 1 VWD is the marked variability in penetrance and expression of the phenotype within families, which makes the use of classic linkage analysis problematic. Therefore much of the knowledge gained in this area has relied on labour-intensive strategies such as direct sequencing of genomic DNA.

Some cases of type 1 VWD have been found to result from heterozygous deletions, frameshifts and nonsense mutations that overlap those documented in the homozygous form of type 3 disease. Compound heterozygosity for a type 1 allele and one of the type 2 variant alleles has also been reported. Recently, a missense mutation (Y1584C) has been found in a significant number of type 1 VWD cases. This, in combination with rarer but well-described dominant-negative mutations in exon 26 (C1130F and C1149R), provides the first opportunity to incorporate genetic testing into the diagnosis of type 1 VWD. Each of these mutations is associated with restriction endonuclease site changes and, consequently, they can be readily assessed in a molecular diagnostic facility.

Less common coagulation factor deficiencies

As the genes for all of the procoagulant proteins have been cloned and characterized, molecular genetic testing should be feasible for inherited deficiency of any of these factors. However, the diagnosis of these disorders (factor XI and X deficiencies and others) remains firmly based in the clinical hemostasis laboratory through the performance of biological clotting assays.

Although specific research laboratories may be interested in determining the disease-causing mutations in these families, primarily as a means to assist in structure and function analysis, the performance of these tests for diagnostic purposes is not usual. An exception is the recent documentation of mutations in the ERGIC-53/LMAN1 gene in patients with inherited combined factor V and VIII deficiencies. Most cases of this rare disorder are caused by one of two point mutations in this intermediate compartment processing protein; thus, documentation of either of these mutations would definitively establish an otherwise unusual diagnosis.

COLOUR PLATES FOR CHAPTERS 3, 4 & 17

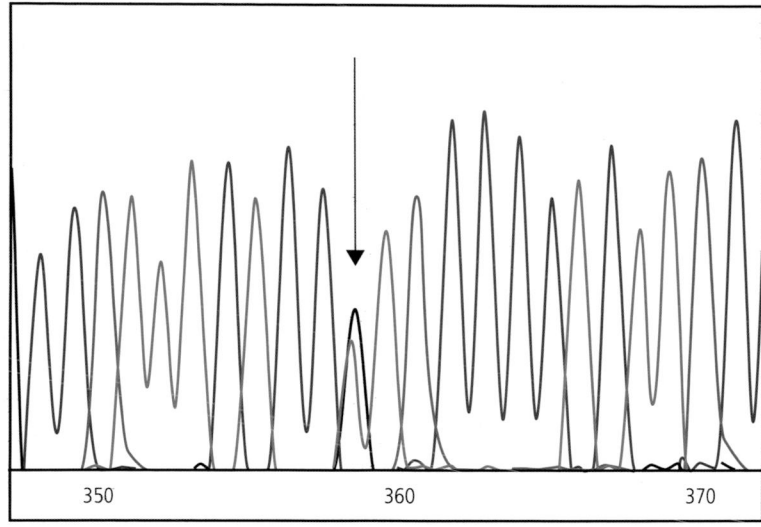

Plate 1 DNA sequence derived from a carrier of hemophilia A. The sequence shows a double peak (G + A) shown by the arrow in the sequencing chromatogram. This woman is heterozygous for a glutamine to premature stop codon mutation in exon 9 of the factor VIII gene.

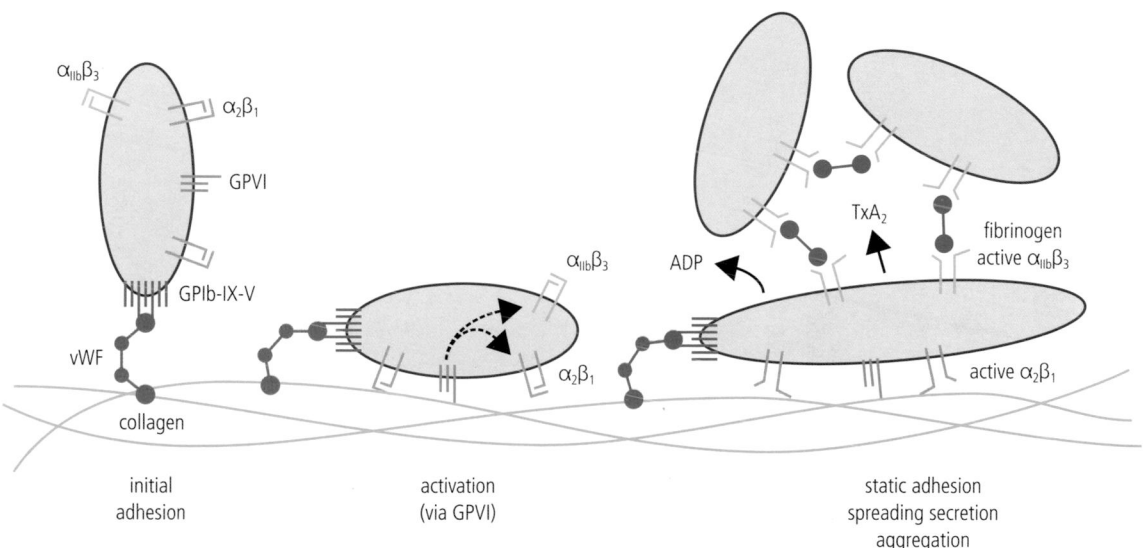

Plate 2 A general diagram showing the phases of hemostatic plug/thrombus formation at medium and high rates of shear. Platelets are initially captured (tethered) by von Willebrand factor (VWF) bound to immobilized collagen. Collagen activates platelets via Gp VI leading to an increase in affinity of the integrins $\alpha_{IIb}\beta_3$ and $\alpha_2\beta_1$ for VWF/fibrinogen and collagen, respectively. This activated state mediates stable platelet adhesion and potentiates activation through further activation of Gp VI and also release of ADP and TxA_2. The formation of a procoagulant surface also supports formation of thrombin. VWF and fibrinogen, in combination with ADP, TxA_2 and thrombin, mediate thrombus formation (aggregation), spreading and stabilization (clot retraction).

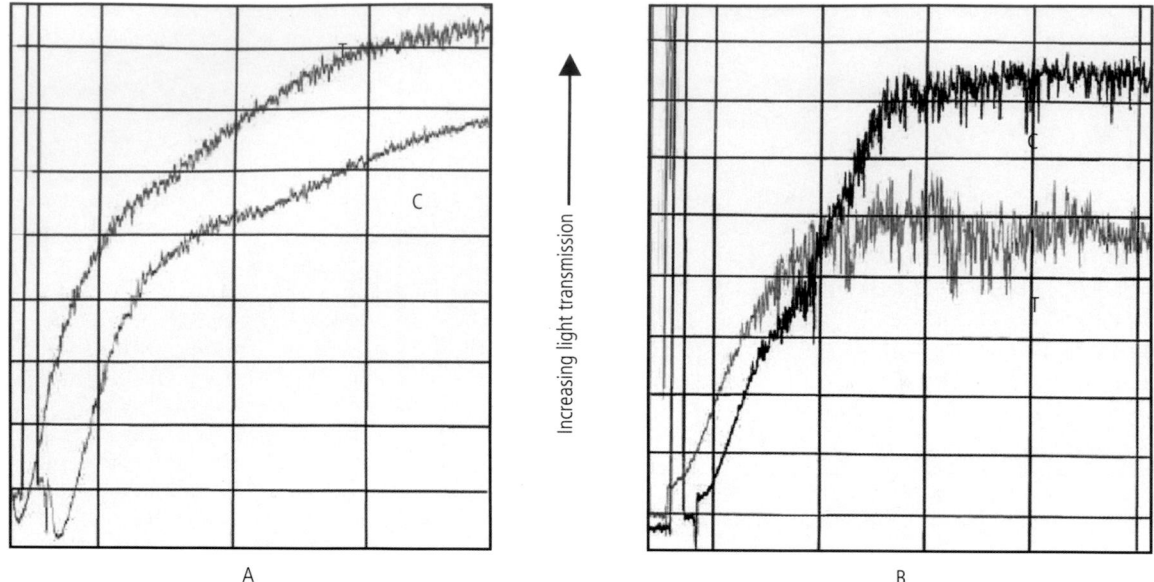

Increasing light transmission

A

B

Plate 3 (a) Platelet aggregation profiles after the addition of 5 μm adenosine diphosphate (ADP) to test (T) and normal control (C) platelet-rich plasma. (b) Platelet aggregation tracings (C, normal control; T, test) after addition of the agonist ristocetin at a concentration of 1 mg/mL.

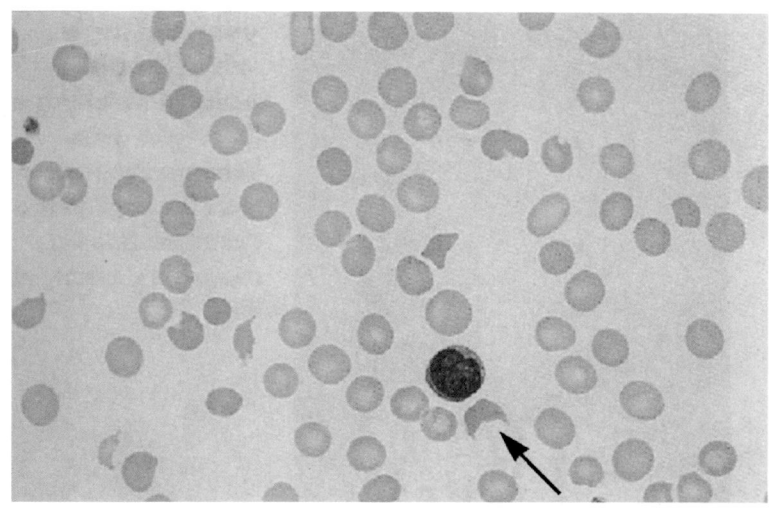

Plate 4 The peripheral blood film in thrombotic thrombocytopenic purpura (TTP) showing schistocytes (arrowed) and thrombocytopenia. Reprinted from *Blood in Systemic Disease* 1e, Greaves and Makris, 1997, with permission from Elsevier.

Inherited platelet disorders

As with the less common coagulation factor deficiencies, the diagnosis of inherited platelet disorders is predominantly by phenotypic analysis. Standard morphology, platelet aggregation studies and an evaluation of platelet receptor density will usually establish or exclude a diagnosis of Bernard–Soulier syndrome or Glanzmann thrombasthenia, the two most frequently encountered, but nevertheless rare, recessive inherited platelet disorders.

In unusual instances, knowledge of the causative mutation in these patients could be useful, perhaps for prenatal testing. In the Bernard–Soulier syndrome, a heterogeneous mutational pattern has been documented, with both homozygous and compound heterozygous mutations identified in the genes encoding Gp Ibα, Ibβ and IX. A variety of different mutations have been found at these loci, including deletions, frameshifts, nonsense and missense changes. To date, no Bernard–Soulier mutations have been identified in the GpV gene.

In Glanzmann thrombasthenia, a similarly varied pattern of mutations has been documented in the genes for Gp IIb and IIIa.

In platelet-type (or pseudo) VWD, the standard coagulation studies are similar to those encountered with type 2B VWD. Here the clarification of this phenotype does require molecular tests and heterozygous dominant missense mutations can be found in the Gp Ibα gene, which have been shown through the analysis of recombinant mutant protein to possess an increased binding affinity for the A1 domain of VWF.

Molecular diagnostics for thrombotic disease

While an inherited tendency for excessive bleeding can often be ascribed to single gene abnormalities, there is ample evidence to suggest that, in contrast, the clinical manifestations of hypercoagulability are the result of adverse interactions between multiple genes and the environment. Thus, the use of molecular diagnostics to document markers of thrombotic risk (thrombophilia) will prove to

Table 3.1 The common thrombophilic states with their prevalence in the general population and the enhanced relative risk for venous thromboembolism.

	Prevalence in the general population (%)	Relative risk for venous thrombosis
Factor V Leiden	4	× 5
Prothrombin gene mutation	2	× 3
MTHFR thermolabile variant	10	× 1.5
Antithrombin deficiency	0.02	× 25–50
Protein C deficiency	0.2	× 10
Protein S deficiency	0.08	× 2–10

be far more challenging than with the inherited hemorrhagic disorders. To further complicate matters, despite the fact that with appropriate testing thrombophilic mutations can be identified in approximately 50% of patients following a first clinical episode of venous thromboembolism, interpretation of these results remains problematic in some cases (Table 3.1).

Inherited resistance to activated protein C: Factor V Leiden

Until 1994, the investigation of patients with clinical evidence of hypercoagulability was usually unproductive. However, with the discovery by Dahlback and Hildebrand of an inherited form of resistance to the proteolytic effects of activated protein C, and the subsequent finding of a common missense mutation in the factor V gene by Bertina's group in Leiden, a major advance was made in the laboratory assessment of thrombotic risk.

The Leiden mutation substitutes a glutamine for an arginine at amino acid residue 506 in factor V, the initial cleavage site for activated protein C. The mutation is readily detected by PCR and restriction analysis because of the alteration of an *Mnl* I restriction site. Between 2 and 5% of individuals in Western populations have been documented to be heterozygous for factor V Leiden. In contrast, the mutation is extremely rare in subjects of Asian and African descent.

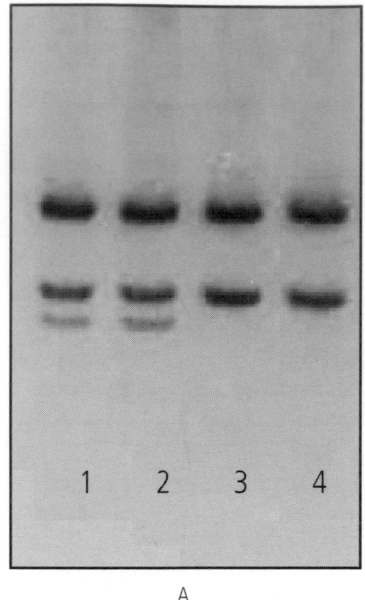

A
Prothrombin gene mutation

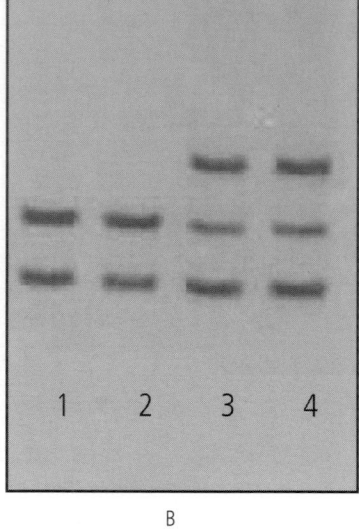

B
Factor V Leiden

Figure 3.6 (a) PCR and restriction enzyme analysis of the prothrombin 20210 gene mutation. Lanes 3 and 4 show the normal restriction pattern while lanes 1 and 2 show the pattern in two DNA samples containing the heterozygous state for the prothrombin 20210 mutation. (b) PCR and restriction enzyme analysis of the factor V Leiden mutation. Lanes 1 and 2 show the normal restriction pattern while lanes 3 and 4 contain DNA with the heterozygous state for the factor V Leiden mutation.

In most laboratories, initial screening for resistance to activated protein C is performed using the prolongation of an activated partial thromboplastin time (APTT) based assay as an indicator; patients testing positive (prolongation in the presence of factor V-deficient plasma) are subsequently evaluated by a PCR assay (Fig. 3.6).

Where large-scale PCR-based molecular analysis is in routine use, some laboratories may choose to proceed directly to the genetic test, as the result is definitive and more than 95% of activated protein C resistance is a result of this single mutation. Rare, alternative factor V mutations have been documented at arginine 306 (Arg to Thr and Arg to Gly), but it seems unlikely that these variants are significant markers of a thrombotic risk.

Persons heterozygous for the factor V Leiden mutation have an approximately five-fold increased relative risk of venous thrombosis. It is found in 15–20% of patients experiencing their first episode of venous thrombosis and in 50–60% of thrombosis patients with a family history of thrombotic disease. The hypercoagulable phenotype associated with factor V Leiden has variable penetrance; some individuals may never manifest a clinical thrombotic event. Coinheritance of other inherited thrombotic risk factors or exposure to environmental risk factors (i.e. oral contraceptives) can dramatically enhance thrombotic risk in carriers of factor V Leiden. Many clinicians test for this disorder in patients with a family history of thrombosis who are about to be exposed to an acquired thrombotic risk factor. Individuals homozygous for the mutation have a 70-fold enhanced relative risk of venous thrombosis.

Prothrombin 20210 3′ non-coding sequence variant

In 1996, Poort et al. described an association between a G to A nucleotide polymorphism at position 20210 in the 3′ untranslated region (UTR) of the prothrombin gene, increased plasma levels of prothrombin and an enhanced risk for venous thrombosis. This polymorphic sequence is at the very end of the 3′ UTR and exerts its effect on prothrombin levels in the heterozygous state. Although the plasma levels of prothrombin in subjects heterozygous for this polymorphism are higher on average than those in individuals with a normal prothrombin genotype, levels are usually still within the normal range. As a consequence, this polymorphism can only be evaluated by genetic testing, which is achieved by a PCR–restriction digest procedure (Fig. 3.6) or through an alternate allele-specific PCR strategy.

As with the factor V Leiden genotype, the prevalence of the prothrombin 20210 G to A variant in the general population is relatively high at 1–5%. This variant is also rare in persons of Asian and African descent. The heterozygous state is associated with a two- to fourfold increase in the relative risk for venous thrombosis.

Thermolabile C677T 5,10-methylenetetrahydrofolate reductase variant

The third, high prevalence genetic variant recently found to be associated with an increased thrombotic risk is the C to T variant at nucleotide 677 (an alanine to valine substitution) in the 5, 10-methylene-tetrahydrofolate reductase (MTHFR) gene. This genotype results in expression of an enzyme with increased thermolability. Homozygosity for the variant is associated with hyperhomocysteinemia, particularly in the presence of folate deficiency. In many populations (southern Europeans and Hispanic Americans), approximately 10% of subjects are homozygous for the C677T variant, a sequence change that can easily be detected by a PCR-based strategy. Unlike the factor V Leiden and prothrombin 20210 variants, the role of the MTHFR C677T polymorphism as an independent risk factor for venous thromboembolism appears minor.

Deficiencies of antithrombin, protein C and protein S

Deficiencies of the major anticoagulant proteins antithrombin, protein C and protein S have long been known to represent individual significant risk factors for the development of venous thromboembolism.

Diagnosis of these three disorders relies on standard functional tests or immunoassays. All three of the deficiency states are associated with significant mutational heterogeneity and routine molecular diagnostic investigation of these mutations is not warranted. However, our understanding of the molecular influences on these conditions is improving, as shown by the recent description of variability within a distinct region on chromosome 1q that influences the level of free protein S in plasma.

The future for diagnostic molecular hemostasis

As the Human Genome Project rapidly advances towards its goal, with its accompanying technological benefits, we can expect that more information will be available for molecular diagnostic testing of hemostatic disorders, and that the assay strategies employed will become more efficient. The development of later generation DNA microarrays represents just one example of the new technologies that will likely influence molecular diagnostic protocols in the near future.

Another area of diagnostic molecular hemostasis where advances are just beginning to become apparent is in the risk assessment for arterial thrombosis. There is no doubt that the genetic factors influencing arterial thrombosis are complex and multiple. However, the recent identification of several platelet receptor polymorphisms that appear to predispose to arterial occlusions suggests that we are beginning to make progress towards this objective.

Further reading

Bertina RM, Koeleman BP, Koster T, *et al*. Mutation in blood coagulation factor V associated with resistance to activated protein C. *Nature* 1994;**369**:64–7.

Fressinaud E, Mazurier C, Mazurier CF, Meyer D. Molecular genetics of type 2 von Willebrand disease. *Int J Hematol* 2002;**75**:9–18.

Giannelli F, Green PM, Sommer SS, *et al*. Haemophilia B: database of point mutations and short additions and deletions, 8th edition. *Nucleic Acids Res* 1998;**26**:265–8.

Gitschier J, Wood WI, Goralka TM, *et al*. Characterization of the human factor VIII gene. *Nature* 1984;**312**:326–30.

Goodeve AC, Peake IR. The molecular basis of hemophilia A: genotype–phenotype relationships and inhibitor development. *Semin Thromb Hemost* 2003;**29**:23–30.

Kurachi K, Davie EW. Isolation and characterization of a cDNA coding for human factor IX. *Proc Natl Acad Sci USA* 1982;**79**:6461–4.

Lakich D, Kazazian HH Jr, Antonarakis SE, Gitschier J. Inversions disrupting the factor VIII gene are a common cause of severe haemophilia A. *Nat Genet* 1993;5:236–41.

Ngo K, Glotz Trifard V, Koziol J, *et al*. Homozygous and heterozygous deletions of the von Willebrand factor gene in patients and carriers of severe von Willebrand disease. *Proc Natl Acad Sci USA* 1988;85:2753–7.

O'Brien LA, James PD, Othman M, *et al*. Founder von Willebrand factor haplotype associated with type 1 von Willebrand disease. *Blood* 2003;**102**:549–57.

Peake IR, Bowen D, Bignell P, *et al*. Family studies and prenatal diagnosis in severe von Willebrand disease by polymerase chain reaction amplification of a variable number tandem repeat region of the von Willebrand factor gene. *Blood* 1990;**76**:555–61.

Poort SR, Rosendaal FR, Reitsma PH, Bertina RM. A common genetic variation in the 3′-untranslated region of the prothrombin gene is associated with elevated plasma prothrombin levels and an increase in venous thrombosis. *Blood* 1996;**88**:3698–703.

Schwaab R, Brackmann HH, Meyer C, *et al*. Haemophilia A: mutation type determines risk of inhibitor formation. *Thromb Haemost* 1995;**74**:1402–6.

Tuddenham EGD, Goldman E, McGraw A, Kernoff PBA. Hemophilia A: carrier detection and prenatal diagnosis by linkage analysis using DNA polymorphism. *J Clin Pathol* 1987;**40**:971–7.

Wacey AI, Kemball-Cook G, Kazazian HH, *et al*. The haemophilia A mutation search test and resource site, home page of the factor VIII mutation database: HAMSTeRS. *Nucleic Acids Res* 1996;**24**:100–2.

Chapter 4
Tests of platelet function

Paul Harrison

Structure of platelets

Human blood platelets are small, anucleated, subcellular fragments that have a critical role in hemostasis and thrombosis. Platelets normally circulate for approximately 10 days, constantly surveying the integrity of the vessel wall. Normal human platelets are small and discoid in shape (0.5×3.0 μm); have a mean volume of 7–11 fL; and circulate in relatively high numbers between 150–400×10^9/L.

A cross-section of a typical discoid platelet is shown in Fig. 4.1.

Function

The small disc shape enables the platelets to be pushed towards the edge of vessels so that the majority circulate adjacent to the vascular endothelial cells that line all blood vessels. Upon detection of vessel wall damage they undergo rapid but controlled adhesion, activation and aggregation to form a hemostatic plug and thus prevent blood loss.

Endothelial cells produce a number of potent antiplatelet substances (e.g. nitric oxide, prostacyclin and CD39) that normally inhibit vessel wall–platelet interactions. Vessel wall damage exposes highly adhesive substrates (e.g. P selectin, Von Willebrand factor [VWF] and collagen, and other extracellular matrix components) which result in:
• Initial adhesion, transient rolling of platelets along the vessel wall and slowing of the cells. Consequently, platelets are more likely to undergo stable adhesion.
• Platelet activation (if there is more extensive damage or stimuli promoting platelet activation).
• Platelet aggregation (see Plate 2, facing p. 24).

The platelets interact with and sense the environment through many types of surface receptors (major receptors and their ligands are summarized in Table 4.1). The net balance between activating or inhibitory stimuli thus controls whether platelets continue to circulate, begin to reversibly interact with the vessel wall or become irreversibly adherent to either the vessel wall or each other.

During adhesion, platelets become activated through signal transduction pathways which mediate shape change, degranulation and spreading upon areas of exposed subendothelium. Activated platelets recruit additional platelets into the growing platelet aggregate or thrombus via a number of positive feedback pathways including release of dense granular adenosine diphosphate (ADP) and generation of thromboxane. Activated platelets also express negatively charged phospholipids on their surface, facilitating the local generation of high amounts of thrombin, which not only further activates other platelets, but also stabilizes the platelet plug through fibrin formation. In this manner, platelets rapidly seal any areas of vessel wall damage and provide a catalytic surface for coagulation to occur, resulting in the formation of a stable hemostatic plug.

Thrombosis is usually the consequence of inappropriate activation of platelets, especially in regions of abnormal vessel wall lesions or damage, e.g. atherosclerotic plaques. The high shear stress that often occurs in these regions also significantly contributes to thrombus formation (via promotion

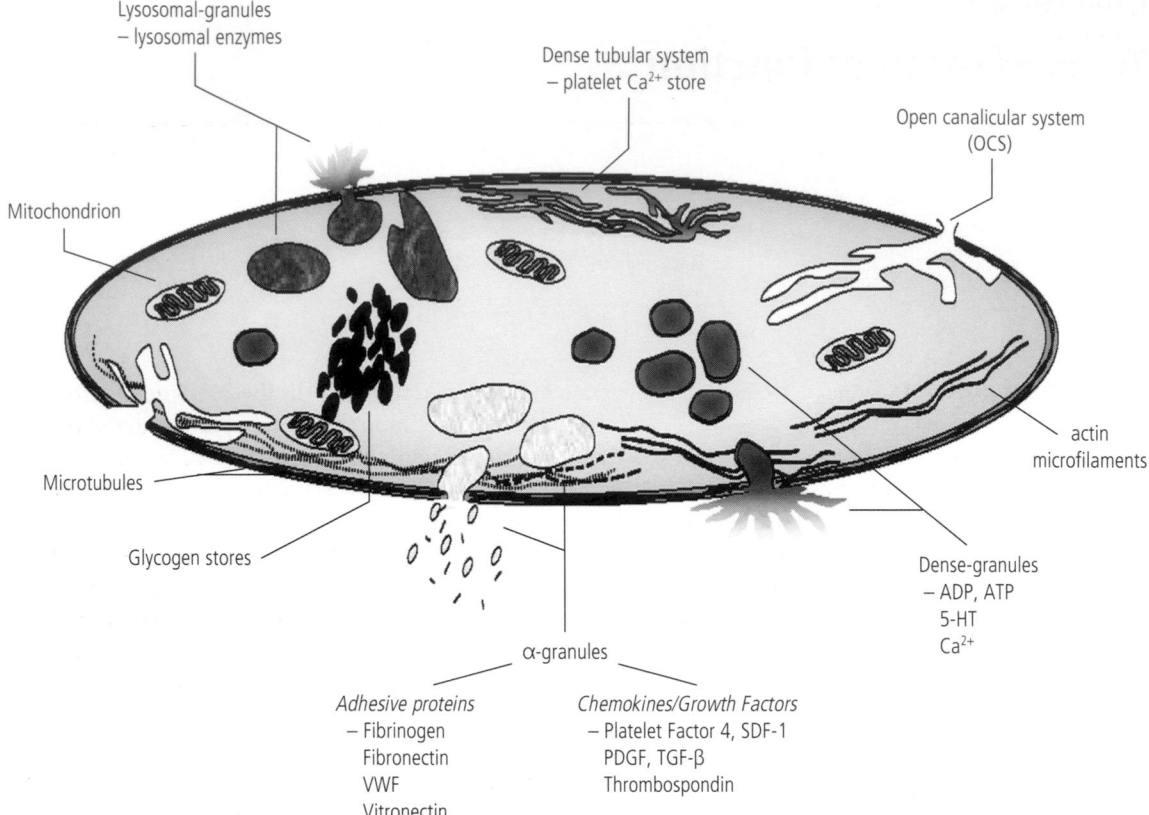

Lysosomal-granules
– lysosomal enzymes

Dense tubular system
– platelet Ca²⁺ store

Open canalicular system
(OCS)

Mitochondrion

actin
microfilaments

Microtubules

Glycogen stores

Dense-granules
– ADP, ATP
5-HT
Ca²⁺

α-granules

Adhesive proteins
– Fibrinogen
Fibronectin
VWF
Vitronectin

Chemokines/Growth Factors
– Platelet Factor 4, SDF-1
PDGF, TGF-β
Thrombospondin

Figure 4.1 Platelet structure and organelles. This diagram summarizes the key structural features of a platelet including the open canalicular system (OCS), the dense tubular system (DTS), actin microfilaments and microtubules, mitochondria, glycogen stores, dense granules, lysosomes and alpha granules. (Reproduced with permission from Watson S and Harrison P. The Vascular function of platelets, page 813, In *Postgraduate Haematology*, 5th Edition (eds Hoffbrand V, Tuddenham E, Catovsky D), Blackwell Publishing, 2005).

of VWF-dependent platelet adhesion and aggregation) along with the events described above.

Antiplatelet drug therapy thus provides an important means to prevent thrombosis in high-risk patients with arterial disease. In contrast, there are also many defects in platelet function that can occur in patients, often resulting in an increased risk of bleeding.

Classification of platelet defects

Platelet abnormalities can be broadly classified into **quantitative** (abnormal in number) and **qualitative** defects (abnormal in function). Defects in number include many types of thrombocytopenia (e.g. caused by immune or non-immune destruction or decreased production) and thrombocytosis (increased platelet number). Functional defects can either be inherited or more commonly acquired (secondary to disease, surgical procedures or drugs, and antiplatelet therapy).

Inherited platelet-related disorders include many abnormalities such as the following:
• defects in various platelet receptors for both adhesive proteins and soluble agonists;
• defects in adhesive proteins that mediate platelet adhesion and aggregation;
• defects in the storage or release of platelet granules;

Table 4.1 Major platelet agonists and their surface receptors. Platelets express a remarkable number and variety of receptors for a wide range of ligands. For many of these receptor–ligand combinations, however, the effect on platelet activation is weak and of uncertain significance. (Reproduced with permission from Watson S and Harrison P, The Vascular function of platelets, page 819, In *Postgraduate Haematology*, 5th Edition (eds Hoffbrand V, Tuddenham E, Catovsky D), Blackwell publications, 2004 (in press)).

Agonist	Receptor	Effect and physiological role
Adhesion molecules		
Collagen	Gp VI	Major signaling receptor for collagen
	$\alpha_2\beta_1$	Supports adhesion by collagen
Fibrinogen	$\alpha_{IIb}\beta_3$	Aggregation, spreading and clot retraction
Fibronectin	$\alpha_5\beta_1$, $\alpha_{IIb}\beta_3$	$\alpha_5\beta_1$ mediates adhesion
Laminin	$\alpha_6\beta_1$	Adhesion
von Willebrand factor	Gp Ib-IX-V, $\alpha_{IIb}\beta_3$	Platelet tethering (also fibrinogen)
Amines		
Adrenaline	α_2	
5-HT	5-HT_{2A}	Mediates vasoconstriction
Cytokines		
TPO	c-Mpl	Maturation of megakaryocytes
Immune complexes		
Fc portion of antibodies	FcγRIIA	Immune-based platelet activation
Lipids		
Lysophospholipids		
PAF	PAF	
Prostacyclin	IP	Endothelial-mediated inhibition
Sphingosine 1-phosphate		
Thromboxanes	TP	Major positive feedback agonist
Nucleotides		
Adenosine	A_{2A}	
ADP	$P2Y_1$	Early role in platelet activation
	$P2Y_{12}$	Major positive feedback receptor
ATP	$P2X_1$	Possible early role in platelet activation
Proteases		
Thrombin	PAR_1, PAR_4	Coagulation-dependent platelet activation
Surface molecules		
CD40 ligand	CD40 and $\alpha_{IIb}\beta_3$	
Tyrosine kinase receptors		
Angiopoietin 1 and 2	Tie-1	
EphrinB1	EphA4 and EphB1	Late events in platelet activation?
Vitamin K-dependent		
Gas6	Sky, Axl and Mer	Supports platelet activation?

- defects in signal transduction pathways;
- defects in exposure of negatively charged phospholipid;
- inherited thrombocytopenias.

Table 4.2 summarizes the classification of inherited platelet function defects.

Platelet function testing

Before platelet function tests are performed, the full clinical history (including family and recent drug-taking history) is obtained and a physical examination of the patient is performed. Platelet

Table 4.2 Classification of inherited platelet defects.

Defect	Disorder
Platelet adhesion	Bernard–Soulier syndrome
	Von Willebrand disease
Platelet aggregation	Glanzmann thrombasthenia
	Congenital afibrinogenemia
Platelet activation (receptor defects)	Collagen receptor defects: $\alpha_2\beta_1$ or Gp VI deficiency
	ADP receptor defects: $P2Y_{12}$ deficiency
	Thromboxane receptor defects
Secretion defects	Storage pool disease
	Hermansky–Pudlak syndrome
	Chédiak–Higashi syndrome
	Grey platelet syndrome
	Quebec platelet disorder
	Wiskott–Aldrich syndrome
Signaling pathways	$G\alpha q$ deficiency
	Cyclooxygenase deficiency
	Phospholipase C deficiency
	Thromboxane synthase deficiency
	Lipoxygenase deficiency
	Calcium mobilization defects
Platelet size	Inherited macrothrombocytopenia
Membrane phospholipids	Scott syndrome

disorders are usually associated with excessive bleeding (especially after trauma) and other classic symptoms including petechiae, epistaxis and menorrhagia. Coagulation protein defects, in contrast, are usually associated with a delayed pattern of bleeding, and the presence of hemarthroses and hematomas.

As many patients present with a transiently acquired defect of platelet function (e.g. caused by aspirin or diet), repeat testing is often necessary to ensure a correct diagnosis. If a hemostatic defect is suspected then laboratories will use a range of initial screening tests. These tests include:
• full blood count and blood film;
• coagulation tests (prothrombin time [PT], activated partial thromboplastin time [APTT] and thrombin time [TT]);
• bleeding time or platelet function analysis with the PFA-100® (as the *in vivo* bleeding time is

considered unreliable, some laboratories are now beginning to use *in vitro* alternatives such as the PFA-100®);
• platelet aggregation (still considered the gold standard although time-consuming);
• factor VIII/VWF levels.

The biggest problems still faced with platelet function testing are a number of quality control issues including anticoagulation, sample quality, sample handling (collection and processing and lack of standardization of methodologies used).

Platelets are not only prone to artefactual *in vitro* activation but also to desensitization. Most functional tests have to be performed relatively quickly (e.g. less than 2 h from sampling). It is also impossible to use standard quality control material apart from freshly drawn blood from normal volunteers.

Global tests of platelet function

Bleeding time

The skin bleeding time has been clinically utilized for almost a century and has been modified several times in attempts to improve reliability. Briefly, a constant blood pressure of 40 mmHg is applied to the upper arm and a disposable, sterile, automated template device is applied to inflict standardized cuts into the forearm. Excess blood is then removed with filter paper at regular intervals and the time for the cessation of bleeding recorded. Normal bleeding times are less than 10 min. Prolonged bleeding times are encountered in patients with severe platelet defects and so the test has been widely utilized as a screening tool.

The clear **advantages** of the bleeding time are that it is a simple test of natural hemostasis including the important contribution of the vessel wall and it also avoids potential anticoagulation artefacts. The **disadvantages** are that bleeding time results can be both poorly reproducible and insensitive to milder forms of platelet dysfunction.

The consensus is that the test does not necessarily correlate well with the bleeding risk and that an accurate clinical history is more valuable. A number of different *in vitro* methods have therefore been devised to try to measure global platelet function within whole blood exposed to conditions that attempt to simulate *in vivo* hemostasis such as the PFA-100®.

Platelet function analyser: PFA-100®

This analyzer, developed by Dade–Behring, is based upon the original principle and prototype instrument described by Kratzer and Born. Widespread experience with the instrument is increasing, but how the test should be utilized within normal laboratory practice remains to be fully defined.

All test components are within disposable cartridges that are loaded into the instrument at the start of the test. Citrated whole blood (800 µL) is pipetted into the cartridge and, after a short incubation period, exposed to high shear (5000–6000/s) through a capillary tube before encountering a membrane with a central aperture of 150 µm diameter. The membrane is coated with collagen and either ADP or epinephrine. The instrument monitors the drop in flow rate as platelets form a hemostatic plug that seals the aperture and stops blood flow. This parameter is recorded as the closure time (CT). The maximal value obtainable is 300 s.

To ensure optimal PFA-100® performance and data interpretation, there are a number of quality control procedures and good practice guidelines that need to be borne in mind:
• Mandatory daily instrument checks, PFA-100® self-test should always be performed.
• Ensuring the quality of blood sampling.
• Ensuring consistency in anticoagulation, 3.8% (0.129 mol/L) or 3.2% (0.105 mol/L) buffered trisodium citrate.
• Checking for cartridge batch variation.
• Testing within 4 h from sampling.
• A control group within each laboratory setting should be established. These individuals should ideally exhibit CTs within the middle of the established laboratory reference range.
• Each laboratory should also ideally establish their own reference ranges on both cartridges utilizing normal volunteers from their institution.

Typical normal ranges obtained with 3.8% trisodium citrate are 58–151 s for collagen/ADP and 94–202 s for collagen/epinephrine. With 3.2% trisodium citrate, typical ranges are 55–112 s for collagen/ADP and 79–164 s for collagen/epinephrine (Oxford Haemophilia Centre, unpublished results).

Within-sample CVs have been reported as approximately 10%, which, although acceptable for a platelet function test, may obviously cause problems with values obtained close to upper normal range cut-off values.

The **advantages** of the test are that it is simple, rapid, does not require specialist training (apart from training in the manipulation of blood samples). It is a potential screening tool for assessing patients with many types of platelet abnormality. Within a typical population of patients tested, the overall negative predictive value of the test is high (more than 90%), although the test is clearly not 100% sensitive to all platelet defects. The test is particularly useful in pediatric settings where the availability of blood is often a limiting factor, particularly for assessing platelet function in non-accidental injury. Given the high shear conditions to which platelets are exposed during the test it is not surprising that the test is highly VWF-dependent and is useful not only for detecting VWD, but also for monitoring therapy, particularly with DDAVP. The instrument thus provides laboratories with a potential screening tool that gives rapid and reliable data with a high negative predictive value.

A number of studies suggest that the PFA-100® is a potential *in vitro* replacement of the bleeding time. The **disadvantages** are that, like the *in vivo* bleeding time, the test is sensitive to both the platelet count and hematocrit and it is therefore crucial that a full blood count is performed to help interpret abnormal results. The test is insensitive to coagulation protein defects including afibrinogenemia, hemophilia A and B and other clotting factors. False-negative results are sometimes obtained; for example, in patients with storage pool disease, primary secretion defects, Hermansky–Pudlak syndrome, type 1 von Willebrand disease (VWD) and the Quebec platelet disorder. Diagnosis of these disorders could therefore be missed if relying on the PFA-100® as a screening test alone. In patients with apparently normal platelet function, the instrument has also been shown to occasionally give false-positive results.

Many studies are also in progress to assess whether the PFA-100® can reliably predict either thrombotic or bleeding complications in different patient groups. As more inter-laboratory experience is gathered, eventually it should be feasible to define the exact role(s) for this instrument in routine laboratory testing.

Platelet aggregation

In the 1960s, the invention of platelet aggregometry revolutionized the analysis of platelet function within routine laboratory testing. Still regarded as the "gold standard," it is the most widely used platelet function test. Citrated platelet-rich plasma (PRP) is normally stirred under conditions of low shear within an incubated cuvette (37°C) between a light source and a photocell. Whole blood may be used in some commercial aggregometers.

The addition of different dosages of a panel of agonists triggers platelet activation, shape change and primary and secondary aggregation events which increase light transmission over time and this is recorded on the aggregation trace (see Plate 3, facing p. 25). By using a panel of agonists at differing concentrations it is possible to detect a number of classic platelet defects. Modern machines usually offer multichannel capability and computer analysis and storage of data, although samples and reagents still have to be prepared manually.

A fully automated and near patient testing aggregation system called the RPFA (Rapid Platelet Function Analyzer), or Ultegra device (Accumetrics), is now available solely for the monitoring of antiplatelet therapy, e.g. Gp IIb/IIIa inhibitors, aspirin and clopidogrel.

The method is as follows:
- Citrated PRP adjusted to 200×10^9/L is added to cuvette at 37°C and preincubated for 5 min.
- The PRP is stirred at the recommended speed (1000 r.p.m.) to allow platelets to come in contact with each other.
- 100% transmission is set with platelet-poor plasma (PPP).
- 0% transmission is set with PRP.
- Agonist is added (10% total volume).
- Aggregation is recorded (10–15 min).

- Calculate percentage aggregation (maximum or final) and slope (rate of aggregation).
- Hemolyzed or very lipemic samples may interfere with light transmission.
- Thrombocytopenic samples are also unsuitable for analysis.

A typical panel of agonists (stored in frozen aliquots) are:
- ADP
- Epinephrine (1.0–10 µmol/L)
- Collagen (1–5 µg/mL), usually mediates a steep aggregation curve but after a characteristic lag phase of more than 1 min
- Aracidonic acid (1.0–2.0 mmol/L)
- Ristocetin (0.5–1.5 mg/mL) is not strictly an agonist but stimulates platelet agglutination through binding of plasma VWF to Gp Ib and therefore will also give abnormal results in VWD
- Thrombin (0.1–0.5 IU/mL).

A typical aggregation curve can sometimes be divided into primary and secondary aggregation responses, the latter being characterized by degranulation and thromboxane generation which mediate irreversible aggregation. Thus, any defects in either thromboxane generation or storage granules will result in a reduced secondary aggregation response.

There are no commercially available quality control kits for platelet function testing. Aggregometers can be checked by using the PRP and PPP to check percentage aggregation settings and dilutions (mixes of PRP and PPP) can be performed to check linearity.

Glanzmann thrombasthenia
There is complete absence of aggregation to agonists such as ADP, but a normal agglutination response to ristocetin.

Bernard–Soulier syndrome
Platelets aggregate to all of the physiologic agonists, but do not agglutinate to ristocetin.

VWD
Patients with VWD will have defective ristocetin-induced agglutination. This can be corrected by addition of normal plasma or cryoprecipitate. A low dose of ristocetin (less than 0.5 mg/mL) will

also only mediate platelet agglutination in type 2B VWD.

Storage pool or release defects

Patients with storage pool or release defects typically show an impaired secondary aggregation response. In order to confirm the diagnosis, platelet nucleotide content should also be measured. Defects in thromboxane generation (e.g. COX-1 deficiency caused by aspirin) will also be characterized by defective arachidonic acid-induced aggregation coupled with impaired secondary aggregation to other agonists.

Flow cytometry

Whole blood flow cytometry offers a very attractive and reliable test for the diagnosis of various platelet receptor, granular and other defects. Flow cytometry can rapidly measure the properties and characteristics of a large number of individual platelets.

The method is as follows:
• Diluted whole blood (preferred, minimizing activation) or PRP preparations are labeled with fluorescently conjugated monoclonal antibodies.
• The diluted suspension of platelets is then analyzed at a rate of 1000–100,000 cells/min through

a focused laser beam within the instrument flow cell.
• The cytometer then detects both scattered and fluorescent light emitted by each platelet. The intensity of each signal is directly proportional to antigen density or the size/granularity of the platelet and usually 5000–20,000 platelet events are collected in total for each sample.
• Only platelets should be analyzed or gated on by the flow cytometer. This is normally achieved by studying the characteristic light scatter pattern that is obtained with platelets which normally allows their resolution from RBCs, WBCs and background "noise" in most samples. However, in some situations where there is an abnormal platelet distribution which overlaps with the RBCs (e.g. macrothrombocytopenia and Bernard–Soulier disease), it is often useful to use a specific identifying antibody (e.g. Gp Ib or IIb/IIIa) to resolve the fluorescent population of platelets from non-fluorescent RBCs/WBCs and debris/noise (Fig. 4.2).
• Double labeling using another antibody with a different fluorophore is also possible.

Care needs to be taken that:
• the subject is rested (20–30 min);
• the venepuncture is clean (discarding the first few milliliters of blood); and

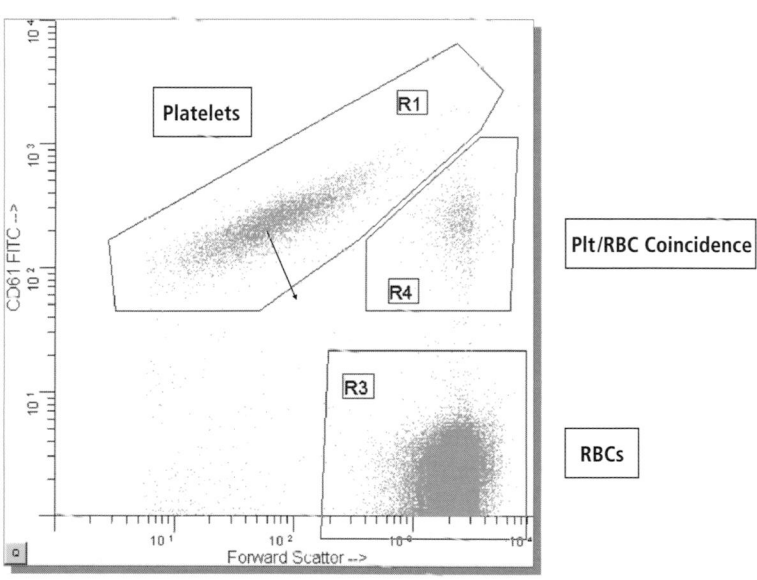

Figure 4.2 A flow cytometry plot using a fluorescent labeled platelet identifying antibody (anti-CD61: glycoprotein IIIa: β_3 integrin). If the instrument is triggered on this fluorescence all other non-platelet events shown below (RBCs) will be eliminated. Optimization of dilution will eliminate the coincident events. (Reproduced with permission from Watson S and Harrison P, The Vascular function of platelets, page 819, in *Postgraduate Haematology*, 5th Edition (eds Hoffbrand V, Tuddenham E, Catovsky D), Blackwell Publishing, 2005).

Blood collected by atruamatic venepuncture into
anticoagulant and used without time delay

Blood (~5 μl) diluted 1:10 in physiological buffer containing directly conjugated antibodies,
agonists and other reagents. Total volume = 50 μl.

Mix by tapping the tube gently and incubate at RT for 20 minutes

Samples diluted in buffer or mild fixative. Total volume = 1000 – 2000 μl.

Analyzed by flow cytometry within 2 hours – collect 10,000 events

Figure 4.3 A typical flow cytometry protocol for the testing and analysis of platelets. Small amounts of blood are incubated with test reagents, diluted and analyzed. New reagents are easily incorporated into this standard procedure.

Diagnosis of platelet defects	Bernard–Soulier syndrome
	Glanzmann thrombasthenia
	Storage pool disease
	HIT
Platelet activation markers	Degranulation markers: CD62p, CD63 and CD40L
	Gp IIb/IIIa conformation
	Platelet–leukocyte conjugates
	Platelet-derived microparticles
Monitoring antiplatelet therapy	Gp IIb/IIIa antagonists
	Clopidogrel and ticlopidine
	Aspirin and COX-1 inhibitors
Measuring platelet production	Reticulated platelets
Accurate platelet counting	Platelet: RBC ratio – new reference method
Platelet associated IgG	ITP
	Alloantibodies
Blood bank tests	Quality control of concentrates
	Leukocyte contamination
	Platelet HPA-1a
	Cross-matching

Table 4.3 Flow cytometric platelet function tests.

HIT, heparin induced thrombocytopenia, ITP, idiopathic thrombocytopenic purpura.

• there are no time delays between sampling and analysis.

It is recommended that daily quality control procedures be performed with stable, fluorescently labeled bead preparations to ensure optimal instrument and laser performance.

The increasing availability of commercial platelet reagents (e.g. antibodies, ligands and probes) has facilitated the development of many types of platelet assay which can be incorporated into a standard protocol (Fig. 4.3).

Table 4.3 summarizes the various types of platelet function that can be tested using a flow cytometer. The most commonly used assay is for the diagnosis of the two major platelet glycoprotein abnormalities: Bernard–Soulier syndrome (Gp Ib deficiency) and Glanzmann thrombasthenia (Gp IIb/IIIa deficiency; Table 4.4). Diagnostic assays

Table 4.4 Mean fluorescent intensity (MFI) and percentage of positive cells showing antibody staining in normal platelets and in platelets from a patient with Glanzmann thrombasthenia (Gp IIb/IIIa deficiency).

Receptor (Mab)	Normal		Patient (LK)	
	Positive cells (%)	MFI	Positive cells (%)	MFI
Mouse IgG (PE)	0.5	–	0.5	–
Gp Ib (anti-CD42b PE)	97.5	557	98.24	851
Mouse IgG (FITC)	0.5	–	0.5	–
Gp IIb (anti-CD41 FITC)	95.99	13.97	1.55	
Gp IIIa (anti-CD61 FITC)	98.42	598	0.8	1.63

are also available for quantifying copy number of any major glycoprotein, studying granular defects (e.g. storage pool disease), heparin-induced thrombocytopenia, and defects in platelet aggregation, secretion or procoagulant activity.

The use of whole blood has several advantages over purified platelet preparations and PRP:

- platelets are analyzed in the presence of erythrocytes and leucocytes;
- only small quantities of blood are required per tube (2–5 µL);
- there is no loss of subpopulations of cells during separation procedures;
- providing the venepuncture is well standardized, minimal manipulation of fresh samples results in little artefactual *in vitro* platelet activation;
- it is possible to study platelets from patients with thrombocytopenia; and
- both the *in vivo* resting activation state and dose–response to classical agonists can be measured with high sensitivity.

When diagnosing any platelet function or receptor defect it is good practice to analyze a normal control sample in parallel to ensure that normal results can be obtained with the test in question. This will also facilitate the eventual calibration of a normal range. Results are normally expressed as mean fluorescent intensity (MFI) or as a percentage of the gated platelet population (Table 4.4). Absolute quantification of receptor density is now possible by using calibrated fluorescent standards, some of which are available in kit form (e.g. Dako, Sigma, Biocytex). The lowest limit of detection by these techniques is quoted as approximately 500 molecules/platelet.

A panel of activation-dependent antibodies (e.g. CD62p, CD63, PAC-1) can be used to assess a patient's platelet response to dose–response curves of agonists that are used for aggregation (e.g. TRAP, ADP, collagen).

Further reading

BSCH Haemostasis and Thrombosis Task Force Guidelines on Platelet Function Testing. *J Clin Pathol* 1988;**41**:1322–30.

Cattaneo M. Inherited platelet-based bleeding disorders. *J Thromb Haemost* 2003;**1**:1628–36.

Favaloro EJ. Clinical application of the PFA-100. *Curr Opin Hematol* 2002;**9**:407–15.

Fressinaud E, Veyradier A, Truchaud F, *et al.* Screening for von Willebrand disease with a new analyzer using high shear stress: a study of 60 cases. *Blood* 1998;**91**:1325–31.

George JN. Platelets. *Lancet* 2000;**355**:1531–9.

Gresele P, Page C, Fuster V, Vermylen J, eds. *Platelets in Thrombotic and Non-thrombotic Disorders*. Cambridge University Press, 2002.

Harrison P. Progress in the assessment of platelet function. *Br J Haematol* 2000;**111**:733–44.

Harrison P, Robinson MS, Mackie IJ, *et al.* Performance of the platelet function analyzer PFA-100 in testing abnormalities of primary haemostasis. *Blood Coagul Fibrinolysis* 1999;**10**:25–31.

Hayward CP. Inherited platelet disorders. *Curr Opin Hematol* 2003;**10**:362–8.

Jackson SP, Schoenwaelder SM. Antiplatelet therapy: in search of the "magic bullet". *Nat Rev Drug Discov* 2003;**2**:775–89.

Jilma B. Platelet function analyzer (PFA-100): a tool to quantify congenital or acquired platelet dysfunction. *J Lab Clin Med* 2001;**138**:152–63.

Michelson AD. Flow cytometry: a clinical test of platelet function. *Blood* 1996;**87**:4925–36.

Rand ML, Leung R, Packham MA. Platelet function assays. *Transfus Apheresis Sci* 2003;**28**:307–17.

Ruggeri ZM. Platelets in atherothrombosis. *Nat Med* 2002;**8**:1227–34.

Schmitz G, Rothe G, Ruf A, *et al*. European Working Group on Clinical Cell Analysis: Consensus protocol for the flow cytometric characterization of platelet function. *Thromb Haemost* 1998;79:885–96.

Yardumian DA, Mackie IJ, Machin SJ. Laboratory investigation of platelet function: a review of methodology. *J Clin Pathol* 1986;39:701–12.

Part 2

The practice of clinical hemostasis and thrombosis

Chapter 5
Hemophilia A and B

Rhona M. Maclean and Michael Makris

Introduction

Hemophilia A and B are bleeding disorders inherited in an X-linked recessive fashion, caused by deficiencies in factor VIII (FVIII) and factor IX (FIX), respectively. The first description of hemophilia is thought to be a passage describing bleeding following circumcision in the Babylonian Talmud of the 2nd century AD, "It was taught by the Tana'im: If she circumcised her first son and he died, and a second son and he died, she must not circumcise a third one."

It was initially thought that hemophilia was caused by abnormalities of the vascular system, and it was not until the late 1800s and early 1900s that a deficiency of a component of the blood was thought to be responsible.

Hemophilia A and B are not confined to those of white ethnic background; all racial groups are equally affected. They are not common, with an incidence of 1 in 5000 live male births for hemophilia A, and 1 in 30,000 live male births for hemophilia B. The clinical symptoms and signs of these two disorders are identical, and specific factor assays are required to distinguish them. With modern management, children with hemophilia today can look forward to a normal life expectancy.

Severity and symptoms

Hemophilia is classified as severe, moderate or mild on the basis of assayed plasma coagulation factor levels. This laboratory classification largely correlates with the clinical bleeding risk (Table 5.1), thus allowing a prediction to be made about individual bleeding risk and outcome.

Table 5.1 Classification of severity of hemophilia.

Classification of severity	Concentration of coagulation factor
Severe	< 0.01 IU/mL or < 1% of normal
Moderate	0.01–0.05 IU/mL or 1–5% of normal
Mild	> 0.05 IU/mL or > 5% of normal

- *Severe disease:* those with severe disease develop spontaneous joint and muscle hematomas, in addition to bleeding after minor injuries, accidents and surgical procedures.
- *Moderate disease:* those with moderate disease do not tend to bleed spontaneously, but develop muscle and joint hematomas after mild trauma. They also bleed excessively after surgery and dental extractions.
- *Mild disease:* individuals with mild hemophilia do not bleed spontaneously. They do, however, bleed after surgery, significant trauma or dental extractions.

Factor VIII synthesis

The FVIII gene at Xq28 spans 186,000 base pairs (bp) of DNA, contains 26 exons and is transcribed in the telomere to centromere direction to produce a mature mRNA of approximately 9 kb. The precursor protein (2351 amino acids) is predominantly synthesized in liver hepatocytes, with a molecular weight of approximately 293,000 Da.

FVIII circulates bound to von Willebrand factor (VWF), with a ratio of approximately one molecule of FVIII to 50 molecules of VWF.

The FVIII gene is unusual in that the intron between exons 22 and 23 (intron 22, or IVS22) contains two additional genes known as F8A and F8B. F8A is transcribed in the opposite orientation to that of the FVIII gene, and an additional two copies of the F8A are found approximately 500 kb telomeric to the FVIII gene.

The most common genetic defect responsible for severe hemophilia A (45% of cases) is caused by the inversion and translocation of exons 1–22 away from exons 23–26 by homologous recombination between the F8A gene within the IVS22 and one of the F8A copies lying outwith the gene. This mutation occurs virtually always in male germ cells; in more than 95% of affected individuals with the intron 22 inversion, their mothers were demonstrated to be carriers.

More recently, a similar inversion involving a sequence within exon 1 of the FVIII gene was described; this is thought to be responsible for the disease in approximately 3% of individuals with hemophilia A. Overall, mutations are identifiable in over 90% of individuals with hemophilia A; the remainder involve point mutations (46% of those with severe disease, 91% of those with mild/moderate disease) and deletions (8% of those with severe hemophilia A).

Factor IX synthesis

The FIX gene is centromeric to the FVIII gene on the X chromosome at Xq27. It is considerably smaller than the FVIII gene; spanning 34 kb of DNA, containing only eight exons, coding for an mRNA of 2.8 kb which translates into a protein of 415 amino acids.

Like FVIII, FIX is predominantly synthesized in the liver. The FIX serine protease requires post-translational γ-carboxylation of its glutamyl (Glu) residues by a vitamin-K dependent process.

The FIX promoter contains binding sites for a number of different regulatory elements. Mutations within the FIX promoter region at bp − 23 to bp + 13 give rise to an unususal form of hemophilia B (hemophilia B Leyden). This presents in affected individuals as severe hemphilia B; but at puberty,

the FIX levels progressively increase, in some to normal levels. It is thought that these mutations introduce a switch in the promoter to an androgen-dependent gene expression.

However, the majority of mutations in the FIX gene responsible for hemophilia B are point mutations (approximately 80%), the remainder being splice site, frameshift or gross deletions/rearrangements (approximately 3–4% each).

Inheritance

Both hemophilia A and B are X-linked recessive inherited disorders, therefore affecting males almost exclusively. It is not uncommon, however, for carrier females to have reductions in FVIII or FIX levels to the extent that they will require treatment prior to any invasive procedure, or following major trauma.

Where the female is a carrier, there is a 50 : 50 chance that either of her sons are affected by hemophilia, or that her daughters are carriers. When the offspring are from a hemophiliac male and a normal female, all sons will be unaffected, but daughters obligate carriers.

Females with markedly reduced FVIII/IX levels

This is possible in the following rare circumstances:
• With extreme lyonization of the FVIII or FIX gene in carriers.
• If there is hemizygosity of the X chromosome (e.g. in Turner (XO) syndrome).
• A female can be affected if she is the offspring of both a hemophiliac male and a carrier female.
• In females with the Normandy variant of von Willebrand disease (VWD) (FVIII deficiency only).
• In females with acquired hemophilia.

Carrier testing

All females who are obligate carriers or possible carriers of hemophilia should be offered genetic counseling to provide them with the information necessary to make informed reproductive choices.

They should have their carrier status determined to allow for the optimal management of their pregnancies. The majority of individuals with hemophilia A and B now have an identifiable mutation. If the mutation within the family is known, it is straightforward to screen the potential carrier. If the mutation is not known, then linkage analysis using informative genetic polymorphisms is usually successful (if sufficient family members are available for testing). If neither of these approaches is suitable, then direct mutation detection can be performed (see Chapter 3).

Prenatal diagnosis

Chorion villus sampling (CVS) can be performed at 11–12 weeks gestation, allowing for first trimester termination if desired. Alternatively, amniocentesis can be performed at 16 weeks. The risks of these procedures are low in experienced centers, with a miscarriage rate of 0.5–1%. Fetoscopy to allow for fetal blood sampling is rarely performed; it can only be performed after 20 weeks' gestation and has a high risk of fetal death (1–6%).

Embryo selection

Following *in vitro* fertilization (IVF) treatment, which involves ovarian stimulation, harvesting of mature oocytes followed by fertilization *in vitro*, it is possible to remove a single embryonic cell at the 8–16-cell stage, and carry out genetic diagnosis as above. Female or unaffected male embryos can then be transferred into the uterus. The advantage of this approach is that the trauma of termination of pregnancy can be avoided.

Making the diagnosis

Following the birth of a male infant to a known carrier of hemophilia, the following tests are performed on the cord blood:
- Prothrombin time (PT).
- Activated partial thromboplastin time (APTT).
- Fibrinogen level.
- FVIII or FIX activity.

- Where there is no family history, if the FVIII level is low, VWF assays for antigen and activity should be performed.

The APTT of an affected infant will usually be prolonged when compared with a gestation-specific normal range. FVIII levels in infants are comparable with those of adults, allowing for an accurate diagnosis. FIX levels in infants are considerably lower than those in adults; however, if the FIX level is less than 1%, a diagnosis of severe hemophilia B can be made. Those with equivocal results should have a repeated test at 6 months of age.

Approximately one-third of individuals with hemophilia have no family history of a bleeding disorder. A diagnosis of hemophilia should be suspected if a child has a history of excessive bruising or bleeding, or presents with a swollen painful joint or muscle hematoma.

The majority of children with moderate or severe hemophilia will present by 4–5 years of age. Where there is no family history, it is important to exclude the diagnosis of VWD, as the Normandy variant of VWD is phenotypically identical to mild hemophilia A (although with autosomal inheritance). If this is suspected, a VWF–FVIII binding assay should be performed to establish the correct diagnosis (see Chapter 6).

Clinical manifestations and their treatment

Bleeding episodes

General principles

Bleeding episodes are treated by increasing the appropriate coagulation factor to hemostatic levels. For mild hemophilia, it is often possible to use desmopressin (DDAVP) for this purpose; an infusion of DDAVP 0.3 µg/kg will increase the FVIII levels (and VWF levels) three- to fivefold. For those with moderate or severe hemophilia A or hemophilia B, infusions of coagulation factor concentrates are required. Pharmacokinetic studies have shown that 1 U FVIII/kg body weight increases the FVIII level on average 0.02 IU/mL, whereas 1 U FIX/kg body weight increases the FIX level 0.01 IU/mL.

Calculating the quantity of FVIII required

$$\text{Units FVIII to be infused} = \frac{(\text{desired level FVIII}^* - \text{actual level FVIII}) \times \text{weight in kg}}{2}$$

For example, if a 70-kg man with severe hemophilia (FVIII less than 1%) has a muscle hematoma and the desired FVIII level is 50% of normal:

$$\text{Units of FVIII to be infused} = \frac{(50 - 0) \times 70}{2}$$

$$= 1750 \text{ U FVIII}$$

Calculating the FIX required

Units FIX to be infused =
(desired level FIX − actual level FIX) × weight in kg

Recombinant FIX has a 30% lower recovery in comparison with plasma-derived FIX. If the product to be used is recombinant FIX, then the result of the above equation should be multiplied by 1.4.

Joint bleeds

Joints are the most common sites of spontaneous bleeding in those with severe hemophilia A and B (Fig. 5.1). The affected joint is painful, warm, swollen, occasionally erythematous and tends to be held in a flexed position. It must be appreciated that early on there may be no abnormal physical signs of a hemarthrosis, but patients often know if a bleed is starting. If treated promptly, levels of 30–50% will usually suffice to treat a minor bleed, together with paracetamol (acetaminophen) for pain. Occasionally, a second dose (8–12 h after the first) may be required. With severe bleeding, several days of treatment with opiate analgesia is required. Table 5.2 shows the distribution of spontaneous bleeds in severe hemophiliacs.

Physiotherapy is important from an early stage to ensure muscle atrophy does not occur and to prevent the development of joint flexures. Recurrent joint bleeds usually benefit from regular coagulation factor infusions (secondary prophylaxis)

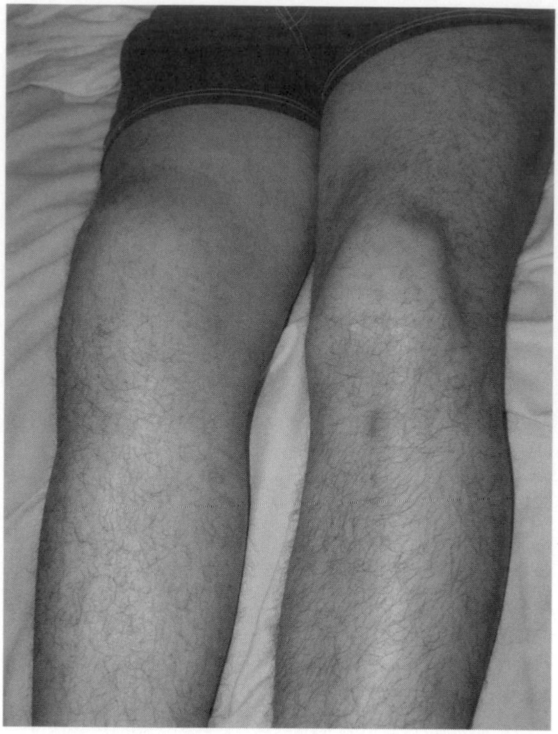

Figure 5.1 Right knee hemarthrosis in a severe hemophilia A patient. Bleeds such as this are unusual in countries where patients have home treatment with clotting factor concentrates. Usually there are no physical signs and the only symptoms are pain and limitation of joint movement.

Table 5.2 Joints most frequently affected by spontaneous bleeds in severe hemophilia.

Knee	45%
Elbow	25%
Ankle	15%
Shoulder	5%
Hip	5%
Other joints	5%

in order to prevent the development of hemophilic arthropathy.

Muscle bleeds

Muscle bleeds within closed fascial compartments can be limb-threatening because of blood vessel and nerve compression. Bleeding into the iliopsoas

* As a percntage or IU/dL.

muscle and retroperitoneum is not uncommon and patients present with:
- groin pain;
- hip flexion; and
- internal rotation.

Blood loss can be significant and femoral nerve compression can occur, resulting in permanent neurologic deficit. Pelvic ultrasound or CT scanning will confirm the diagnosis and treatment is required to raise the coagulation factor level to 100% for several days.

Intracranial hemorrhage

This is the most common cause of death from bleeding in hemophiliacs, and can occur spontaneously as well as after trauma. If suspected, or if thought to be possible following head trauma, coagulation factor concentrates should be administered to raise the coagulation factor level to 100% prior to any diagnostic tests.

Hematuria

Spontaneous hematuria is relatively common in severe hemophiliacs. It tends to be painless unless clots form within the ureters, and is usually self-limiting. Treatment of the hematuria predominantly consists of maintaining adequate hydration. If the hematuria fails to settle within a few days it may be necessary to raise coagulation factor levels to 50% of normal. Antifibrinolytic agents should never be given as these increase the likelihood of intraureteric clot formation and clot colic. The aetiology of this hematuria is usually unknown, but other causes, such as infection, renal calculi and neoplastic disease should be considered. One of the HIV protease inhibitor drugs (indinavir) induces crystalluria and calculi formation which can lead to hematuria.

Gastrointestinal bleeding

Gastrointestinal bleeding tends to be caused by anatomical lesions rather than coagulation factor deficiency and should be fully investigated. Raising the coagulation factor level to more than 50% is usually sufficient. Antifibrinolytics are helpful in mucosal bleeding.

Pseudotumours

These are now rare in countries with ready availability of clotting factor concentrates. Repeated bleeding episodes at a single site result in the development of an encapsulated hematoma. This progressively enlarges, erodes and invades surrounding structures, hence the name pseudotumour. Surgical removal is difficult and is associated with a significant morbidity/mortality.

Dental treatment

Minor dental work (scaling and polishing) can be performed without factor replacement but dental blocks or extractions require factor concentrates or DDAVP administered as appropriate. Antifibrinolytic agents (such as tranexamic acid as a mouthwash) should be provided for 3–5 days after any dental work.

Surgery

For major surgical procedures, coagulation factor levels should be maintained at 50–100% for 7–10 days to ensure adequate hemostasis and wound healing. This can be achieved either by bolus injections, one dose to bring level to 100% then once daily FIX, twice daily for FVIII, or by continuous infusion after initial bolus dose, as guided by coagulation factor assays.

Continuous infusions have the advantage of:
- eliminating the "peaks and troughs" seen with bolus factor administration;
- less factor concentrate consumption for the same procedure;
- less cost; and
- more convenient for staff to administer.

One disadvantage is that these infusions tend to cause venous irritation, but this can be reduced by an infusion of saline in tandem through the same cannula.

Intramuscular injections and non-steroidal anti-inflammatory drugs should be avoided.

Primary prophylaxis

Primary prophylaxis was first introduced in Sweden in the late 1950s and early 1960s. The rationale was that moderate hemophiliacs do not have spontaneous hemarthroses, and they also have significantly less joint arthropathy compared with those with coagulation factor levels of less than 1%.

It has since been conclusively shown that converting a severe hemophiliac to one with moderate disease by regular infusions of coagulation factor concentrate reduces the number of spontaneous joint bleeds, reduces the resulting joint damage and is now recommended for all children with severe disease.

In the UK, prophylaxis tends to be introduced after one or two spontaneous joint bleeds, and the dose and frequency of administration is titrated to prevent spontaneous bleeding events. FVIII (20–40 IU/kg) is given ideally three times weekly by intravenous infusion, FIX (25–40 IU/kg) usually only needs to be given twice weekly.

Initially, prophylaxis is given by staff based at the hemophilia center, while training the parents (and later the child) to take over this role. In many children it is possible to manage with peripheral venous access, but in some it is necessary to use central venous access devices (e.g. Port-A-Caths). More recently, internal arteriovenous fistulae in the forearm have been utilized for venous access because of complications of infection and thrombosis associated with central venous access devices.

Treatment

Clotting factor replacement

A landmark in the treatment of patients with bleeding disorders was the introduction of fresh frozen plasma in the 1940s which, because it contained all clotting factors, could be used to treat all clotting factor deficiencies. Over the last 70 years, the number of different concentrates – as well as their purity – has increased significantly and in the last 10 years molecular technology has produced both FVIII and FIX as recombinant proteins.

Plasma derived

Human plasma-derived concentrates are made from pools with each containing up to 30,000 plasma donations. Table 5.3 lists currently available concentrates.

Transfusion transmitted infection is the major potential complication of plasma-derived clotting factor concentrates. Because of this, all plasma-derived concentrates undergo viral inactivation by at least one and preferably two different viral inactivation procedures. Table 5.4 lists some of the currently used viral inactivation procedures. Although in the past some of the procedures were not very effective in eliminating all pathogenic viruses, the currently used ones are highly efficient in this respect.

Table 5.3 Currently available clotting factor concentrates.

Factor concentrate	Type available
Fibrinogen	Plasma derived
Factor VII	Plasma derived and activated recombinant
Factor VIII	Plasma derived and recombinant
Porcine FVIII	Porcine plasma derived
von Willebrand factor	Plasma derived
Factor IX	Plasma derived and recombinant
Factor XI	Plasma derived
Factor XIII	Plasma derived
Prothrombin complex	Plasma derived
Activated prothrombin complex	Plasma derived

Table 5.4 Viral inactivation and removal techniques.

Heat treatment
    Dry heat at 80°C for 72 h
    Heat in solution at 60°C for 10 h (pasteurization)
    Vapour heat at 60°C for 10 h, 1160 mb pressure
Solvent detergent treatment
    TNBP and Tween
    Triton X-100
    Cholate
Nanofiltration
Chromatographic purification
    Monoclonal antibody
    Heparin affinity
    Ion exchange

Recombinant products

Recombinant clotting factors are produced by the insertion of the relevant gene into a cell line. Following cell culture, the clotting factor is secreted into and harvested from the culture medium. Recombinant concentrates are currently available for factors VIII, IX and VIIa. Early preparations of recombinant concentrates contained human albumin as a stabilizer and used animal proteins during the manufacturing process (first-generation products). Second-generation recombinant clotting factors are stabilized without the addition of human albumin but have albumin in the cell culture medium. In third-generation products, human and animal proteins have been removed from the culture media. As for plasma-derived products, all recombinant clotting factor concentrates undergo viral inactivation.

Other hemostatic agents

Cryoprecipitate and fresh frozen plasma

Hemophilia care should be delivered from hemophilia centers with access to plasma-derived, virally inactivated clotting factor concentrates. In underdeveloped countries and in developed countries in an emergency (if FVIII concentrate is unavailable), cryoprecipitate can be used as the source of FVIII, but it must be appreciated that each cryoprecipitate unit contains only 80–100 IU of FVIII and it is not virally inactivated. In the absence of FIX con-

centrates, fresh frozen plasma (preferably virally inactivated) should be used for hemophilia B patients.

DDAVP

Desmopressin (DDAVP) is a vasopressin analogue that can release FVIII and VWF from endothelial cells. It can be given intravenously (0.3 µg/kg as an infusion over 30 min), subcutaneously or intranasally. It is useful in the management of mild hemophilia A, type 1 VWD and some platelet defects. DDAVP can be repeated over a short period but efficacy will then decrease because of tachyphylaxis. However, a few days later the endothelial stores are replenished, and original efficacy is re-established.

Common adverse effects include a mild headache, flushing and fluid retention so patients should be advised to reduce their fluid intake in the subsequent 12–24 h. Because of the problem with fluid retention, DDAVP should be avoided in children under the age of 2 years.

Tranexamic acid

Tranexamic acid is an antifibrinolytic agent that can be given orally or intravenously. It is very useful where there is mucosal bleeding and should be routinely administered to hemophiliacs having dental extractions.

Complications of treatment

Despite the success of concentrate treatment, a number of complications occur and these are summarized in Table 5.5.

Table 5.5 Complications of clotting factor therapy.

Allo-antibody formation – inhibitor development
Infections
    HIV
    Hepatitis A, B, C, D, G
    Parvovirus B19
    ?vCJD
Immune modulation
Thrombosis
Anaphylaxis

vCJD, variant Creutzfeldt–Jakob disease.

Inhibitor development

Allo-antibodies develop in up to 30% of children with severe hemophilia A who receive treatment with FVIII concentrate. They are rare in hemophilia B patients (less than 3%). These antibodies are more likely to develop:

- before the age of 5 years;
- within the first 50 treatment days;
- where there is a family history of inhibitor development; or
- in patients with FVIII/IX gene deletions.

They are usually suspected when a previously effective treatment is no longer sufficient to achieve hemostasis. The prolonged APTT does not normalize *in vitro* after the addition of normal plasma and confirmation is with the Bethesda assay.

The treatment of acute bleeding of hemophiliacs with inhibitors is difficult and expensive. It depends on the level of the inhibitor and whether it is a low or a high responding one.

High responding patients develop a rapidly increasing antibody level each time they are exposed to human FVIII. The two main types of treatment of acute bleeding in these patients are:
1 activated prothrombin complex concentrates such as FEIBA or Autoplex; and
2 recombinant FVIIa (NovoSeven).
Porcine FVIII concentrate is also useful in patients without a cross-reacting antibody to porcine FVIII, but it is currently not widely available.

In every patient with an inhibitor, the possibility of elimination through immune tolerance should be considered. There are three immune tolerance protocols available:
1 *high-dose protocol*: administers FVIII daily;
2 *low-dose protocol*: alternate daily administration; or
3 *Malmo protocol*: FVIII is combined with intravenous immunoglobulin, cyclophosphamide and immunoabsorption or plasmapheresis.
The reported success rates from small reported series are 30–80%. Once an inhibitor has been eliminated the chance of it recurring is 15%.

Infections

The viral inactivation of concentrates introduced in 1985 was highly effective in eliminating most transfusion-transmitted viruses. The risk of infection in patients treated prior to 1985 were 25–70% for HIV, 100% for hepatitis C and 50% for hepatitis B.

Approximately two-thirds of the HIV-infected hemophiliacs have now died but of those alive, the use of highly active antiretroviral therapy (HAART) has allowed near normal existence with immune reconstitution and a dramatically reduced mortality.

Hepatitis C

- 15% of patients infected cleared the virus naturally (antibody-positive but PCR-negative).
- 85% were chronically infected (persistence more than 6 months).
- Approximately 20–30% of infected patients have evidence of cirrhosis.
- 5–10% have developed liver failure or hepatocellular carcinoma.

Factors accelerating liver disease progression include:
- time since infection;
- older age at infection;
- HIV coinfection; and
- higher alcohol consumption.

Treatment with pegylated interferon and ribavirin achieves cure of hepatitis C in 30% of those infected with HCV genotype 1 and 70% of those infected with genotype 2 or 3.

Hepatitis B

Approximately 50% of hemophiliacs treated with pooled plasma products prior to viral inactivation were infected with hepatitis B virus, but most clear the virus spontaneously, with less than 5% showing chronic hepatitis B virus infection. All non-immune hemophiliacs should be vaccinated against this virus.

Parvovirus B19

This causes fifth disease in childhood and most adults show evidence of past infection. Although the disease itself is relatively minor, its importance lies in the fact that the virus is resistant to all currently used viral inactivation techniques. The implication of this is that unknown viruses can theoretically be transmitted by all currently available plasma-derived concentrates, and this is one of the main reasons for the introduction of recombinant concentrates in countries where alternative "safe" plasma-derived concentrates exist.

Variant Creutzfeldt–Jakob disease

vCJD is a prion disease that is the human equivalent of the bovine spongiform encephalopathy (BSE), which was endemic in the British cow population in the late 1980s and early 1990s. A significant number of UK hemophiliacs have been exposed to plasma from donors who subsequently developed vCJD. At this stage none of the UK hemophiliacs have shown evidence of the disease and no hemophiliac worldwide has ever developed classic or variant CJD. It has, however, prompted the Department of Health in the UK to recommend that plasma products be sourced from non-UK donors.

Immune modulation

In vitro it is possible to show that concentrates exert an immunosuppressive effect. This has been observed and reported in hemophiliacs but this phenomenon could have been a result of the chronic hepatitis C affecting the hemophiliacs studied.

Thrombosis

Thrombosis is a rare complication that was well recognized when prothrombin complex concentrates were used to cover surgery in patients with hemophilia B, prior to the addition of antithrombin and heparin to the product. It is still seen in patients treated with activated prothrombin complex concentrates, especially when the daily dosage exceeds 200 IU/kg.

Anaphylaxis

Allergic reactions to concentrates are now very rare because of the higher purity of the concentrates. There are two situations where this can still occur and it can be very severe:
1 porcine FVIII when used in patients with hemophilia A and inhibitors; and
2 recombinant factor IX concentrate in hemophilia B patients with FIX gene deletions.

Acquired hemophilia A

Acquired hemophilia is a rare bleeding disorder caused by the development of specific autoantibodies that are capable of inhibiting the action of naturally occurring FVIII. Its incidence is 2 per million population per year. It is largely a disease of the elderly. Patients with malignancy or autoimmune disorders are more likely to be affected. Less than 10% of all cases occur in the postpartum period.

Patients present with prominent subcutaneous hematomas as well as bleeding elsewhere (Fig. 5.2). Unlike classic hemophilia, hemarthroses are rare. There is prolongation of the APTT, which does not correct following the *in vitro* addition of normal plasma. The FVIII level is reduced, but rarely to less than 2%. The Bethesda assay demonstrates an inhibitor but the degree of bleeding is often more severe than suggested by the inhibitor level.

Treatment is aimed at stopping the acute bleeding and eliminating the inhibitor. Acute bleeds are treated with activated prothrombin complex concentrates, porcine FVIII or recombinant FVIIa. DDAVP and high doses of FVIII concentrate are rarely helpful in acquired hemophilia. The most common method used to eliminate the inhibitor is through the use of high-dose steroids (1 mg/kg/day), intravenous immunoglobulin (0.4 mg/kg/day for 5 days) plus low-dose cytotoxic therapy (cyclophosphamide or azathioprine).

Recently, the monoclonal anti-CD20 antibody rituximab has been shown to be effective in the elimination of acquired inhibitors, but its precise role in practice remains to be established.

Most patients with acquired hemophilia die within 1–2 years of diagnosis, from comorbid conditions rather than bleeding, which is actually a rare cause of death in this condition.

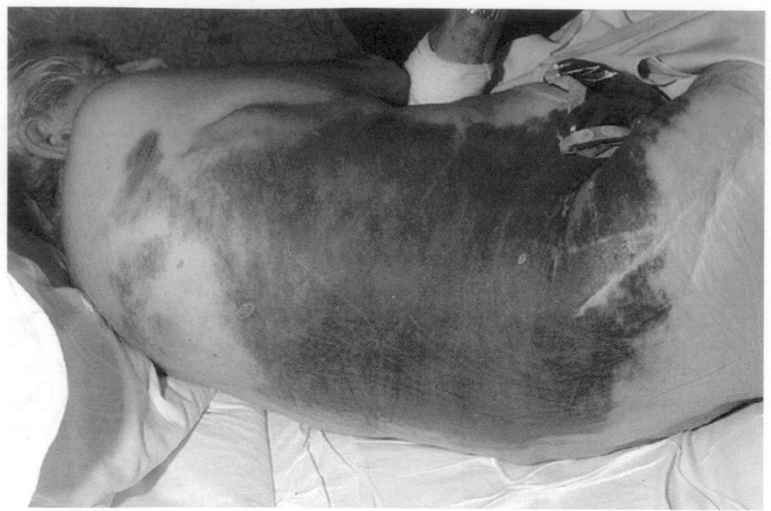

Figure 5.2 Extensive spontaneous subcutaneous hematoma in a patient with acquired hemophilia A. In contrast to congenital hemophilia, these patients often present with extensive subcutaneous bleeds and rarely have hemarthroses.

The future

Undoubtedly, hemophilia care is currently the best it has ever been and the clotting factor concentrates have never been safer. A number of advances are currently under development and are likely to enter clinical practice and perhaps become routinely available within the next decade:

• Recombinant clotting factors with no human or animal proteins used in the manufacturing process.
• Recombinant factors for the rarer deficiencies, e.g. FX and FXI.
• Modified recombinant clotting factors with longer half-lives.
• Recombinant porcine FVIII for use in inhibitor patients.
• Recombinant VWF concentrate.
• Agents to be coadministered with DDAVP to improve its efficacy (e.g. interleukin 11).
• Embryo selection in female hemophilia carriers to exclude implantation of male hemophilic embryos.
• Gene therapy where a normal FVIII or FIX gene is introduced in patients with hemophilia.

Further reading

Hay CR, Baglin TP, Collins PW, Hill FG, Keeling DM. The diagnosis and management of factor VIII and IX inhibitors: a guideline from the UK Haemophilia Centre Doctors' Organization. *Br J Haematol* 2000;**111**:78–90.

Ljung R. Paediatric care of the child with hemophilia. *Haemophilia* 2002;**8**:178–82.

Mannucci PM. Hemophilia and related bleeding disorders: a story of dismay and success. *Hematology (Am Soc Hematol Educ Program)* 2002:1–9.

Mannucci PM, Tuddenham EG. The hemophilias: from royal genes to gene therapy. *N Engl J Med* 2001;**344**:1773–9.

UK Haemophilia Centre Doctors' Organization. Guidelines on the selection and use of therapeutic products to treat hemophilia and other hereditary bleeding disorders. *Haemophilia* 2003;**9**:1–23.

Chapter 6
Von Willebrand disease

Giancarlo Castaman, Alberto Tosetto and Francesco Rodeghiero

Genetics

Von Willebrand disease (VWD) is caused by a deficiency and/or abnormality of von Willebrand factor (VWF) and represents the most frequent inherited bleeding disorder. VWF is synthesized by endothelial cells and megakaryocytes. Its gene includes approximately 178 kilobases (kb) with 52 exons and is located at chromosome 12p13.2. The primary product of VWF gene is a 2813 amino acid protein comprising a signal peptide of 22 amino acids (also called prepeptide), a large propeptide of 741 amino acids (also called propeptide) and a mature VWF subunit of 2050 amino acids. Four types of repeated molecular domains (D1, D2, D', D3, A1, A2, A3, D4, B, C1, C2) of cDNA are responsible for the different binding functions of the propeptide.

Proteomics

The building block of VWF multimers is a dimer of two single-chain pro-VWF molecules, joined through disulfide bonds at the C-terminal region. This reaction occurs after the cleavage of the signal peptide and the subsequent translocation and glycosylation of the precursor molecules into the endoplasmic reticulum. The pro-VWF dimers are then transported to the Golgi apparatus, where, after further post-translational modifications including processing of high mannose oligosaccharides, they are polymerized into very large molecules up to a molecular weight of $20,000 \times 10^3$ through disulfide bonds, connecting the two N-terminal ends of each dimer. After polymerization, pro-VWF multimers move to the trans-Golgi network where the propeptide (also called VWAgII) is cleaved off by a paired amino acid-cleaving enzyme (PACE or furin), and remains, at least within the cell, non-covalently associated with VWF.

VWF is secreted from the cell via a *constitutive* and a *regulated* pathway. The regulated pathway is used for a rapid stimuli-induced release (e.g. by desmopressin through its binding on vasopressin V2 receptor of endothelial cells). The regulated pathway is from specialized storage organelles of endothelial cells known as Weibel–Palade bodies which (like alpha granules in platelets) contain fully processed and functional VWF with "unusually large" multimers.

There is a specific plasma protease in the circulation which acts on VWF multimers released from the cell, cleaving the VWF subunit at the bond between Tyr 1605 and Met 1606 (Tyr 842 and Met 843 of the mature subunit), to create the full spectrum of circulating VWF species, ranging from the single dimer to multimers made of up to 20 dimers in each VWF multimer, removing the very large variants.

In addition to endothelial cells, megakaryocytes and platelets, VWF is present in the subendothelial matrix, where it is bound, through specific regions in its A1 and A3 domains, to different types of collagen.

Physiology

VWF is essential for platelet–subendothelium adhesion and platelet–platelet cohesion and aggregation in vessels with elevated shear stress. This function is partially explored *in vivo* by measuring the bleeding time. Adhesion is promoted by the interaction of a region of the A1 domain of VWF with platelet glycoprotein (Gp) Ib. It is thought that high shear stress is able to activate the A1 domain of the collagen-bound VWF by stretching VWF multimers into their filamentous form. The interaction between Gp Ib and VWF can be mimicked by the addition of the antibiotic ristocetin, which promotes the binding of VWF to Gp Ib to fresh or formalin-fixed platelet suspension. Aggregation of platelets within the growing hemostatic plug is promoted by the interaction with a second receptor on platelets, the Gp IIb-IIIa (or integrin $\alpha_{IIb}\beta_3$) which, after activation, binds to VWF and fibrinogen, recruiting more platelets into a stable plug. Both these binding activities of VWF are highest in the largest VWF multimers.

VWF is the carrier of factor VIII (FVIII) in plasma. VWF protects FVIII from proteolytic degradation, prolonging its half-life in circulation and efficiently localizing it at the site of vascular injury. Each monomer of VWF has one binding domain, located in the first 272 amino acids of the mature subunit (D′ domain) able to bind one FVIII molecule. *In vivo*, however, only 1–2% of available monomers are occupied by FVIII. This explains why high molecular weight multimers are not essential for the carrier function of FVIII, although one would expect that molecules of the highest molecular weight should be most effective in localizing FVIII at the site of vascular injury. In any case, any change in plasma VWF level is usually associated with a concordant change in FVIII plasma concentration.

Classification of von Willebrand disease

The current nomenclature of factor VIII–VWF complex, as recommended by the International Society on Thrombosis and Hemostasis, is summarized in Table 6.1. The current revised classification of VWD identifies two major categories:
1 *Quantitative*: type 1 partial loss and type 3 with total loss of VWF.
2 *Qualitative*: type 2, VWF defects (Table 6.2).

In type 2, four subtypes have been identified reflecting different pathophysiological mechanisms:

Table 6.1 Recommended nomenclature of factor VIII–von Willebrand factor complex.

Factor VIII	
Protein	VIII
Antigen	VIII:Ag
Function	VIII:C
Von Willebrand factor	
Mature protein	VWF
Antigen	VWF:Ag
Ristocetin cofactor activity	VWF:RCo
Collagen binding capacity	VWF:CB
Factor VIII binding capacity	VWF:FVIIIB

Table 6.2 Classification of von Willebrand disease. (Modified from Sadler 1994)

Quantitative deficiency of VWF
Type 1 Partial quantitative deficiency of VWF
Type 3 Virtually complete deficiency of VWF

Qualitative deficiency of VWF
Type 2 Qualitative deficiency of VWF
Type 2A Qualitative variants with decreased platelet-dependent function associated with the absence of high and intermediate molecular weight VWF multimers
Type 2B Qualitative variants with increased affinity for platelet Gp Ib, with the absence of high molecular weight VWF multimers
Type 2M Qualitative variants with decreased platelet-dependent function not caused by the absence of high molecular weight VWF multimers
Type 2N Qualitative variants with markedly decreased affinity for factor VIII

1 Classic type 2A is characterized by the absence of high and intermediate molecular weight (HMW) multimers of VWF in plasma.
2 Type 2B is characterized by an increased affinity of VWF for platelet Gp Ib causing removal of HMW multimers from plasma.
3 Type 2M is a variant with decreased platelet-dependent function and the presence of normal multimers on gel electrophoresis.
4 Type 2N (Normandy) shows a full array of multimers because the defect lies in the N-terminal region of the VWF where the binding domain for FVIII resides. The subtype is phenotypically identified only by tests exploiting FVIII–VWF binding.

Molecular biology of von Willebrand disease

The first mutations observed in patients with VWD were detected in exon 28 of the VWF gene, which codes for A1 and A2 domains of mature VWF, responsible for the interaction with platelet receptor Gp Ib.

Type 2A

Most are caused by missense mutations in the A2 domain, with R1597W or Q or Y and S1506L representing 60% of cases. Expression experiments have demonstrated two possible mechanisms:

1 *Group I mutations:* show impaired secretion of HMW multimers, caused by secondary defective intracellular transport.

2 *Group II mutations:* show normal synthesis and secretion of a VWF which is probably more susceptible to *in vivo* proteolysis.

Usually, these are autosomal dominant with high penetrance and expressivity.

Type 2B

The vast majority are caused by missense mutations in the A1 domain; 90% of cases are a result of R1306W, R1308C, V1316M and R1341Q mutations. Usually, these are autosomal dominant with high penetrance and expressivity.

Type 2M

A few heterogeneous mutations are responsible for type 2M. One recurrent mutation (type 2M Vicenza) has been recently reported in families from Europe (R1205H), with a second (M740I) exclusively identified in families from the Vicenza area.

Type 2N

Missense mutations in FVIII-binding domain at N termini of VWF are responsible for type 2N. The R854Q mutation is the most frequent mutation observed, found in approximately 2% of the Dutch population. This mutation may cause symptoms only in homozygous or compound heterozygous states. Type 2N is suspected in presence of a marked reduction of FVIII in comparison to VWF (pseudo-hemophilia) and is confirmed by assessing FVIII–VWF binding. Its identification is important for genetic counseling to exclude hemophilia A carrier status.

Type 1

Type 1 VWD is usually autosomal dominant, with variable expressivity and penetrance. However, three distinct groups can be identified pointing to different genetic backgrounds (Table 6.3):

Table 6.3 Type 1 VWD: heterogencity of clinical and laboratory phenotype.

	Group A	*Group B*	*Group C*
Symptoms	Manifest bleeding	Intermediate bleeding	Mild or very mild bleeding
Linkage	Cosegregation with low VWF	Cosegregation with low VWF variable	Cosegregation with low VWF inconsistent
VWF level	Approx. 10% in all affected	Approx. 30% in most affected; propositus may have lower values	40–50%
Diagnosis	Easy	Repeated testing needed	Not always possible; blood group-adjusted range?
Molecular basis	Dominant negative effect; other mechanisms?	Largely unknown? Compound heterozygote	Largely unknown? Modifiers outside VWF gene

• *Group A:* comprises cases displaying high penetrance and expressivity. Linkage with a VWF allele is usually clear. In this group, missense mutations have been described, resulting in a dominant negative mechanism. In this model, mutant wild-type heterodimers are retained in the endoplasmic reticulum and only wild-type homodimers are released into circulation.

• *Group B:* characterized by intermediate reduction of VWF, with variable penetrance and expressivity. This heterogeneity may indeed be explained in some cases by the inheritance of two different VWD alleles. For example, coinheritance of R854Q mutation with a null mutation increases the severity of bleeding within a given family, so that simple heterozygotes show only minor bleeding symptoms and greater VWF levels. Null alleles may be caused by frameshifts, nonsense mutations or deletions that overlap with those identified in type 3 VWD.

• *Group C:* comprises cases with borderline VWF levels and mild symptoms. In some of these families, linkage studies have failed to establish a relationship between the phenotype and a given VWF allele, so we must assume that a major effect of one or more gene(s) outside the VWF gene and other non-genetic factors are contributing to the expression of a bleeding phenotype. One example is the ABO blood group which explains up to 60% of the variation in VWF plasma levels, type O subjects having VWF levels 25–35% lower than in non-O individuals.

Type 3

Partial or total gene deletions have been reported in addition to mechanisms shared with some type 1 cases (see above). In general, mutations may be scattered over the entire gene, but some mutations (e.g. 2435delC or R2535X) are particularly recurrent in northern Europe. Several stop codons, either in homozygotes or compound heterozygotes, have also been reported. Homozygosity for gene deletions is associated with the appearance of antibodies against VWF, which may then render replacement therapy ineffective as well as stimulating anaphylactic reactions upon treatment.

Prevalence and frequency of subtypes of von Willebrand disease

Until the late 1980s, the prevalence of VWD was based on the number of patients registered at a specialized center, with figures ranging from 4 to 10 cases/100,000 inhabitants. It is generally assumed the number of persons with symptomatic VWD, requiring specific treatment, to be at least 100 per million.

A few studies estimated the prevalence of VWD by screening of small populations using formal standardized criteria. A prevalence approaching 1% has been demonstrated, without ethnic differences. However, the large majority of cases diagnosed by population studies appear to have mild disease, and most of these subjects were never referred for detailed hemostatic evaluation, so it remains unknown what proportion of these cases were a result of the effect of a gene(s) outside the VWF gene influencing the circulating level of VWF.

Approximately 70% of VWD cases appear to have type 1 by center series. These estimates are obviously biased because it is expected that many type 1 cases without major symptoms are not referred and that almost all severe type 3 are followed at a specialized center. In contrast to the above reported percentages, in population studies almost all cases were represented by type 1.

Clinical manifestations

Clinical expression of VWD is usually mild in type 1 with increasing severity in type 2 and type 3. However, in some families, variable severity of bleeding manifestations is evident, underlying the different molecular basis responsible for the diverse phenotypes of disorder and its variable penetrance. In general, the severity of bleeding correlates with the degree of the reduction of FVIII:C, but not with the magnitude of BT prolongation or with ABO blood type of the patient. Mucocutaneous bleeding (epistaxis, menorrhagia) is a typical, prominent manifestation of the disease and may affect quality of life. VWD may be highly prevalent in patients with isolated menorrhagia. Females with VWD may require treatment with antifibrinolytics, iron supplementation or estro-progestinic pill to control heavy menses. Bleeding after dental extraction is the most frequent postoperative bleeding manifestation. Because FVIII:C is usually only mildly reduced, manifestations of a severe coagulation defect (hemarthrosis, deep muscle hematoma) are rarely observed in type 1 VWD and are mainly post-traumatic. In type 3, the severity of bleeding may sometimes be similar to that of hemophilia. Bleeding after delivery in type 1 is rarely observed because FVIII–VWF levels tend to correction at the end of pregnancy in mild type 1 cases. However, a few cases fail to normalize their FVIII–VWF levels and need prophylaxis with DDAVP or FVIII–VWF concentrates before delivery. Females with types 2A, 2B and 3 disease usually need replacement therapy postpartum to prevent immediate or late bleeding. Postoperative bleeding may not occur even in more severely affected type 1 patients, whereas in type 3 prophylactic treatment is always required. Usually, the distribution of different types of bleeding (apart from joint bleeding) is similar among the different subtypes.

Laboratory diagnosis of von Willebrand disease

The diagnosis of VWD, and in particular of type 1, may require several laboratory assessments. The diagnostic work-up of VWD can be divided into three steps:

1 Identification of patients suspected for VWD, on the basis of data from personal and family clinical history and results of the screening tests of hemostasis.

2 Diagnosis of VWD with identification of its type.

3 Characterization of the subtype.

Table 6.4 summarizes the practical approach for diagnosing and typing VWD.

Table 6.4 Practical approach to the diagnosis of von Willebrand disease (VWD).

1 VWD diagnosis should be considered within the context of an appropriate personal and/or familial bleeding history

2 Other common hemostatic defects should be excluded by performing BT, platelet count, APTT and PT

3 If personal and/or familial bleeding history is significant, VWF:RCo assay should be carried out at this stage. If not possible, VWF:Ag assay or VWF:CB assay should be performed. VWF:Ag < 3 IU/dL suggests type 3 VWD

4 If any of these tests is below the normal range, the diagnosis of VWD should be considered. The clinical usefulness of separate reference ranges for ABO has not been demonstrated

5 In mild deficiencies, the assay should be repeated on a second occasion to confirm the diagnosis or to increase the sensitivity of the procedure in the case of a normal test in a patient with a high diagnostic suspicion

6 Other family members with possible bleeding history should be evaluated. Finding another member with bleeding and reduced VWF strongly confirms the diagnosis

7 VWF:Ag and VWF:RCo and FVIII:C should be measured on the same sample to assess the presence of reduced ratio VWF:RCo to VWF:Ag (a ratio < 0.7 suggests type 2 VWD) or FVIII:C to VWF:Ag (a ratio < 0.7 suggests type 2N VWD) to be confirmed by binding study of FVIII:C to patient's VWF

8 Aggregation of patient platelet rich plasma in the presence of increasing concentration of ristocetin (0.25, 0.5, 1.0 mg/mL, final concentration) should be assessed. Aggregation at low concentration (≤ 0.5 mg/ml) suggests type 2B VWD

9 Multimeric pattern using a low-resolution gel should be evaluated. Lack of high molecular weight multimers suggests type 2A and/or 2B disease. Presence of full complement of multimers suggests type 1 (or 2N, 2M). Absence of multimers in type 3

10 If bleeding history is clinically significant, carry out a test infusion with desmopressin. FVIII–VWF measurements should be evaluated at baseline, 60, 120 and 240 min from the start of intravenous infusion or subcutaneous injection. BT (or PFA-100 if available) should be measured at 60 and 240 min

APTT, activated partial thromboplastin time; BT, bleeding time; PT, prothrombin time; VWF:Ag, von Willebrand factor antigen; VWF:CB, von Willebrand factor collagen activity; VWF:RCo, ristocetin cofactor activity.

Screening tests

These tests are usually applied to patients with suspected bleeding tendency. The **platelet count** is usually normal, but mild thrombocytopenia may occur in patients with type 2B. The **bleeding time (BT)** is usually prolonged, but may be normal in patients with mild forms of VWD especially when platelet VWF content is normal. The **prothrombin time (PT)** is normal whereas the **partial thromboplastin time (PTT)** may be prolonged to a variable degree, depending on the plasma FVIII levels.

Identification of the type

VWF antigen (VWF:Ag) is unmeasurable in type 3 VWD, whereas it may be low in type 1 and low or normal in type 2 VWD.

The assay for **ristocetin cofactor activity (VWF:RCo)** explores the interaction of VWF with the platelet Gp Ib/IX/V complex and is still the standard method for measuring VWF activity. It is based on the property of the antibiotic ristocetin to agglutinate formalin-fixed normal platelets in the presence of VWF. In patients with a normal VWF structure (type 1 VWD), values of VWF:RCo are similar to those of VWF:Ag.

Factor VIII coagulant activity (FVIII:C) plasma levels are very low (1–5%) in patients with type 3 VWD. In patients with type 1 or type 2 VWD, FVIII:C may be decreased to a variable extent but sometimes is normal.

The multimeric pattern of VWF can be analyzed by agarose gel electrophoresis. Low-resolution agarose gels distinguish VWF multimers, which are conventionally indicated as high, intermediate and low molecular weight. In type 1 VWD all multimers are present, whereas in type 2A and 2B high and intermediate or high molecular weight multimers, respectively, are missing.

Characterization of the subtype

For a correct diagnosis of patients with VWD and their correct treatment, other assays are necessary to define specific subtypes.

Ristocetin-induced platelet agglutination (RIPA) is measured by mixing increasing concentrations of ristocetin and patient platelet-rich plasma (PRP) in the aggregometer. Results are expressed as the concentration of ristocetin (mg/mL) able to induce 30% of agglutination. Most VWD types and subtypes are characterized by hyporesponsiveness to ristocetin, at variance with type 2B, which is characterized by hyper-responsiveness to ristocetin, because of a higher than normal affinity of VWF for platelet Gp Ib/IX/V complex.

VWF multimeric analysis with high-resolution agarose gels can allow better identification of type 1 and 2 VWD subtypes.

Platelet VWF has an important role in primary hemostasis, because it can be released from alpha granules directly at the site of vascular injury. On the basis of its measurement, type 1 VWD may be classified in three subtypes:

- *Type 1 "platelet normal"*: with a normal content of functionally normal VWF.
- *Type 1 "platelet low"*: with low concentrations of functionally normal VWF.
- *Type 1 "platelet discordant"*: containing dysfunctional VWF in platelets.

Factor VIII binding assay measures the affinity of VWF for FVIII. This assay allows type 2N VWD to be distinguished from mild to moderate hemophilia A.

In general, a proportionate reduction of both VWF:Ag and VWF:RCo with RCo : Ag ratio > 0.7 suggests diagnosis of type 1. The ratio between FVIII and VWF:Ag is always ≥ 1 and the severity of type 1 VWD phenotype can usually be evaluated by performing platelet VWF measurements. If the VWF:RCo : Ag ratio is < 0.7 a type 2 VWD might be present.

According to the RIPA method, type 2B VWD can be diagnosed in the case of an enhanced RIPA (< 0.8 mg/mL), while types 2A and 2M are characterized by reduced RIPA (> 1.2 mg/mL).

Multimeric analysis in plasma is necessary to distinguish between type 2A VWD (lack of the largest and intermediate multimers) and type 2M VWD (all the multimers present as in normal plasma).

Type 2N VWD can be suspected in case of discrepant values between FVIII and VWF:Ag (ratio < 0.7) and diagnosis should be confirmed by a specific test of VWF–FVIII binding capacity (VWF–FVIIIB).

Additional tests used in VWD diagnosis include the **closure time (CT)** and assays of VWF activity based on binding to collagen (VWF:CB). The evaluation of CT with PFA-100® (Platelet Function Analyzer) allows rapid and simple determination of VWF-dependent platelet function at high shear stress. This system was demonstrated to be sensitive and reproducible for the screening of VWD, even though the CT is normal in type 2N VWD. However, its utility in the clinical setting remains to be demonstrated.

Assays for VWF:CB are also available and the ratio of VWF:CB to VWF:Ag levels appears to be useful for distinguishing between type 1 and 2 VWD. These relatively new assays have not been properly standardized yet and are not officially recommended by the Scientific Standardization Committee of the International Society of Thrombosis and Hemostasis.

A new ELISA test exploiting the interaction of VWF with plate-immobilized Gp Ib in the presence of ristocetin seems to be very promising in replacing VWF:RCo; however, its validation remains still to be fully ascertained. Tables 6.5 and 6.6 summarize the diagnostic tests and their significance.

Management of patients with von Willebrand disease

Desmopressin and transfusional therapy with blood products represent the two treatments of choice in VWD. Other forms of treatment can be considered as adjunctive or alternative to these (Fig. 6.1).

Table 6.5 Basic and discriminating laboratory assays for the diagnosis of VWD.

Test	Pathophysiologic significance	Diagnostic significance
Ristocetin cofactor (VWF:RCo) using formalin-fixed platelets and fixed ristocetin concentration (1 mg/mL)	VWF–Gp Ib interaction as mediated by ristocetin *in vitro* (ristocetin, normal platelets, patient's plasma)	"Functional test"; most sensitive screening test
Immunological assay with polyclonal antibody (VWF:Ag)	Antigen concentration	Correlates with VWF:RCo in type 1; reduced VWF:RCo/VWF:Ag (< 0.7) suggests type 2 VWD; level < 3 IU/dL suggests type 3 VWD
FVIII:C level (one-stage assay)	FVIII–VWF interaction	Not specific, but useful for patient management; disproportionately reduced compared with VWF in type 2N VWD
Bleeding time	Platelet–vessel wall VWF-mediated interaction	Not specific; correlates with platelet VWF content in type 1 VWD
Ristocetin-induced platelet aggregation (RIPA) using patient platelets	Threshold ristocetin concentration inducing patient's platelet-rich plasma aggregation	Allows the discrimination of type 2B, characterized by reduced threshold; absent in type 3 at every ristocetin concentration
Multimeric analysis (low-resolution gel)	Multimeric composition of VWF	Presence of full range of multimers in type 1; high and intermediate molecular weight multimers absent in type 2A and high in type 2B; multimers absent in type 3
Platelet VWF	Reflects endothelial stores	Useful to predict responsiveness to desmopressin in type 1
Binding of VIII:C to VWF	Interaction of normal FVIII with patient plasma VWF	Allows the identification of type 2N, characterized by low binding values

Table 6.6 Other tests proposed for VWD diagnosis.

Test	Pathophysiologic significance	Diagnostic significance
Binding of VWF to collagen	VWF–collagen interaction	Correlates with VWF:RCo in type 1 VWD; some collagen preparations more sensitive to high molecular weight multimers; not yet well standardized
Closure time PFA-100	Simulates primary hemostasis after injury to a small vessel	More sensitive than BT in screening for VWD; not tested in bleeding subjects without specific diagnosis; specificity unknown; more data needed before recommendation for clinical laboratory
Monoclonal antibody-based ELISA	Moab against an epitope of VWF involved in the interaction with Gp Ib	Correlation with VWF:RCo not confirmed; not to be used in place of VWF:RCo
ELISA-based "VWF:RCo"	Measure interaction between VWF and captured rGp Ibα fragment in the presence of ristocetin	Promising new test proposed as a substitute for VWF:RCo; validation on larger patient series required

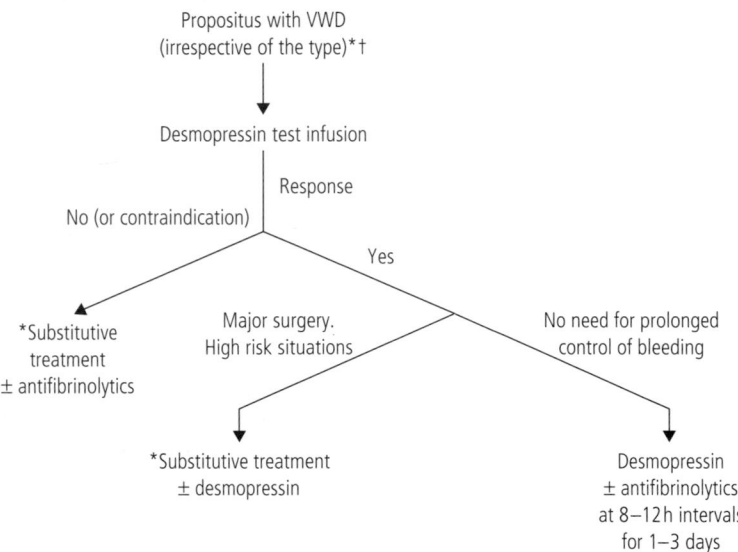

* Platelet count fall in type 2B, but not clinical symptoms; exclusion of type 2B with RIPA desirable.
† Response to desmopressin is consistent over time in the same individual and within the family.

Figure 6.1 Flow chart of a practical approach to the treatment of von Willebrand disease.

Desmopressin

Desmopressin (1-deamino-8-D-arginine vaso-pressin, DDAVP) is a synthetic analog of vaso-pressin originally designed for the treatment of diabetes insipidus. DDAVP increases FVIII and VWF plasma concentrations without relevant side-effects when administered to healthy volunteers or patients with mild hemophilia A and VWD.

DDAVP has become widely used for the treatment of these diseases. It is relatively inexpensive and carries no risk of transmitting blood-borne viruses. DDAVP is usually administered intravenously at a dosage of 0.3 µg/kg diluted in 50–100 mL saline infused over 30 min. The drug is also available in concentrated form for subcutaneous or intra-nasal administration, which can be convenient for home treatment. This treatment increases plasma

FVIII–VWF three to five times above basal levels within 30–60 min. In general, high FVIII–VWF concentrations last for 6–8 h. Infusions can be repeated every 12–24 h depending on the type and severity of the bleeding episode. However, most patients treated repeatedly with DDAVP become less responsive to therapy (tachyphylaxis).

Side-effects of DDAVP include mild tachycardia, headache and flushing, which are attributed to the vasomotor effects of the drug, often attenuated by slowing the rate of infusion. Hyponatremia and volume overload resulting from the antidiuretic effects of DDAVP are relatively rare but have been described, mainly in young children who received closely repeated infusions. Even though no venous thrombotic episodes have been reported, this drug should be used with caution in elderly patients with atherosclerotic disease, as myocardial infarction and stroke have occurred in hemophiliacs and uremic patients given DDAVP.

Patients with type 1 VWD, especially type 1 "platelet normal," are the best candidates for DDAVP treatment. In these patients, FVIII, VWF and the BT are usually corrected within 30 min and remain normal for 6–8 h. In other VWD subtypes, responsiveness to DDAVP is variable. In type 2A, FVIII levels are usually increased by DDAVP but the BT is shortened in only a minority of cases.

Desmopressin is best avoided in type 2B, because of the transient appearance of thrombocytopenia. However, there have been reports on the clinical usefulness of DDAVP in some type 2B cases. In any case, platelet count should be checked during test infusion to unravel possible non-classic type 2B cases with thrombocytopenia occurring after infusion.

In type 2N, relatively high levels of FVIII are observed following DDAVP, but released FVIII circulates for a shorter time period in patients' plasma because the stabilizing effect of VWF is impaired.

Patients with type 3 VWD are usually unresponsive to DDAVP, even though in some patients an increase of FVIII:C to effective hemostatic levels may occur.

Other non-transfusional therapies

Two other types of non-transfusional therapies are used in the management of VWD: antifi-brinolytic amino acids and estrogens. **Antifibrinolytic amino acids** are synthetic drugs that interfere with the lysis of newly formed clots by saturating the binding sites on plasminogen, thereby preventing its attachment to fibrin and making plasminogen unavailable within the forming clot. ε-Aminocaproic acid (50 mg/kg q.i.d.) and tranexamic acid (15–25 mg/kg t.i.d.) are the most frequently used antifibrinolytic amino acids and can be administered orally, intravenously or topically. They are useful alone or as adjuncts in the management of oral cavity bleeding, epistaxis, gastrointestinal bleeding and menorrhagia. They carry a potential risk of thrombosis in patients with an underlying prothrombotic state and are contraindicated in the management of urinary tract bleeding.

Estrogens increase plasma VWF levels, but the response is quite variable and unpredictable, so that they are not widely used for therapeutic purposes. It is common clinical experience that the continued use of oral contraceptives is very useful in reducing the severity of menorrhagia in women with VWD, even in those with type 3, despite the fact that FVIII–VWF levels are not modified.

Transfusional therapies

Transfusional therapy with blood products containing FVIII–VWF is currently the treatment of choice in patients who are unresponsive to DDAVP. Cryoprecipitate has been the mainstay of VWD therapy for many years. However, at present its role remains significant only in developing countries and should be prepared from virus-inactivated plasma by using simple physical methods such as methylene blue inactivation. In developed countries, virus-inactivated concentrates, originally developed for the treatment of hemophilia A, are the treatment of choice for VWD patients unresponsive to DDAVP.

Concentrates obtained by immunoaffinity chromatography on monoclonal antibodies (FVIII more than 2000 IU/mg) contain very small amounts of VWF and are therefore unsuitable for VWD management.

A chromatography-purified concentrate particularly rich in VWF and with a very low content of

Type of bleeding	Dose (IU/kg) (FVIII units)	Number of infusions	Objective
Major surgery	50	Once a day or every other day	Maintain factor VIII > 50 IU/dL for at least 7 days
Minor surgery	30	Once a day or every other day	Factor VIII > 30 IU/dL for at least 5–7 days
Dental extractions	20–40	Single	Factor VIII > 30 IU/dL for up to 6 h
Spontaneous or post-traumatic bleeding	20–40	Single	

Table 6.7 Regimens of factor VIII–VWF concentrates recommended in VWD patients unresponsive to desmopressin.

FVIII has been produced (very high purity VWF concentrate) and has been effective when tested in a small cohort of type 3 VWD cases. Sometimes it is necessary to infuse an initial dose of purified FVIII concentrate, until the infused VWF has had time to stabilize the endogenously synthesized FVIII.

The regimens of concentrates recommended for the control of bleeding episodes are summarized in Table 6.7. Because commercially available intermediate and high purity FVIII–VWF concentrates contain large amounts of FVIII and VWF, high postinfusion levels of these moieties are consistently obtained with a higher than predicted rise in the next 24 h. Deep vein thrombosis has been reported in patients with VWD receiving repeated infusions of FVIII–VWF concentrates.

These FVIII–VWF products are not always effective in correcting the BT because no concentrate contains a completely functional VWF, as tested *in vitro* by evaluating the multimeric pattern.

Conclusions

Von Willebrand disease is the most common inherited bleeding disorder. Definite diagnosis and characterization usually requires an array of tests and should be reserved for patients with a significant bleeding history. Nowadays, several safe and effective therapeutic options are easily available to prevent or control bleeding episodes, thus improving patients' quality of life. For some subjects (group C individuals, see Table 6.3), the benefit of a definite diagnosis of VWD versus the social burden of receiving the stigma of a congenital disorder and the related personal or familial anxiety should be carefully considered. For these cases, simply reassuring the patient that she or he does not have a severe bleeding disorder and offering the possibility of consultation in case of need is the preferred choice. Most clinicians would administer DDAVP to control bleeding in these subjects despite the lack of a definite diagnosis.

Further reading

Castaman G, Eikenboom JCJ, Bertina R, Rodeghiero F. Inconsistency of association between type 1 von Willebrand disease phenotype and genotype in families identified in an epidemiologic investigation. *Thromb Haemost* 1999;**82**:1065–70.

Castaman G, Federici AB, Rodeghiero F, Mannucci PM. Von Willebrand's disease in the year 2003: towards the complete identification of gene defects for correct diagnosis and treatment. *Haematologica* 2003;**88**:94–108.

Castaman G, Rodeghiero F. Current management of von Willebrand's disease. *Drugs* 1995;**50**:602–14.

Eikenboom JCJ, Reitsma PH, Peerlinck KMJ, Briet E. Recessive inheritance of von Willebrand's disease type 1. *Lancet* 1993;**341**:982–6.

Eikenboom JCJ. Congenital von Willebrand disease type 3: clinical manifestations, pathophysiology and molecular biology. *Clin Haematol* 2001;**14**:365–79.

Kouides PA. Females with von Willebrand disease: 72 years as the silent majority. *Haemophilia* 1998;**4**:665–76.

Mannucci PM. Treatment of von Willebrand's disease. *N Engl J Med* 2004;**351**:683–94.

Mohlke KL, Ginsburg D. Von Willebrand disease and quantitative variation in von Willebrand factor. *J Lab Clin Med* 1997;**130**:252–61.

Nichols WC, Ginsburg D. Von Willebrand disease. *Medicine* 1997;**76**:1–20.

Rodeghiero F, Castaman G. Congenital von Willebrand disease type 1: definition, phenotypes, clinical and laboratory assessment. *Clin Haematol* 2001;**14**: 321–35.

Rodeghiero F, Castaman G, Dini E. Epidemiological investigation of the prevalence of von Willebrand's disease. *Blood* 1987;**69**:454–9.

Rodeghiero F, Castaman G, Mannucci PM. Clinical indications for desmopressin (DDAVP) in congenital and acquired von Willebrand disease. *Blood Rev* 1991;**5**:155–61.

Ruggeri ZM. Structure of von Willebrand factor and its function in platelet adhesion and thrombus formation. *Clin Haematol* 2001;**14**:257–79.

Sadler JE. A revised classification of von Willebrand disease. *Thromb Haemost* 1994;**71**:520–3.

Sadler JE, Mannucci PM, Berntorp E, *et al*. Impact, diagnosis and treatment of von Willebrand disease. *Thromb Haemost* 2000;**84**:160–74.

UKHCDO guidelines: The diagnosis of VWD. *Haemophilia* 2004;**10**:199–217.

UKHCDO guidelines: Management of VWD. *Haemophilia* 2004;**10**:218–31.

Chapter 7
The rarer inherited coagulation disorders

Paula Bolton-Maggs and Jonathan Wilde

Introduction

The inherited coagulation disorders hemophilia A and B and von Willebrand disease are well characterized. However, inherited abnormalities of all the other coagulation factors have been recognized, but are not so well known.

All are inherited autosomally and most, with the exception of factor XI, are associated with few or no symptoms in heterozygote individuals. Most of the factor deficiencies are caused by abnormalities in the gene encoding for the particular factor. There are two interesting exceptions:

1 Combined FV and FVIII deficiency is caused by a defect in a protein involved in hepatic cell processing.

2 Combined deficiencies of the vitamin K-dependent factors is a disorder caused by mutations in genes encoding enzymes involved in vitamin K-dependent carboxylation.

As these disorders are rare (Table 7.1), most hematologists will usually have very limited experience and therefore it is essential that the individuals are registered with a hemophilia center.

Rare coagulation disorders

Rare bleeding disorders have certain features in common, which can be considered together.

Genetics

These disorders are autosomal recessive conditions and most commonly occur in individuals whose parents are related, so are much more common in ethnic groups in which consanguineous marriage

Table 7.1 The estimated prevalence and chromosome location of the different defects.

Deficiency	Estimated prevalence of severe deficiency (factor level < 10%)	Gene on chromosome
Factor VIII	133 in 1,000,000[†] males	X
Factor IX		
Fibrinogen	1 in 1,000,000	4
Prothrombin	1 in 2,000,000	11
Factor V	1 in 1,000,000	1
Combined V and VIII	1 in 1,000,000	18
Factor VII	1 in 500,000	13
Factor X	1 in 100,000	13
Factor XI	1 in 1,000,000*	4
Factor XIII	1 in 2,000,000	6 (subunit A)
		1 (subunit B)

* Higher in Ashkenazy Jews where the prevalence of severe deficiency is estimated to be 1 in 190 and 8.1% of the population are heterozygotes. (Seligsohn and Peretz 1994).
† Combined factor VIII and IX data, all severity.
Adapted from Peyvandi F, Dugan S, *et al* Rare coagulation deficiencies. *Haemophilia* 2002;**8**:308–321.

is customary, as in many Asian and Arabic communities. Factor XI deficiency (not recessive, as symptoms occur in a proportion of heterozygotes) is particularly common in Ashkenazi Jews.

As they are autosomal disorders, both males and females are affected; menorrhagia is a common feature of all these disorders, and many are associated with hemorrhage related to childbirth.

Clinical features

Severely deficient infants with these disorders (except factor XI) are particularly at risk from intracranial hemorrhage and need to be identified quickly so that appropriate treatment is rapidly available for serious bleeding.

In general, bleeding manifestations in these disorders tend to be more variable and less predictable than in hemophilia A and B. Some of the deficiencies are also associated with thrombosis, probably as a consequence of particular molecular defects.

Treatment

Treatment products for most of these conditions are generally not licensed but are available in an emergency situation in most hospitals.

If fresh frozen plasma (FFP) is used, either because it is the only treatment option or in an emergency while awaiting a specific concentrate, it should be virally inactivated (either by solvent-detergent or methylene blue treatment). As plasma products are used for treatment in most of these disorders, affected individuals should be vaccinated against both hepatitis A and B using the subcutaneous route in order to avoid the risk of muscle hematoma associated with the intramuscular route.

Antifibrinolytic therapy such as tranexamic acid is a useful adjunct to blood products, particularly for mucous membrane bleeding, but must be used with caution in those disorders with an associated risk of thrombosis.

Recent guidelines covering treatment products have been published and should be consulted for further information (UKHCDO 2003).

Pregnancy

Pregnancy and delivery should be carried out in an obstetric unit with an associated hemophilia center, or at least in close liaison with a hemophilia center specialist.

Women with severe deficiency of fibrinogen, factors VII, X and XIII are at risk of miscarriage if not treated prophylactically during pregnancy.

Good communication between obstetric, hemophilia unit and pediatric staff is essential in order to optimize treatment for the mother and to rapidly identify and plan replacement therapy for an affected neonate.

Investigation

Accurate laboratory testing is important in the identification of these disorders. Sampling of neonates and young infants can be particularly difficult. It is vital to establish that a sample has been properly taken in order to interpret the results. The use of appropriate normal ranges for infants is also essential. Vitamin K deficiency will affect the levels of factors II, VII, IX and X. This may need to be taken into account in interpretation of results. Normal adult population ranges should be defined for each assay by the local laboratory. The lower limit of normal for many of these factors is higher than the frequently used 50 u/dL.

Individual deficiencies

Fibrinogen

Hereditary defects of the fibrinogen gene result in three phenotypes:

1 *Impaired production:* hypofibrinogenemia or afibrinogenemia, depending upon severity.
2 *Synthesis of abnormally structured molecules:* dysfibrinogenemia.
3 *Reduced production of an abnormal molecule:* rare (hypodysfibrinogenemia).

Afibrinogenemia

This defect is associated with variable bleeding tendency; people with severe deficiency may have infrequent bleeding while others have marked mucosal and intramuscular bleeding. Neonates may present with umbilical cord bleeding, and they may have intracranial hemorrhage. Mucosal and muscle bleeding may occur, and wound healing may be impaired. Women are at risk of recurrent miscarriage, and both antenatal and postnatal hemorrhage. Paradoxically, thrombosis has also been reported in severe deficiency not in relation to therapy or other provoking events.

The diagnosis of afibrinogenemia depends upon demonstrating absence of fibrinogen by both functional and antigenic assays.

Individuals with hypofibrinogenemia are also at risk of bleeding with less severe manifestations such as bleeding after surgery rather than spontaneous events.

Dysfibrinogenemia

This is a collection of disorders with variable clinical features (over 300 variants have been described). Some patients have a mild bleeding disorder. Some molecular defects are unequivocally associated with thrombosis. The diagnosis may be difficult as the pattern of abnormalities can be quite variable. Family studies can be extremely helpful. The personal and family history of bleeding and thrombosis will help in guiding management.

For therapy of both disorders, two unlicensed concentrates are available in the UK and are preferred to cryoprecipitate as they are treated to reduce risks of viral transmission. The half-life of fibrinogen is 3–5 days, and a level of more than 0.5 g/L is associated with a reduced risk of bleeding.

Prothrombin

Prothrombin deficiency is extremely rare. Complete deficiency is not recorded and is probably incompatible with life (as demonstrated in mice). The two phenotypes are:
- quantitative (hypoprothrombinemia); or
- qualitative (dysprothrombinemia).

Individuals with hypoprothrombinemia may suffer from joint and muscle bleeds and also mucosal bleeding. The recommended treatment is to use either three-factor (II, IX, X) or four-factor (II, VII, IX, X) prothrombin complex concentrates, originally developed for treatment of hemophilia B patients.

Factor V deficiency

Factor V deficiency presents in childhood with bruising and mucous membrane bleeding. Infants with severe deficiency are at risk of intracranial haemorrhage, which may occur antenatally.

Reported cases appear to have a high risk of inhibitor development associated with replacement therapy. Affected children should also have a factor VIII assay performed to exclude combined deficiency. Treatment is with fresh frozen plasma, preferably a virally inactivated product. Large volumes may be required, leading to a risk of fluid overload. The minimum level of factor V required for hemostasis is approximately 15 u/dL.

Combined deficiency of factors V and VIII

This interesting disorder is caused by defects in the gene for a protein responsible for intracellular transport (ERGIC-53). Levels of both factors are most commonly between 5 and 20 IU/dL. Spontaneous bleeding is relatively uncommon; bleeding after surgery is a risk.

Treatment is with both factor VIII concentrate (as for hemophilia A) and FFP (as for FV deficiency).

Factor VII deficiency

This is the most common of the rare disorders (excluding FXI). People with mild deficiency (heterozygotes) do not usually have a bleeding problem. Generally bleeding is confined to individuals with very low levels (< 2 u/dL), but the correlation of level with bleeding is not close; some individuals with very low levels do not bleed, whilst those with higher levels do. Mucous membrane bleeding is particularly common. Menorrhagia is common in women. Thrombosis has also been reported. Neonates with severe deficiency are at risk of intracranial hemorrhage.

There is a heterogeneity of molecular defects and the thromboplastin used in the laboratory assay can profoundly affect factor VII levels recorded (e.g. FVII Padua). This may explain the lack of correlation of level with bleeding history.

The recommended treatment is recombinant activated factor VII (rVIIa), or a plasma-derived concentrate. The half-life of factor VII is particularly short (6 h) but, despite this, prophylaxis (where indicated) 1–3 times a week may be sufficient.

Factor X deficiency

Severe factor X deficiency (FX < 1 IU/dL) is associated with a significant risk of intracranial hemorrhage in the first weeks of life and umbilical stump bleeding. Mucosal hemorrhage is a particular feature, with severe epistaxis being common at any level of deficiency. Menorrhagia occurs in half of the women. Severe arthropathy may occur as a result of recurrent joint bleeds. Mild deficiency is defined by FX levels of 6–10 IU/dL; these individuals are often diagnosed incidentally but may experience easy bruising or menorrhagia.

Antifibrinolytic therapy is particularly useful for mucous membrane bleeding.

Factor X is present in intermediate purity factor IX concentrates (prothrombin complex concentrates). Factor X levels should be monitored as caution is required because of the known prothrombotic properties of these concentrates. The long half-life of factor X (20–40 h) means that in those children with recurrent joint bleeds prophylaxis can be successful given once or twice a week.

Prior experience with FFP suggests that in severe deficiency an FX level of 20–35 IU/dL is sufficient for hemostasis postoperatively in severe deficiency, but it is likely that levels lower than this (e.g. down to 5 IU/dL) may be sufficient.

Factor XI deficiency

The role of factor XI in the coagulation mechanism has recently been revised; it is physiologically activated by traces of thrombin and serves to potentiate the propagatory pathway once coagulation has been initiated via the tissue factor pathway. This serine protease is unique in being a dimer. Although factor XI deficiency is particularly common in Ashkenazi Jews, it is found in all ethnic groups; however, the mutations in Jewish patients are restricted with two being particularly common. Overall, the prevalence of severe deficiency is approximately 1 in 1 million, but mild deficiency is much more common. In the UK, mild factor XI deficiency is currently being reported at a frequency similar to that of hemophilia B. This is partly because current activated partial thromboplastin time (APTT) reagents are sensitive to mild FXI deficiency and there is a greater readiness to investigate these mildly prolonged APTTs levels.

Factor XI deficiency is unlike most of the other rare coagulation disorders in that heterozygotes may have a significant bleeding tendency that is poorly predicted by the factor XI level. Spontaneous bleeding is extremely rare, even in those with undetectable FXI levels. Bleeding is provoked by injury and surgery, particularly in areas of high fibrinolytic activity (mouth, nose and genitourinary tract). Women both with severe or mild deficiency may suffer menorrhagia and postpartum hemorrhage. The bleeding tendency varies both within a family and an individual at different times. This may be related to mild variation in other factors, such as von Willebrand factor. This makes the management of surgery in FXI deficiency more complicated. Babies with severe deficiency do not bleed spontaneously (intracranial hemorrhage has not been reported), but are at risk of excessive bleeding at circumcision.

Oral antifibrinolytic therapy is very useful for the management of mucosal bleeding (menorrhagia) and is sufficient for the management of dental extractions, even in people with severe deficiency.

Two factor XI concentrates are available, but both have been associated with thrombotic events in some individuals, particularly those with additional risk factors such as older age, the presence of cardiovascular disease or malignancy. Because of this, antifibrinolytic drugs should not accompany them, and peak levels of more than 100 u/dL should be avoided.

FFP can be used, but in people with severe deficiency it is difficult to produce a sufficient rise (to more than 30 u/dL) without the risk of fluid overload.

More recently, activated factor VII, which is a recombinant product, has been used. This is particularly useful in severely deficient patients with factor XI inhibitors.

In the case of circumcision, the factor XI level should be checked and if less than 10 u/dL at birth, the procedure should be delayed and the level checked at six months. If still below 10 u/dL, the circumcision should be performed in hospital with FFP or concentrate cover, and the religious requirements discussed with the family. If the level is more than 10 u/dL, antifibrinolytics will usually suffice.

The management of people with heterozygous deficiency and a bleeding history (FXI of approximately 20–60 u/dL) is more difficult and is dependent upon the bleeding history of the individual patient and the hemostatic challenge.

Factor XIII deficiency

Factor XIII cross-links and stabilizes fibrin. Severe deficiency, with undetectable factor XIII, is associated with:
- a serious bleeding disorder, usually presenting in infancy;
- bleeding from the umbilical stump in 80% of patients;
- intracranial hemorrhage;
- joint and muscle bleeds;
- miscarriages and bleeding after delivery or surgery; and
- delayed wound healing.

For these reasons, usually once severe deficiency is detected, an individual is treated with prophylaxis for life. Individuals with levels of 1–4 u/dL are also likely to have bleeding symptoms and rarely bleeding is reported in people with levels above 5 u/dL.

The diagnosis is suspected when the coagulation screen is normal. Clot solubility in urea or acetic acid will be abnormal, and the defect is confirmed by a factor XIII assay. Difficulties in the screening tests were noted in the UKNEQAS exercises. Because this is not a routine in most laboratories, it is advisable to send the sample to a specialist center.

Factor XIII has a long half-life of 7–10 days and, in practice, regimens with 4–6-weekly intervals have proved effective for prophylaxis. It is suggested that levels of 4–10 u/dL are sufficient to prevent hemorrhage.

In the emergency situation (e.g. when presented with an infant with a serious bleeding diathesis), once blood has been taken for testing, either FFP or cryoprecipitate is effective treatment. However, plasma-derived concentrates are available and are the treatment of choice.

Combined deficiencies of the vitamin K-dependent factors: II, VII, IX and X

Combined deficiency of all the vitamin K-dependent factors is a rare but important bleeding disorder to recognize. By 2000, only 13 families had been reported. The inheritance is autosomal recessive. Mucocutaneous and postoperative-related bleeding have been reported. Severe cases may present with intracranial hemorrhage or umbilical cord bleeding in infancy.

The clinical picture and response to vitamin K is variable, some responding to low-dose oral vitamin K but others non-responsive even to high-dose intravenous replacement. In those non-responsive to vitamin K, Prothrombin Complex Concentrates (PPCs) are the product of choice. Levels of the factors range from < 1 to 50 u/dL. Some individuals have associated skeletal abnormalities (probably related to abnormalities in bone vitamin K-dependent proteins such as osteocalcin). Genetic defects have been reported in the enzymes associated with vitamin K metabolism (e.g. in γ-glutamyl carboxylase).

Illustrative case histories

Case 1

A 13-month-old infant presented with a 2-cm diameter swelling on his head and a swollen thigh caused by running into a door 2 weeks previously. He was thought to be suffering from non-accidental injury and was admitted. Ultrasound examination confirmed a muscle hematoma. Coagulation screening demonstrated a prolonged prothrombin time (PT) of 25.4 s (normal range [NR] 11.5–15) and APTT of 80 s (NR 27–39). His factor X level was < 1 IU/dL. Both parents had prolonged coagulation tests and low factor X levels; both were asymptomatic. He was treated for the acute bleed with an intermediate purity factor IX concentrate with monitoring of factor X levels. Over the next 3 years he had repeated muscle and joint bleeds and is now being treated with once weekly prophylaxis. His concentrate dose is determined by regular dose–response and half-life analysis.

Comment

This case illustrates a picture similar to severe hemophilia A. Non-accidental injury is unfortunately more common than bleeding disorders so that unless appropriate investigations are undertaken, diagnosis may be delayed or missed.

Case 2

A baby boy developed massive bilateral cephalohematomas 24 h after spontaneous vaginal delivery. He was otherwise well, with normal, unrelated parents. Blood tests showed a profound anemia (Hb 7.0 g/dL) and incoagulable blood with undetectable fibrinogen. Liver disease was excluded and he was not septic. Cranial ultrasound confirmed that there was no evidence of intracranial hemorrhage. Both parents (and both maternal grandmothers) were noted to have low fibrinogen levels and prolonged thrombin times. He was transfused with red cells and treated with regular cryoprecipitate until fibrinogen concentrate could be obtained. He was treated prophylactically, requiring a central venous access device, but by 9 months of age was noted to have subclavian vein thrombosis related to this. Magnetic resonance scanning demonstrated extensive thrombosis of the upper body venous system. It was not possible to determine if therapy had contributed to the thrombotic risk. Prophylaxis was stopped for 5 months during which time he had several bruises and was treated for minor bumps to the head, but had no serious bleeding. When he began to walk and fall, his mother was anxious for regular prophylaxis to be resumed. It is unclear whether this is necessary in the long term.

Comment

In the absence of mutation detection it was impossible to be sure that this child did not have compound heterozygosity for hypo- and dysfibrinogenemia, which might have increased his risk of thrombosis. Mutation detection can be helpful in predicting the clinical picture in fibrinogen disorders, and will probably also prove useful in factor VII and X deficiency where the clinical picture can be variable.

Case 3

A 12-year-old girl was admitted after a heavy third menstrual period. She had been bleeding for 10 days, fainted at school, and on admission was found to have severe anemia with Hb 6.0 g/dL.

Coagulation testing demonstrated a normal APTT and a PT of 41 s. Her factor VII level was 2.2 IU/dL. She had been adopted, and had no other bleeding problems; she had not bled excessively after being bitten by a dog requiring open reduction of a fracture of the forearm nor after being knocked down by a car. Once her periods had become established and controlled with hormone therapy, she did not have any other bleeding problems and by the age of 18 had defaulted from follow-up.

Comment

This case illustrates that individuals with severe factor VII deficiency may have very few problems and contrasts with the next case.

Case 4

An Asian baby with parents who were first cousins was delivered by cesarean section. He was noted to have nasal bleeds twice on day 3 and a blood-stained discharge from the umbilical cord on day 5. He was admitted with irritability on day 18 and collapsed on admission with Hb 8 g/dL, PT 32 s, APTT 39 s. CT scanning of the head showed intracranial hemorrhage (ICH) in the posterior fossa. His FVII level was 4 IU/dL. He was treated initially with FFP (which did not shorten the PT) until a FVII concentrate was available. He was treated symptomatically over this acute event. However, further episodes of ICH occurred over the next 2 months, leading to cerebral atrophy and predictable developmental delay. He was started on prophylaxis twice a week at the age of 6 months via a venous access device. At 4½ years he had a mental age of 2½, epilepsy, no speech and no vision on the right side as a consequence of his previous ICHs. At the age of 5½ years he was noted to have severe iron deficiency (Hb 6.9 g/dL, mean corpuscular volume [MCV] 59), common in children of Asian origin (dietary), compounded by developmental problems and his bleeding disorder.

Comment

Where ICH occurs in relation to a severe congenital factor deficiency it needs to be recognized and treated early and intensively to try to avoid long-term developmental problems. Iron deficiency is very common in the Asian community as a result of dietary deficiency.

Case 5

A Pakistani child with related parents was referred at the age of 1 year. She had easy bruising and bleeding from minor cuts which lasted several hours. Her PT was 45 s and the APTT was 92 s. Factor V was < 1 u/dL. At the age of 15 and 18 months she had recurrent mouth bleeds from trauma associated with walking and was treated prophylactically twice weekly with FFP. At 2 years she had a retroperitoneal hemorrhage. At 3 years there were concerns about her neurological development, and at 5½ years imaging supported the occurrence of a possible ICH in the past. At 3 years there was evidence of an inhibitor and regular FFP infusions were stopped. She had recurrent muscle bleeds leading to shortening and wasting, and the necessity for tendon-lengthening surgery at the age of 7 years by which time her inhibitor had disappeared. She continued to have recurrent muscle and joint bleeds treated symptomatically with FFP infusions (the inhibitor having resolved). Menarche occurred aged 13 but her periods have not been heavy.

Comment

Factor V deficiency is difficult to manage and may be associated with the development of inhibitors as in this case.

Conclusions

The rare coagulation disorders may present with serious and life-threatening bleeding. Prompt investigation and recognition of these disorders is essential so that the appropriate treatment can be instigated. ICH is a serious risk in many of these disorders and may have catastrophic consequences.

Hematologists need to work closely with pediatricians to recognize these disorders. In communities where consanguinity is common there needs to be a heightened awareness of the risk of these potentially serious bleeding disorders.

Acknowledgements

This chapter is based upon guidelines published by members of the Rare Haemostatic Disorders Working Party of the United Kingdom Haemophilia, Centre Doctors' Organization (Bolton-Maggs *et al.* 2004).

Further reading

Bolton-Maggs PHB, Perry DJ, Chalmers EA, Parapia LA, Wilde JT, Williams MD, Collins PL, Kitchen S, Dolan G, Mumford AD (2004). The Rare Coagulation Disorders – review with guidelines for management. *Haemophilia*, 10(5):593–628.

Brenner B. Hereditary deficiency of vitamin K-dependent coagulation factors. *Thromb Haemost* 2000;84:935–6.

Ginsburg D, Nichols WC, Zivelin A, Kaufman RJ, Seligsohn U. Combined factors V and VIII deficiency: the solution. *Haemophilia* 1998;4:677–82.

Haverkate F, Samama M. Familial dysfibrinogenemia and thrombophilia. Report on a study of the SSC Subcommittee on Fibrinogen. *Thromb Haemost* 1995;73:151–61.

Mannucci PM, Duga S, Peyvandi F. Recessively inherited coagulation disorders. *Blood* 2004;104:1243–52.

Peyvandi F, Duga S, Akhavan S, Mannucci PM. Rare coagulation deficiencies. *Haemophilia* 2002;8:308–21.

Seligsohn U, Peretz H. Molecular genetics aspects of factor XI deficiency and Glanzmann thrombasthenia. *Haemostasis* 1994;24:81–5.

UK Haemophilia Centre Doctors' Organization (2003). "Guidelines on the selection and use of therapeutic products to treat haemophilia and other hereditary bleeding disorders". *Haemophilia*, 9(1):1–23.

UK Haemophilia Centre Doctors' Organization. *National Haemophilia Database. Report on Annual Returns for 2000 and 2001*. Manchester: UK Haemophilia Centre Doctors' Organization, 2003.

Williams MD, Chalmers EA, Gibson BE. The investigation and management of neonatal haemostasis and thrombosis. *Br J Haematol* 2002;119:295–309.

Chapter 8
Quantitative platelet disorders

Walter H.A. Kahr and Victor S. Blanchette

Introduction

The etiology of thrombocytopenia is dependent on the patient's age and clinical presentation. The most probable cause of thrombocytopenia in a newborn infant is different from that of an older child or adult, or that of a pregnant woman. Ranking of the most likely causes of a low platelet count will also depend on whether the patient is well or not. This chapter focuses on a practical approach in the assessment and management of inherited and acquired quantitative platelet disorders. Qualitative platelet disorders are covered in Chapter 9 and are not discussed here.

Definition of thrombocytopenia

Thrombocytopenia is defined by a platelet count of less than 150×10^9/L (the normal range is 150–400×10^9/L). Increased bleeding purely as result of a reduction of platelets does not usually occur until the count drops below 50×10^9/L. Platelet counts of less than 20×10^9/L increase the risk of life-threatening bleeding (e.g. central nervous system or gastrointestinal). However, a prospective assessment of bleeding in adults with leukemia revealed that serious bleeding was similar using a 10×10^9/L or 20×10^9/L threshold for prophylactic platelet transfusions, suggesting that life-threatening bleeding increases significantly only when the platelet count drops below 10×10^9/L.

Platelet production

Platelets are shed from megakaryocytes through the action of thrombopoetin (TPO) and other cytokines, which stimulate pluripotent hematopoietic stem cells to form mature megakaryocytes in bone marrow. The average life span of human platelets is 7–10 days. A daily turnover of approximately 40×10^9 platelets/L blood is required to maintain a constant platelet count. Newly formed or young platelets are thought to be more functional in hemostasis than older platelets. However, some antibodies observed in neonatal alloimmune thrombocytopenia (NAIT) may impede platelet function of young platelets by specific interaction with the fibrinogen receptor GP IIb/IIIa (thought to explain the higher incidence of serious bleeding in NAIT compared to immune thrombocytopenia [ITP] at equivalent low platelet counts). Aspirin (ASA) inhibits platelets irreversibly, thus at least 7 days are required to remove ASA-exposed platelets from the circulation.

Patient history

Immediate (rather than delayed) bleeding is typical of thrombocytopenia, similar to other primary hemostatic defects, platelet function defects and von Willebrand disease (VWD). Common features include:
- petechiae;
- mucocutaneous bleeding;
- epistaxis;
- menorrhagia;
- hemarthroses and intramuscular hematomas are rare.

A careful history assessing the response to trauma, surgical challenges including circumcision, dental extraction, tonsillectomy, menses, and

Disorder	Gene (chromosome)
X-linked disorders	
Wiskott–Aldrich syndrome (WAS)	*WAS* (Xp11.23-p11.22)
X-linked thrombocytopenia	*WAS* (Xp11.23-p11.22)
X-linked macrothrombocytopenia with dyserythropoiesis	*GATA1* (Xp11.23)
Autosomal dominant disorders	
Mediterranean thrombocytopenia/ Bernard–Soulier syndrome carrier	*GPIbα* (17p12)
MYH9-related thrombocytopenia	*MYH9* (22q11)
May–Hegglin anomaly	
Sebastian syndrome	
Fechtner syndrome	
Epstein syndrome	
Familial platelet disorder with associated myeloid leukemia	*AML1/CBFA2/RUNX1* (21q22.2)
Thrombocytopenia with radio-ulnar synostosis	*HOXA11* (7p15-p14.2)
Velocardiofacial (VCF) & DiGeorge syndrome	*GPIbβ* (22q11)
Platelet-type (pseudo) von Willebrand disease	*GPIbα* (17p13)
Paris–Trousseau thrombocytopenia & Jacobsen syndrome	*FLI1* (11q23)
Autosomal dominant thrombocytopenia with linkage to chromosome 10	*FLJ14813* (10p12-11.2)
Quebec platelet disorder	Unknown
Montreal platelet syndrome	Unknown
Macrothrombocytopenia with platelet expression of glycophorin A	Unknown
Autosomal recessive disorders	
Gray platelet syndrome (can be dominant)	Unknown
Bernard–Soulier syndrome	*GPIbα* (17p13)
	GPIbβ (22q11)
	GPIX (3q21)
Congenital amegakaryocytic thrombocytopenia	*MPL* (1p34)
Thrombocytopenia with absent radii	Unknown

Table 8.1 Genetics and inheritance pattern of congenital thrombocytopenias. (Adapted from Balduini *et al.* 2003 and Drachman 2004.)

postpartum hemorrhage can be useful in defining the presence of a primary hemostatic defect.

Bleeding since birth or early childhood is suggestive of an inherited condition, whereas symptoms in older patients are more likely to be caused by an acquired defect.

Family history

A family history of bleeding and thrombocytopenia suggests an inherited condition. Table 8.1 lists some congenital thrombocytopenias and their mode of inheritance.

Medication history

A careful medication history is important, because many drugs can cause thrombocytopenia, as shown in Table 8.2. Platelet-inhibiting drugs such as ASA, non-steroidal anti-inflammatory drugs (NSAIDs), ticlopidine, clopidogrel, dipyridamole and GP IIb/IIIa antagonists (abciximab, tirofiban,

Table 8.2 Drugs causing thrombocytopenia. (Adapted from George *et al.* 1998 and Aster 2002.)

Drug	Mechanism
Immune-mediated	
Acetaminophen	
Aminoglutethimide	
Aminosalicylic acid	
Amiodarone	
Amphotericin B	
Carbamazepine	May also induce marrow aplasia
Cimetidine	
Chlorothiazide/hydrochlorothiazide	
Danazol	
Diatrizoate meglumine (Hypaque)	
Diclofenac	
Digoxin	
Gold/gold salts	May also induce marrow aplasia
IFN-α	May also inhibit megakaryocyte proliferation
Levamisole	
Meclofenamate	
Methyldopa	
Nalidixic acid	
Oxprenolol	
Procainamide	
Quinidine and quinine	
Ranitidine	
Rifampin	
Sulfasalazine	
Sulfisoxazole	
Trimethoprim-sulfamethoxazole	
Vancomycin	
Unique antibody-mediated process	
Heparin	PF4-heparin-antibody causes HIT by platelet activation
Abciximab, eptifibatide and tirofiban	GP IIb/IIIa (integrin $\alpha_{IIb}\beta_3$) antagonist; or peptide derivative
Suppression of platelet production	
Anagrelide	Inhibits megakaryocyte maturation
Valproic acid	Inhibits megakaryocyte maturation; common and dose-related; may also induce marrow aplasia
Suppression of all hematopoietic cells	
Chemotherapeutic agents	
Thrombotic thrombocytopenic purpura	
Ticlopidine	Incidence 1 in 5000; may also induce marrow aplasia
Clopidogrel	Incidence 1 in 15,000
Mitomycin C	
Cyclosporine and FK506 (tacrolimus)	

eptifibatide), should also be identified when evaluating a bleeding patient. Particular attention should be paid to whether the patient is receiving heparin (including exposure to heparin in line flushes) because heparin-induced thrombocytopenia (HIT; see below) needs to be excluded. Non-prescription (e.g. herbal) medications should also be documented, as they may contribute to thrombocytopenia and/or platelet dysfunction. For instance, patients and physicians may not be aware that tonic water (as in "gin and tonic") contains quinine, an extract from cinchona tree bark which can be associated with thrombocytopenia.

Medical history

Infection

One of the most common causes of thrombocytopenia is infection. Infectious causes of thrombocytopenia include human immunodeficiency virus type 1 (HIV), influenza, varicella zoster virus, rubella virus, Epstein–Barr virus (EBV), cytomegalovirus (CMV), hantavirus, mycoplasma, mycobacteria, malaria, trypanosomiasis, *Rickettsiae* and *Ehrlichiae*. Patients at risk for HIV infection, such as intravenous drug users and individuals who practice high-risk sexual activities (e.g. unprotected sex with multiple partners), may have HIV-associated thrombocytopenia. Children receiving live viral vaccines often have a transient thrombocytopenia. Infection-associated hemolytic uremic syndrome (HUS) caused by *Escherichia coli* (serotype O157:H7), *Shigella*, *Salmonella* and *Campylobacter jejuni* can follow an acute diarrheal illness and is characterized by thrombocytopenia with schistocytes seen on a blood film. Severe sepsis resulting from bacterial infection leading to disseminated intravascular coagulation (DIC) results in thrombocytopenia and associated coagulopathy (see below).

Systemic diseases

Systemic diseases involving the bone marrow, such as aplastic anemia, myelofibrosis, leukemia, lymphoma or metastatic cancers infiltrating the bone marrow often result in thrombocytopenia, but this

is often manifested as a pancytopenia involving all three cell types: platelets, erythrocytes and leukocytes.

Other systemic illnesses such as renal and liver disease not only affect platelet function, but also are often accompanied by mild to moderate thrombocytopenia.

Other causes

Poor nutritional intake, such as can occur in the elderly or alcoholics, may result in decreased intake of vitamin B_{12} and folate resulting in megaloblastic anemia and thrombocytopenia. In addition, excessive alcohol intake has direct inhibitory effects on platelet production.

Pregnancy is commonly (approximately 7% of pregnant women) associated with thrombocytopenia, usually appearing during the third trimester; multiple etiologies need to be considered (see below).

Transfusion history

Previous transfusions may place an individual at risk of developing post-transfusion purpura, in which severe thrombocytopenia can appear 5–10 days after the transfusion of a blood product.

Physical examination

The clinical appearance of the patient is an important first clue to the etiology of thrombocytopenia. A sick patient in the intensive care unit may have a number of possible etiologies, including severe sepsis, DIC, drug-induced, post-transfusion purpura, massive blood transfusion and systemic illness. In contrast, a well patient with newly diagnosed isolated thrombocytopenia may have an inherited thrombocytopenia, ITP or, in a neonate, auto- or alloimmune thrombocytopenia.

Certain congenital thrombocytopenias are accompanied by typical physical findings such as skeletal abnormalities, facial dysmorphologies, hearing deficiencies and cataracts, as described in Table 8.3. Evidence of an enlarged spleen or other systemic findings (e.g. fever, jaundice, adenopathy,

Table 8.3 Diagnostic features of congenital thrombocytopenias. (Adapted from Balduini *et al.* 2003 and Drachman 2004.)

Disorder	Platelet size	Clinical and laboratory features
Wiskott–Aldrich syndrome (WAS)	Small	Moderate–severe thrombocytopenia; immunodeficiency; eczema; reduced/absent WAS protein in lymphocytes detected by Western blot
X-linked thrombocytopenia	Small	As WAS except mild/absent immunodeficiency + eczema
X-linked macrothrombocytopenia with dyserythropoiesis	Large	Dysmegakaryocytopoiesis and dyserythropoiesis with severe thrombocytopenia and variable anemia; confirm by analysis of *GATA1* gene
Mediterranean thrombocytopenia/Bernard–Soulier carrier	Large	Mild thrombocytopenia; common in Mediterranean region; equivalent to heterozygote Bernard–Soulier syndrome
MYH9-related thrombocytopenia	Large	Non-muscle myosin heavy-chain IIA immunocytochemistry in neutrophils
May–Hegglin anomaly		Neutrophil inclusions
Sebastian syndrome		Neutrophil inclusions
Fechtner syndrome		Neutrophil inclusions; sensorineural hearing loss; nephritis; cataracts
Epstein syndrome		Sensorineural hearing loss; nephritis
Familial platelet disorder with associated myeloid leukemia	Normal	Predisposition for acute myeloid leukemia
Thrombocytopenia with radio-ulnar synostosis	Normal	Reduced/absent megakaryocytes; radio-ulnar synostosis ± other malformations
Velocardiofacial & DiGeorge syndrome	Large	Cardiac abnormalities; parathyroid and thymus insufficiencies; learning disabilities; facial dysmorphology
Platelet-type (pseudo) von Willebrand disease	Large	Increased platelet aggregation with low-dose ristocetin caused by mutation in GP Ibα
Paris–Trousseau thrombocytopenia and Jacobsen syndrome	Large	Cardiac and facial abnormalities; cognitive disabilities; giant platelet granules
Autosomal dominant thrombocytopenia with linkage to chromosome 10	Normal	Small megakaryocytes with hypolobulated nuclei; putative kinase mutation
Quebec platelet disorder	Normal	Delayed-onset bleeding unresponsive to platelet transfusions; urokinase in platelets detected (Western blot)
Montreal platelet syndrome	Large	Spontaneous platelet aggregation *in vitro*
Macrothrombocytopenia with platelet expression of glycophorin A	Large	Platelets express glycophorin A (flow cytometry); decreased platelet aggregation with arachidonic acid
Gray platelet syndrome	Large	Pale appearing platelets in blood film; reduced/absent alpha granules in TEM
Bernard–Soulier syndrome	Large	Absent platelet aggregation with ristocetin; homozygous defect in GP Ib/IX/V
Congenital amegakaryocytic thrombocytopenia	Normal	Isolated hypomegakaryocytic thrombocytopenia evolving into aplastic anemia; severe thrombocytopenia; TPO receptor mutation
Thrombocytopenia with absent radii	Normal	Shortened or absent forearms caused by bilateral radial aplasia ± other skeletal anomalies; severe thrombocytopenia at birth

Platelet size according to mean platelet volume (MPV): Small platelets (MPV < 6 fL); normal platelets (MPV 7–11 fL); large platelets (MPV > 11 fL). TEM, transmission electron microscopy; TPO, thrombopoietin; VWF, von Willebrand factor.

cachexia) can be helpful in deciding whether an underlying illness is the likely cause for the thrombocytopenia.

Petechiae consisting of small (< 2 mm), red, flat, discrete lesions, occurring most frequently in the dependent areas on the ankles and feet, represent extravasated red cells from capillaries and are the hallmark of a primary hemostatic disorder. They are non-tender and do not blanch under pressure. Purpura (< 1 cm) and ecchymoses (> 1 cm) represent larger areas of bleeding, and when observed in mucous membranes such as the oropharynx are described as wet purpura. These findings are in contrast to delayed bleeding into joints or muscle, which suggest a coagulation disorder rather than a platelet or von Willebrand factor (VWF) problem.

Laboratory evaluation

Laboratory tests are discussed in detail in Chapter 4, so only selected points are emphasized here. Modern technology has greatly facilitated laboratory evaluation and reporting of clinical tests.

Blood film

The importance of examining a blood film in a patient with newly diagnosed thrombocytopenia cannot be overemphasized (Fig. 8.1). For example:

- Visualization of schistocytes (red blood cell [RBC] fragments) could be indicative of thrombotic thrombocytopenic purpura/hemolytic uremic syndrome (TTP/HUS) or DIC.
- Evidence of platelet clumps would suggest pseudothrombocytopenia.
- Megathrombocytes with Döhle-like bodies in neutrophils could be indicative of MYH9-related diseases.
- Pale agranular-appearing platelets could represent gray platelet syndrome.
- Blasts suggest the diagnosis of leukemia or myeloproliferative disorder.

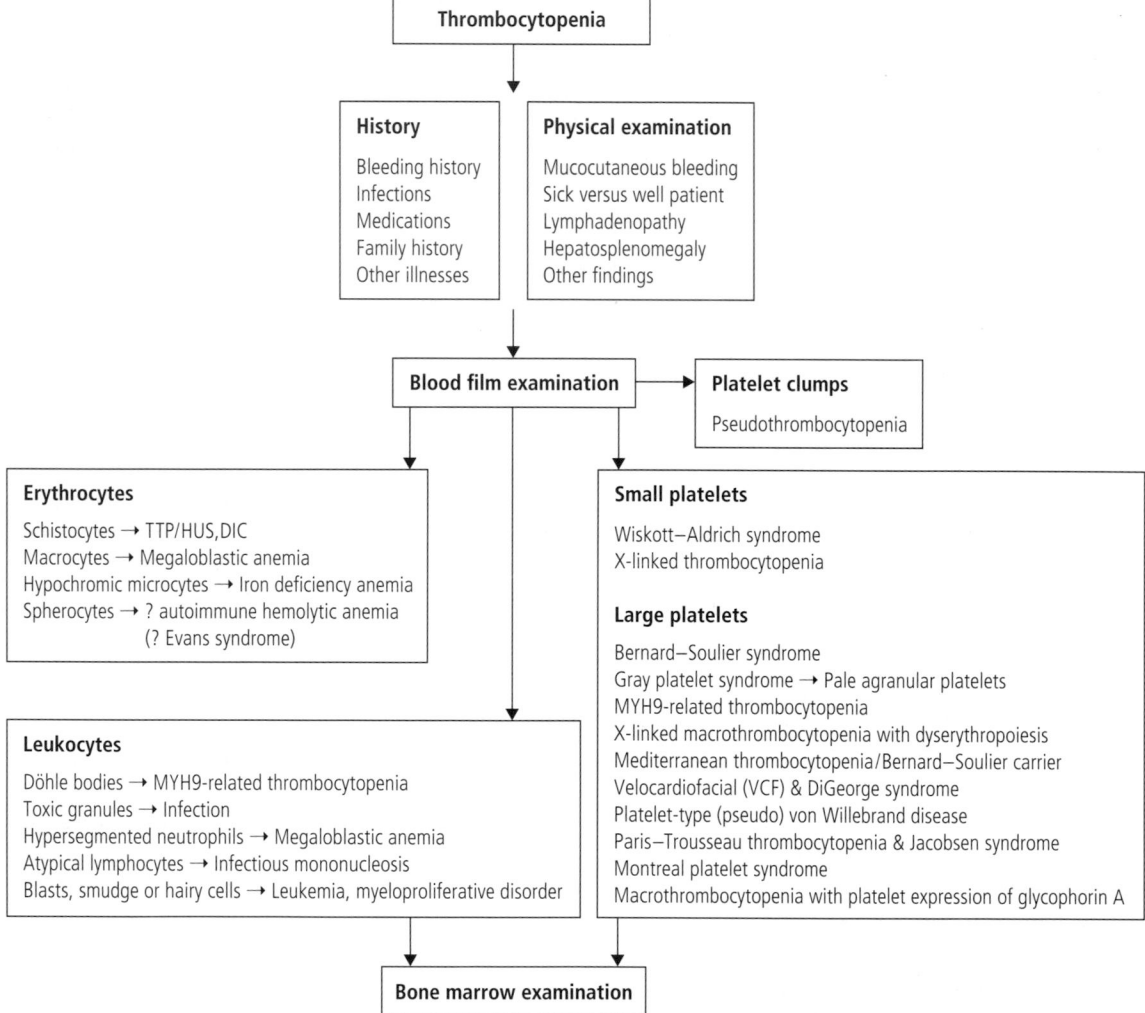

Figure 8.1 Diagnostic strategy for evaluating thrombocytopenia in a "well" child or adult.

- Macrocytes with hypersegmented neutrophils suggests megaloblastic anemia.
- Toxic granulation indicates infection.
- Spherocytes may be observed in Evans syndrome (coexisting autoimmune hemolytic anemia and ITP).

Pseudothrombocytopenia resulting from EDTA-induced platelet clumping can often be overcome by obtaining a heel prick sample from an infant or blood collected into citrate or heparin anticoagulants. Tests for VWD may be useful in the diagnosis of a patient who has type 2B VWD or platelet-type VWD because in these conditions the thrombocytopenia is accompanied by decreased VWF.

Bone marrow examination

For a typical presentation of ITP, a bone marrow examination is not required in patients under the age of 60 years. However, a bone marrow aspirate and biopsy is recommended in:
- patients before splenectomy;
- those with additional cytopenias;
- patients with lassitude, protracted fever, bone or joint pain;
- those with unexplained macrocytosis;
- patients with no response to treatment; and
- children before treatment with steroids, because acute lymphoblastic leukaemia may rarely present with thrombocytopenia and steroids would result in an inadequately treated malignancy.

Mean platelet volume

For inherited causes of thrombocytopenia, a useful diagnostic algorithm is based on the platelet size or mean platelet volume (MPV), as shown in Table 8.3. One caveat of this approach is that not all automated counters are able detect very small platelets (as in e.g. Wiskott–Aldrich syndrome) or very large platelets (as in e.g. Bernard–Soulier syndrome), resulting in underestimation of the platelet count. This emphasizes the importance of examining the blood film.

Specialized platelet function tests (see Chapter 4)

Specialized tests that may be indicated in order to diagnose specific congenital thrombocytopenias include:

- platelet function analyzer (PFA-100®);
- platelet aggregation;
- flow cytometry using antibodies labeling GP Ib (for Bernard–Soulier syndrome);
- platelet electron microscopy (for gray platelet syndrome);
- specialized immunocytochemistry (for MYH9-related diseases);
- Western blot for protein analyses (for Quebec platelet disorder); and
- DNA analysis.

Mechanisms of thrombocytopenia in children and adults

Thrombocytopenia can be classified according to increased platelet sequestration, the presence of decreased platelet production and increased platelet destruction (Table 8.4). Some of the more common causes will be highlighted. A diagnostic strategy for evaluating thrombocytopenia in a "well" child or adult is shown in Fig. 8.1.

Platelet sequestration

In healthy individuals, splenic pooling (sequestration) accounts for approximately one-third of the total platelet mass, but may be as high as 90% in individuals with massive splenomegaly. The platelet count from an enlarged spleen rarely drops below 50×10^9/L (unless there is massive splenomegaly) and, because there is usually no increased risk of bleeding, no treatment is warranted.

Decreased platelet production

Because platelets originate from megakaryocytes, inhibition of megakaryocytes or their precursors is often reflected by reduced numbers of megakaryocytes in a bone marrow biopsy, resulting in underproduction of platelets.

A number of viruses cause thrombocytopenia by inhibition of megakaryocytopoiesis, including measles, HIV, varicella, mumps, EBV, rubella, CMV, parvovirus and dengue infection. The platelet count usually recovers once the virus has cleared.

Table 8.4 Causes of thrombocytopenia in children and adults.

Increased platelet sequestration
Hypersplenism

Decreased platelet production
Aplastic anemia (idiopathic or drug-induced)
Myelodysplastic syndrome
Marrow infiltrative process
Infection (bacterial; viral: HIV-1, CMV, hepatitis C virus)
Osteopetrosis
Paroxysmal nocturnal hemoglobinuria
Nutritional deficiencies (iron, folate, vitamin B$_{12}$)
Drug or radiation-induced thrombocytopenia (chemotherapeutic agents, anagrelide, valproic acid, alcohol)
Congenital platelet disorders (see Table 8.3)

Increased platelet destruction
Immune mediated thrombocytopenias
Acute and chronic ITP
Autoimmune diseases with ITP (SLE, Evans syndrome, autoimmune lymphoproliferative disorders, lymphoma, antiphospholipid antibody syndrome)
Infection-related (viral, bacterial, protozoan)
HIV-associated thrombocytopenia
NAIT
Post-transfusion purpura
Drug-induced thrombocytopenia

Non-immune-mediated thrombocytopenias
DIC
Kasabach–Merritt syndrome
Thrombotic thrombocytopenic purpura
Hemolytic uremic syndrome
Catheters, prostheses, cardiopulmonary bypass
Familial hemophagocytic lymphohistiocytosis
Congenital platelet disorders (see Table 8.3)

Miscellaneous
Liver disease, renal disease, thyroid disease
Massive transfusions, exchange transfusions, extracorporeal circulation
Allogeneic bone marrow transplantation, graft-versus-host disease
Heat or cold injury

CMV, cytomegalovirus; DIC, disseminated intravascular coagulation; ITP, immune thrombocytopenic purpura; NAIT, neonatal alloimmune thrombocytopenia; SLE, systemic lupus erythematosus.

Drug-induced thrombocytopenia is common in cancer patients who have been treated with bone marrow suppressing chemotherapy or radiation. Although the mechanisms are poorly understood,

a number of drugs have been implicated in aplastic anemia, including anticonvulsants, NSAIDs, sulfonamides and gold salts. Some drugs known to affect megakaryocytopoiesis are listed in Table 8.2. Anagrelide, used in the treatment of thrombocythemia in patients with myeloproliferative diseases, can cause severe thrombocytopenia. Valproic acid, commonly used in seizure disorders and for psychiatric patients, has been associated with thrombocytopenia resulting from direct bone marrow suppression. Chronic alcohol intake has a direct effect on thrombopoiesis and may also be accompanied by vitamin deficiencies and splenic sequestration in alcoholics, all contributing to the thrombocytopenia. Drug-induced thrombocytopenias usually resolve after removal or lowering of the dosage of the offending drug.

Marrow infiltration (myelophthisis) by leukemia, solid tumors, storage diseases and disseminated Langerhans' cell histiocytosis can inhibit platelet production. Other causes of thrombocytopenia resulting from inhibition of megakaryocytopoiesis and other hematopoietic cells include myelodysplastic syndromes, aplastic anemia, paroxysmal nocturnal hemoglobinuria and osteopetrosis. Osteopetrosis can be diagnosed by imaging studies and the other conditions with a bone marrow aspirate and biopsy.

Nutritional deficiencies of iron, folate or vitamin B$_{12}$ resulting in megaloblastic anemia are often accompanied by thrombocytopenia because of abnormal platelet production. The condition is completely reversible with appropriate supplementation.

Thrombocytopenia resulting from congenital platelet disorders (Table 8.3) may be caused either by inadequate platelet production (megakaryocyte defect) or by the increased clearance of platelets because of inherent structural defects. Treatment modalities depend on the severity of the bleeding diathesis, and include DDAVP, tranexamic acid, platelet transfusion and, during life-threatening bleeding episodes, recombinant factor VIIa.

Increased platelet destruction

Platelet destruction can be mediated by immunological mechanisms involving T-cell cytotoxicity, autoantibodies, alloantibodies and drug-dependent antibodies, or by non-immune processes (Table 8.4).

Immune thrombocytopenia

ITP is probably the most common immune destructive thrombocytopenia in children and adults, occurring in approximately 1 in 10,000 persons/ year. ITP is an immune disorder in which autoantibodies are produced against platelet surface antigens resulting in increased clearance of platelets from the circulation. Both children and adults are affected; in adults it is more often a chronic disorder, whereas in children it tends to be a self-limiting condition. There is a two- to threefold female predominance in adults, while young boys and girls are affected equally. Although the etiology of ITP is poorly understood, infections appear to play a part because, in the case of childhood ITP, the onset is often preceded by a viral infection. Secondary causes of ITP are also observed in patients with:
- systemic lupus erythematosus (SLE);
- autoimmune lymphoproliferative syndrome;
- Evans syndrome;
- antiphospholipid antibody syndrome; and
- neoplasia-associated immune thrombocytopenia.

The diagnosis of primary ITP is suggested by the presence of isolated thrombocytopenia in an otherwise well patient in the absence of other causes. The patient may present with evidence of mucocutaneous bleeding, or after a routine complete blood count (CBC) in an asymptomatic individual. Systemic causes and drug-induced thrombocytopenias as well as congenital thrombocytopenias (e.g. positive family history, abnormal blood film) need to be ruled out. Bone marrow biopsy is recommended in adults over 60 years old to rule out a myelodysplastic syndrome. Platelet autoantibody measurements are not sensitive nor specific enough to be clinically useful. Plasma TPO levels are usually normal or mildly elevated in ITP, but are greatly elevated in amegakaryocytic states (e.g. as in amegakaryocytic thrombocytopenia and aplastic anemia) and therefore may be useful if available.

In adults, treatment of ITP consists of glucocorticoids (prednisone 1 mg/kg/day p.o.), IV immunoglobulin (IVIG; 1 g/kg/day i.v. for 2 days) or IV anti-D (75 µg/kg) in Rh(D)-positive patients with intact spleens. With major bleeding episodes or if the platelet count is less than 10×10^9/L, glucocorticoids can be given together with either IVIG or IV anti-D. In the presence of intracranial hemorrhage (ICH), platelet transfusions are also indicated.

The natural course of acute ITP in children is that most will recover completely within a few weeks without any treatment. The major concern is ICH, which can occur when platelets fall below 20×10^9/L but usually only when they fall below 10×10^9/L. The incidence of ICH is estimated to be between 0.2 and 1%. Platelet-inhibiting drugs such as ASA and other NSAIDs should be avoided. If the child presents with wet purpura or evidence of major bleeding and/or platelet counts below 20×10^9/L, then oral prednisone (3–4 mg/kg/day), IV methylprednisolone (5–30 mg/kg/day), IVIG (0.8–1 g/kg/day), or IV anti-D (75 µg/kg) in Rh(D)-positive children can be given depending on the urgency. As for adults, platelet transfusions are reserved for life-threatening bleeding and ICH. For the treatment of relapsed and chronic ITP, see the review by Cines and Blanchette.

Pregnancy-associated thrombocytopenia

Thrombocytopenia during pregnancy can be difficult to diagnose:
- *Gestational thrombocytopenia* (incidental or benign thrombocytopenia of pregnancy): accounts for approximately 73% of cases.
- *Hypertensive disorders of pregnancy* (chronic hypertension, gestational hypertension, pre-eclampsia/eclampsia): accounts for approximately 21% of cases.
- *ITP/SLE:* accounts for approximately 4% of the causes of thrombocytopenia during pregnancy.

Gestational thrombocytopenia is a diagnosis of exclusion, but can be attributed more than 95% of the time to an asymptomatic pregnant patient with a platelet count between 70×10^9/L and 149×10^9/L. Thrombocytopenia develops in approximately 50% of patients with pre-eclampsia where the HELLP syndrome (haemolysis, elevated liver enzymes, low platelets) can be a serious complication.

The microangiopathic hemolytic anemias TTP/HUS may be difficult to discern from pre-eclampsia or the HELLP syndrome in a pregnant woman, and plasma exchange may be required despite an uncertain diagnosis (see below). ITP occurs in 1–2 per 1000 pregnancies and represents approximately 3% of the causes of thrombocytopenia during pregnancy. A pregnant patient with ITP can be treated with IVIG (1 g/kg prepregnant weight) and/or prednisone (1 mg/kg prepregnant weight) in the acute setting to raise the platelet count to above 10×10^9/L. The reader is referred to recent reviews for details of the management of ITP during pregnancy.

Post-transfusion purpura

Post-transfusion purpura is a rare disorder, which usually presents with severe thrombocytopenia within 1 week after transfusion of a blood product. It is caused by the formation of alloantibodies, most commonly against the platelet alloantigen HPA-1a epitope (also known as PL[A1] or Zw[a]) where the platelet GP IIIa contains a leucine at position 33. Polymorphisms of GP IIIa result in alloantigen HPA-1a and alloantigen HPA-1b (PL[A2] or Zw[b]; proline at position 33 of GP IIIa), which occur at a frequency of approximately 86% and 13% in white people, respectively. Most frequently, the affected patient is a homozygous HPA-1b multiparous woman or a person with a previous blood transfusion who has produced alloantibodies against HPA-1a, which paradoxically cause destruction of autologous platelets through poorly understood mechanisms. Treatment consists of IVIG, corticosteroids or plasmapheresis. Platelet transfusions are contraindicated except in rare circumstances, when HPA-1a negative platelets may be used for life-threatening bleeding complications.

HIV-associated thrombocytopenia

HIV-related thrombocytopenia can be caused by increased platelet destruction, commonly during early-onset HIV, as well as to decreased platelet production more often seen later on in patients with acquired immunodeficiency syndrome (AIDS).

The immune-mediated platelet destruction in HIV is indistinguishable from ITP with respect to increased destruction of antibody-coated platelets and the response to prednisone, IVIG and splenectomy. It differs from classic ITP with respect to:
- male predominance;
- markedly elevated platelet-associated IgG, IgM, and complement C_3, C_4;
- presence of circulating immune complexes; and
- antibody-mediated peroxide lysis of platelets.

Treatment with antiretroviral therapy tends to improve the defective thrombopoiesis in HIV-infected patients. TTP is also found more frequently in HIV-infected patients and can be treated accordingly (see below).

Drug-induced thrombocytopenia

Drug-induced thrombocytopenia may be caused by immune- or non-immune-mediated platelet destruction or suppression of platelet production. The distinction is not always readily apparent; however, some drugs can be categorized to fall under one or more of these mechanisms. In addition, there are different mechanisms of drug-induced immune-mediated platelet destruction:
- Drugs that bind to platelet glycoproteins forming a "compound epitope" include penicillin, quinidine, quinine and sulfonamide. The antibody binding to such platelets is dependent on the presence of the offending drug.
- Gold salts and procainamide, on the other hand, can induce true autoantibodies which subsequently can bind to platelets in the absence of the original offending drug.
- Antiplatelet agents such as tirofiban, eptifibatide and abciximab, which specifically target the GP IIb/IIIa receptor on platelets, cause thrombocytopenia in 1–5% of cardiac patients via antibody-mediated processes.

Heparin-induced thrombocytopenia

HIT differs from other thrombocytopenias in that it is a hypercoagulable state rather than a bleeding condition, manifesting as venous and/or arterial thrombosis. This is discussed in more detail in Chapter 17.

Non-immune destructive thrombocytopenias

Non-immune destructive thrombocytopenias include DIC, Kasabach–Merritt syndrome, TTP, HUS and other conditions listed in Table 8.4.

Disseminated intravascular coagulation

The diagnosis of DIC is usually apparent because the most common causes in adults and older children are infections with septicemia, acute trauma (especially involving brain) and cancer. Obstetrical causes include placental abruption, fetal demise, amniotic fluid embolism and pre-eclampsia. Some neonatal causes of DIC include infection, birth asphyxia, abruptio placentae, major vessel thrombosis, necrotizing enterocolitis, brain injury and purpura fulminans (protein C, protein S deficiency). The pathophysiology of DIC involves the generation of thrombin leading to platelet activation and fibrin formation within the microvasculature, resulting in the consumption of platelets and coagulation factors.

Laboratory indicators of DIC are:
- a falling platelet count;
- concomitant prolongation of the prothrombin time (PT; or international normalized ratio [INR]) and activated partial thromboplastin time (aPTT);
- decreased fibrinogen and elevated fibrinogen degradation products (FDPs) or D-dimers on serial measurements; and
- red blood cell fragments (schistocytes) may be seen on the blood film.

Treatment consists of reversing the underlying systemic illness, with transfusion of platelets, fresh frozen plasma or cryoprecipitate in a bleeding patient when levels fall below critical values. Infusion of activated protein C in critically ill septic patients may improve survival.

Kasabach–Merritt syndrome

Kasabach–Merritt syndrome (Fig. 8.2) is a thrombocytopenia noted most commonly in a newborn infant with a hemangioma of infancy of the histopathologic subtype kaposiform hemangioendothelioma or tufted hemangioma. Although poorly understood, the pathogenesis is thought to be caused by platelet trapping and activation within the abnormal endothelium of the hemangioma resulting in thrombocytopenia and laboratory evidence of DIC, including hypofibrinogenemia and increased D-dimers. Kasabach–Merritt hemangiomas tend to grow rapidly for several months followed by spontaneous regression in the first few years of life. However, individualized treatment using vascular ligation, embolization, corticosteroids, α-interferon (IFN-α) or vincristine may

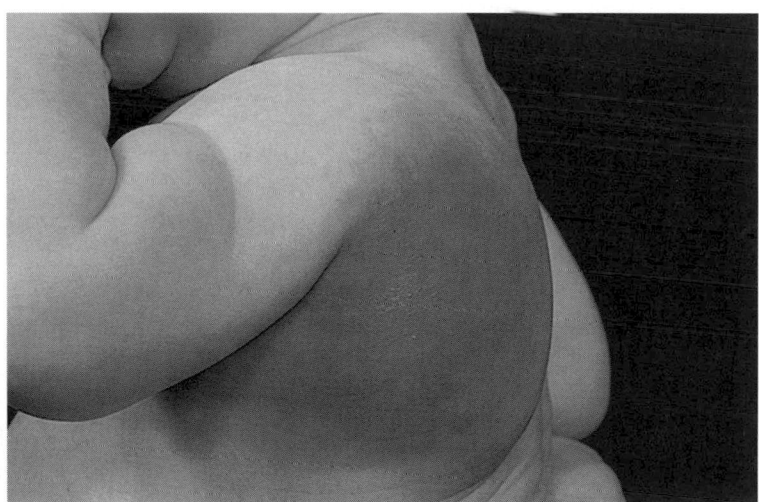

Figure 8.2 Kasabach–Merritt syndrome. Reprinted from *Blood in Systemic Disease* 1e, Greaves and Makris, 1997, with permission from Elsevier.

be required in some cases of life-threatening thrombocytopenia and coagulopathy.

Thrombotic thrombocytopenic purpura

TTP is a syndrome characterized by platelet aggregation in the microcirculation. Patients present with thrombocytopenia, microangiopathic hemolytic anemia, fever, renal dysfunction and neurologic deficits. TTP is discussed in more detail in Chapter 17.

Hemolytic uremic syndrome

HUS is another microangiopathic hemolytic condition that is closely related to TTP but has some unique clinical characteristics. HUS is frequently seen in infants and young children, occurring in approximately 1 in 100,000 annually, but may also affect the elderly. HUS usually follows an acute diarrheal illness often resulting from enterohemorrhagic *Escherichia coli* O157:H7, or *Shigella*, *Salmonella*, or *Campylobacter jejuni*. HUS is frequently accompanied by renal failure and may be the leading cause of acute renal failure in infants and young children. Although a prodromal bloody diarrhea is most common, approximately 10% of pediatric patients do not have antecedent diarrhea. The clinical presentation is sometimes difficult to distinguish from TTP, and some experts classify TTP and HUS as one disease entity, TTP/HUS. However, there are some distinct differences because in HUS the pathogenesis often involves a Shiga-like toxin, resulting in endothelial cell death in vessels of the intestinal submucosa and renal microvasculature, explaining the common clinical intestinal and renal findings in typical HUS. Also, children with HUS resulting from *E. coli* O157:H7 infection tend to have normal plasma levels of ADAMTS13, suggesting an alternative microangiopathic mechanism. Most importantly, the treatment of HUS in children is distinct from adults in that supportive care is the mainstay in children. Transfusion may be required for symptomatic anemia as well as dialysis when necessary. Antimotility agents may worsen the clinical manifestations of infectious HUS, whereas the role of antibiotics is unresolved. Because of the potentially high morbidity and mortality in TTP/HUS and the often difficult clinical distinction between TTP and HUS, children with atypical HUS, familial HUS and all adults with HUS should be treated with plasma exchange.

Thrombocytopenia in the newborn infant

A useful approach in determining the etiology of thrombocytopenia in a newborn is to distinguish the sick premature infant from a well term infant. The incidence of thrombocytopenia in healthy newborn infants is approximately 1–2%. Approximately 22% of all neonates admitted to neonatal intensive care units develop thrombocytopenia. In 20% of these thrombocytopenic patients the platelet count drops below 50×10^9/L.

Common causes of thrombocytopenia in a sick preterm infant include:
- bacterial or viral sepsis;
- DIC;
- necrotizing enterocolitis;
- respiratory disease syndromes;
- meconium and amniotic fluid aspiration;
- asphyxia reflecting precipitating fetomaternal or neonatal conditions; and
- alloimmune or autoimmune thrombocytopenias.

Treatment of non-immune-mediated thrombocytopenia in neonates consists of platelet transfusion according to transfusion threshold guidelines reviewed by Roberts and Murray.

Neonatal alloimmune thrombocytopenia

NAIT is often the most likely cause of thrombocytopenia in the well-appearing full-term infant, while other causes include:
- maternal ITP;
- SLE;
- aortic or renal vein thrombosis; and
- congenital thrombocytopenic.

In NAIT, the destruction of fetal or neonatal platelets results from transplacental passage of maternal platelet-specific alloantibodies. In contrast to neonatal ITP, where the platelet count is low in both the mother and the neonate or fetus, NAIT is not associated with maternal thrombocytopenia, making it a useful laboratory distinction. The most frequent platelet antigen polymorphism in white populations causing NAIT is the HPA-1a epitope (also known as PL[A1] or Zw[a]) where the platelet GP IIIa contains a leucine at position 33. Alloantibodies (anti-HPA-1a) can form if the mother is homozygous for HPA-1b (PL[A2] or Zw[b]; proline at position 33 of GP IIIa) with a significantly increased risk of developing NAIT if the mother also has HLA class-II DRB3*0101.

It is estimated that NAIT affects 1 in 1000–2000 live births and that serious complications such as ICH occur in 10–20% of affected neonates.

Because ICH frequently occurs antenatally and as NAIT can present during the first pregnancy, this often makes it difficult to alter the clinical course of these patients. However, a history of a previously affected infant can be predictive for diagnosing NAIT in a subsequent fetus, with the potential of antenatal intervention. Such intervention may involve either weekly infusions of IVIG with or without corticosteroids given to the mother, or repeated *in utero* fetal platelet transfusions.

A definitive diagnosis of neonatal alloimmune thrombocytopenia requires the demonstration of fetomaternal incompatibility for a platelet antigen, and presence in the maternal serum of a platelet antibody reactive with platelets from the infant and/or biologic father but non-reactive with maternal platelets. However, these serologic tests may not be readily available and neonates with suspected NAIT and severe thrombocytopenia should be managed as emergency cases. The treatment of choice is compatible antigen-negative platelets harvested from the mother or a donor known to be compatible. If such a product is not available, a trial of high-dose IVIG (1 g/kg for 2 days) is warranted; in extreme situations, plasma exchange should be considered. Corticosteroids are not beneficial in this clinical setting, in contrast to neonatal autoimmune thrombocytopenia where first-line therapy for severely thrombocytopenic babies consists of high-dose IVIG with or without added corticosteriods. Exchange transfusion is invasive and is rarely indicated in such infants.

Thrombocytosis

Thrombocytosis is defined by a rise in platelet count of more than 500×10^9/L. Reactive thrombocytosis (RT; secondary thrombocytosis) is much more frequent (85% of cases) than primary thrombocytosis in both children and adults. A variety of clinical conditions can lead to RT, including:

- infection;
- malignancy;
- blood loss;
- inflammation;
- rebound thrombocytosis;
- tissue damage; and
- splenectomy.

Primary thrombocytosis (PT) may be a result of rare cases of familial thrombocytosis caused by an autosomal dominant gain-of-function mutation in the TPO gene resulting in overproduction of TPO. More commonly, PT is caused by clonal proliferation of megakaryocyte precursors seen in essential thrombocythemia (ET), polycythemia vera (PV), chronic myelogenous leukemia (CML), myelofibrosis, and myelodysplastic syndrome (MDS; observed least frequently). In MDS, thrombocytosis may be associated with deletion of the long arm of chromosome 5 (5q-). The clinical distinction between primary and secondary thrombocytosis is often difficult and requires identification or exclusion of potential underlying secondary causes. It is important to distinguish PT from RT because patients with PT are at increased risk for digital or cerebrovascular ischemia, large-vessel arterial or venous thrombosis and bleeding complications. Splenomegaly may be present in PT but not in RT. Elevated erythrocyte or leukocyte counts suggest PT in association with a chronic myeloid disorder. In the case of isolated thrombocytosis, previous medical records may be useful because persistent thrombocytosis is suggestive of PT. Giant platelets are frequently observed in PT whereas platelet size is normal in RT. Platelet function measured by platelet aggregation is often abnormal (decreased) in PT whereas platelet aggregations are normal in RT.

If RT cannot be confirmed based on the above considerations, a bone marrow examination may be useful, because in RT the bone marrow appears normal whereas it is often abnormal in PT (typical features in myelofibrosis, MDS, and CML; in ET, giant dysplastic megakaryocytes with increased ploidy may be evident). Future diagnostic tests may include colony-forming assays (autonomous growth in the absence of specific growth factors) as well as TPO receptor (cMpl) expression assays in megakaryocytes and platelets (reduced in PT).

Treatment of RT consists of treating the underlying disease whereas in PT treatment depends on the presence or absence of symptoms, risk stratification and whether the platelet count is greater than 1500×10^9/L. Asymptomatic patients with elevated platelet counts ($> 1500 \times 10^9$/L) require cytoreduction using anagrelide or hydroxyurea (or IFN-α during pregnancy or childbearing years). Asymptomatic patients older than 60 years, or with cardiovascular risk factors and/or prior thrombosis, require cytoreduction and daily ASA. Symptomatic patients with active cerebrovascular or digital ischemia require immediate platelet pheresis together with cytoreduction and ASA treatment. Platelet transfusions are indicated in life-threatening bleeding because the patient's own platelets are often dysfunctional.

Further reading

Abrams CS, Cines DB. Thrombocytopenia after treatment with platelet glycoprotein IIb/IIIa inhibitors. *Curr Hematol Rep* 2004;**3**:143–7.

Aster RH. Drug-induced thrombocytopenia. In: Michelson AD, ed. *Platelets*. San Diego: Academic Press, 2002:593–606.

Balduini CL, Cattaneo M, Fabris F, *et al.* Inherited thrombocytopenias: a proposed diagnostic algorithm from the Italian Gruppo di Studio delle Piastrine. *Haematologica* 2003;**88**:582–92.

Birchall JE, Murphy MF, Kaplan C, Kroll H. European collaborative study of the antenatal management of feto-maternal alloimmune thrombocytopenia. *Br J Haematol* 2003;**122**:275–88.

Blanchette VS, Johnson J, Rand M. The management of alloimmune neonatal thrombocytopenia. *Baillieres Best Pract Res Clin Haematol* 2000;**13**:365–90.

Chong BH. Heparin-induced thrombocytopenia. *J Thromb Haemost* 2003;**1**:1471–8.

Cines DB, Blanchette VS. Immune thrombocytopenic purpura. *N Engl J Med* 2002;**346**:995–1008.

Drachman JG. Inherited thrombocytopenia: when a low platelet count does not mean ITP. *Blood* 2004;**103**:390–8.

Frevel T, Rabe H, Uckert F, Harms E. Giant cavernous haemangioma with Kasabach–Merritt syndrome: a case report and review. *Eur J Pediatr* 2002;**161**:243–6.

George JN. How I treat patients with thrombotic thrombocytopenic purpura–hemolytic uremic syndrome. *Blood* 2000;**96**:1223–9.

George JN, Raskob GE, Shah SR, *et al.* Drug-induced thrombocytopenia: a systematic review of published case reports. *Ann Intern Med* 1998;**129**:886–90.

Kaushansky K. Thrombopoietin: the primary regulator of platelet production. *Blood* 1995;**86**:419–31.

Levi M, Ten Cate H. Disseminated intravascular coagulation. *N Engl J Med* 1999;**341**:586–92.

Levy GG, Nichols WC, Lian EC, *et al.* Mutations in a member of the ADAMTS gene family cause thrombotic thrombocytopenic purpura. *Nature* 2001;**413**:488–94.

McCrae KR. Thrombocytopenia in pregnancy: differential diagnosis, pathogenesis, and management. *Blood Rev* 2003;**17**:7–14.

Rebulla P, Finazzi G, Marangoni F, *et al.* The threshold for prophylactic platelet transfusions in adults with acute myeloid leukemia. Gruppo Italiano Malattie Ematologiche Maligne dell'Adulto. *N Engl J Med* 1997;**337**:1870–5.

Roberts I, Murray NA. Neonatal thrombocytopenia: causes and management. *Arch Dis Child Fetal Neonatal Ed* 2003;**88**:F359–64.

Schafer AI. Thrombocytosis. *N Engl J Med* 2004;**350**:1211–19.

Tsai HM, Chandler WL, Sarode R, *et al.* Von Willebrand factor and von Willebrand factor-cleaving metalloprotease activity in *Escherichia coli* O157:H7-associated hemolytic uremic syndrome. *Pediatr Res* 2001;**49**:653–9.

Chapter 9
Qualitative platelet disorders

Marco Cattaneo

Introduction

Abnormalities of platelet function are associated with a heightened risk for bleeding, proving that platelets have an important role in hemostasis. Typically, patients with platelet disorders have mucocutaneous bleeding of variable severity and excessive hemorrhage after surgery or trauma.

In this chapter, the main inherited and acquired qualitative platelet defects are reviewed. Abnormalities of platelet function resulting from defects of plasma proteins (e.g. von Willebrand disease, afibrinogenemia) will not be considered here as they are discussed in Chapters 6 and 7.

Inherited qualitative platelet defects

Inherited disorders of platelet function are generally classified according to the functions or responses that are abnormal. However, because platelet functions are intimately related, a clear distinction between disorders of platelet adhesion, aggregation, activation, secretion and procoagulant activity is in many instances problematic. For this reason, a classification of the inherited disorders of platelet function is proposed based on abnormalities of platelet components that share common characteristics (Table 9.1):

- platelet receptors for adhesive proteins;
- platelet receptors for soluble agonists;
- platelet granules;
- signal-transduction pathways;
- procoagulant phospholipids; and
- miscellaneous disorders (less well characterized).

Table 9.1 Inherited platelet defects.

Abnormalities of the platelet receptors for adhesive proteins
Gp Ib/V/IX complex (Bernard–Soulier syndrome, platelet-type von Willebrand disease, Bolin–Jamieson syndrome)
Gp IIb/IIIa (α_{IIb}/β_3) (Glanzmann thrombasthenia)
Gp Ia/IIa (α_2/β_1)
Gp VI
Gp IV

Abnormalities of the platelet receptors for soluble agonists
Thromboxane A_2 receptor
α_2-Adrenergic receptor
$P2Y_{12}$ receptor

Abnormalities of the platelet granules
δ-Granules (δ-storage pool deficiency, Hermansky–Pudlak syndrome, Chédiak–Hygashi syndrome, thrombocytopenia with absent radii syndrome, Wiskott–Aldrich syndrome)
α-Granules (gray platelet syndrome, Quebec platelet disorder, Paris–Trousseau syndrome, Jacobsen syndrome)
α- and δ-granules (α,δ-storage pool deficiency)

Abnormalities of the signal-transduction pathways
Abnormalities of the arachidonate–thromboxane A_2 pathway, $G\alpha q$ deficiency, partial selective PLC-β2 isoenzyme deficiency, defects in pleckstrin phosphorylation, defective Ca^{2+} mobilization, hyper-responsiveness of platelet $Gs\alpha$

Abnormalities of membrane phospholipids
Scott syndrome
Stormorken syndrome

Miscellaneous abnormalities of platelet function
Primary secretion defects
Other platelet abnormalities (Montreal platelet syndrome, osteogenesis imperfecta, Ehlers–Danlos syndrome, Marfan syndrome, hexokinase deficiency, glucose-6-phosphate deficiency)

Abnormalities of the platelet receptors for adhesive proteins

GP Ib/V/IX complex (von Willebrand factor [VWF] binding site)

The Bernard–Soulier syndrome (BSS) is characterized by:
- autosomal recessive inheritance (with one exception of autosomal dominant inheritance);
- prolonged bleeding time;
- thrombocytopenia;
- giant platelets (often not detected on automatic counters);
- decreased platelet survival; and
- lack of platelet agglutination with ristocetin.

The lack of ristocetin-induced agglutination is not corrected by the addition of normal plasma. The platelet responses to physiologic agonists are normal, with the exception of low concentrations of thrombin, because Gp Ibα (one of the two components of Gp Ib) has a critical role in the platelet aggregatory, secretory and procoagulant responses to thrombin.

Bleeding events, which may be very severe in homozygous BSS, can be controlled by platelet transfusion. Most heterozygotes do not have a bleeding diathesis but are the most common cause of macrothrombocytopenia in some parts of the world.

BSS is caused by defects in the genes for Gp Ibα, Ibβ or IX, but not Gp V. The molecular defects that are responsible for BSS (frameshifts, deletions, point mutations) are summarized at http://www.bernard-soulier.org/mutations.

Platelet-type, or pseudo, von Willebrand disease (VWD) is not caused by defects of VWF, but to a gain-of-function phenotype of the platelet Gp Ibα. This abnormal receptor has an increased avidity for VWF, leading to the binding of the largest VWF multimers to resting platelets and their clearance from the circulation. Because the high molecular weight VWF multimers are the most hemostatically active, their loss is associated with an increased bleeding risk, as in type 2B VWD, (which is caused by a gain-of-function abnormality of the VWF molecule). Platelet-type VWD is an autosomal dominant disease caused by gain-of-function

missense mutations of Gp Ibα and associated with amino acid substitutions occurring within the disulfide-bonded double loop region of Gp Ibα (G233V, G233S and M239V).

Bolin–Jamieson syndrome is a rare, autosomal-dominant, mild bleeding disorder associated with a larger form of Gp Ibα in one allele. It has been proposed that it is associated with a large multimer form of the size polymorphism occurring in the mucin-like domain.

Abnormalities of Gp IIb/IIIa (α_{IIb}/β_3)

Glanzmann thrombasthenia (GT) is an autosomal recessive disease caused by lack of expression or qualitative defects of one of the two glycoproteins forming the integrin α_{IIb}/β_3 (in activated platelets these adhesive glycoproteins bridge adjacent platelets, securing platelet aggregation). The diagnostic hallmark is the lack, or severe impairment, of platelet aggregation induced by all agonists. Platelet clot retraction is defective and GT platelets bind to the subendothelium but they fail to spread.

The disease is associated with bleeding manifestations that are similar to those of patients with BSS, although of less severity. GT patients are grouped into three types, according to the severity of α_{IIb}/β_3 deficiency on their platelet membranes:
- Type I patients: < 5% (characterized by lack of fibrinogen in platelet α-granules).
- Type II patients: 10–20%.
- Type III (variant) patients: 50–100%.

The GT defect is caused by mutations or deletions in the genes encoding one of the two glycoproteins forming the α_{IIb}/β_3 integrin. In GT caused by mutations in the β_3 integrin, the levels of the platelet vitronectin receptor (α_v/β_3) are also decreased, but the phenotype of these patients is no different from that of the other GT patients. Details of the molecular defects that are responsible for GT are available at http//med.mssn.edu/glanzmanndb.

Abnormalities of Gp Ia/IIa (α_2/β_1)

Two patients with mild bleeding disorders associated with deficient expression of the platelet receptor for collagen Gp Ia/IIa (α_2/β_1) and selective impairment of platelet responses to collagen have been described. Their platelet defect spontaneously recovered after the menopause, suggesting that α_2/β_1 expression is under hormonal control.

Abnormalities of Gp VI

A selective defect of collagen-induced platelet aggregation was also described in another mild bleeding disorder, characterized by the deficiency of the platelet Gp VI, a member of the immunoglobulin superfamily of receptors, which mediates platelet activation by collagen. The molecular defects that are responsible for the platelet abnormality have not been characterized in the patients described so far. The possibility should be explored that the molecular abnormality lies in the gene encoding for the Fcγ receptor, which is the signaling subunit of Gp VI.

Abnormalities of Gp IV

Gp IV binds collagen, thrombospondin and probably other proteins. Its physiological role is unclear, because its deficiency, common in healthy individuals from Japan and other East Asian populations, is not associated with an abnormal phenotype.

Abnormalities of the platelet receptors for soluble agonists

Thromboxane A₂ receptor

In 1993, a patient with a mild bleeding disorder was described whose platelets had a defective response to the TxA$_2$ analog U46619, albeit having a normal number of TxA$_2$ binding sites and normal equilibrium dissociation rate constants. Despite the normal number of TxA$_2$ receptors, the TxA$_2$-induced IP3 formation, Ca^{2+} mobilization and GTPase activity were abnormal, suggesting that the abnormality in these platelets was impaired coupling between the TxA$_2$ receptor, G protein and PLC. This patient was subsequently found to have an Arg 60 to Leu mutation in the first cytoplasmic loop of the TxA$_2$ receptor, affecting both isoforms of the receptor.

α₂-Adrenergic receptors

Subjects with a selective impairment of platelet response to epinephrine, a decreased number of the platelet α_2-adrenergic receptors and mildly prolonged bleeding times have been described. However, the relationship between this defect and bleeding manifestations still needs to be defined.

P2Y₁₂ receptor for ADP

Human platelets express three distinct P2 receptors stimulated by adenosine nucleotides:
- P2X$_1$.
- P2Y$_1$ receptor for ADP with a role in the initiation of platelet activation.
- P2Y$_{12}$ receptor for ADP essential for a sustained, full aggregation response to ADP.

The concurrent activation of both P2Y receptors is necessary for full platelet aggregation induced by ADP. P2Y$_{12}$ also mediates the potentiation of platelet secretion by ADP and the stabilization of thrombin-induced platelet aggregates.

Only patients with congenital defects of the platelet P2Y$_{12}$ receptors have been described. The first patient (V.R. described in 1992 by Cattaneo *et al.*) had a lifelong history of excessive bleeding, a prolonged bleeding time and abnormalities of platelet aggregation similar to those observed in patients with defects of platelet secretion (reversible aggregation in response to weak agonists and impaired aggregation in response to low concentrations of collagen or thrombin), except that the aggregation response to ADP was severely impaired.

Other measures of platelet function found in this patient were:
- No inhibition by ADP of PGE$_1$-stimulated platelet adenylyl cyclase.
- Normal shape change and normal (or mildly reduced) mobilization of cytoplasmic ionized calcium induced by ADP.
- Presence of approximately 30% of the normal number of platelet binding sites for [^{33}P]2MeSADP or [^{3}H]ADP.

Three additional patients with very similar characteristics were later described. All these patients displayed base pair deletions in the P2Y$_{12}$ gene, shifting the reading frame for several residues before introducing a premature stop codon, causing an early truncation of the protein.

A fifth patient (A.C.) with a congenital bleeding disorder associated with abnormal $P2Y_{12}$-mediated platelet responses to ADP has more recently been characterized. The platelet phenotype is very similar to that of patients with $P2Y_{12}$ deficiency, except that the number and affinity of $[^{33}P]$-2MeSADP binding sites was normal. Analysis of the patient $P2Y_{12}$ gene revealed, in one allele, a G to A transition changing the codon for Arg 256 in the sixth transmembrane domain to Gln and, in the other allele, a C to T transition changing the codon for Arg 265 in the third extracellular loop to Trp. Neither mutation interfered with receptor surface expression but both altered function, suggesting that the structural integrity of these regions corresponding to the extracytoplasmic end of TM 6 and EL 3 is necessary for the normal function of this G protein-coupled receptor.

The study of the children of patient M.G. and patient A.C. allowed the characterization of patients with a heterozygous $P2Y_{12}$ defect whose platelets do not secrete normal amounts of ATP after stimulation with different agonists. This secretion defect was not caused by impaired production of thromboxane A_2 or low concentrations of platelet granule contents, and is therefore very similar to that described in patients with an ill-defined group of congenital defects of platelet secretion, sometimes referred to by the general term "primary secretion defect" (PSD; see below), which is the most common congenital disorder of platelet function.

$P2Y_{12}$ deficiency is probably much more common than currently recognized; it is therefore important to emphasize that this condition should be suspected when ADP, even at relatively high concentrations (10 μM or higher), induces a slight and rapidly reversible aggregation which is preceded by normal shape change. The confirmatory diagnostic test is based on the ability of ADP to inhibit the platelet adenylyl cyclase after its stimulation by prostaglandins or forskolin.

Abnormalities of the platelet granules

Abnormalities of the δ-granules (δ-storage pool deficiency)

The term δ-storage pool deficiency (δ-SPD) defines a congenital abnormality of platelets characterized by deficiency of dense granules in megakaryocytes and platelets. It may present as an isolated platelet function defect or associate with a variety of congenital disorders. Between 10% and 18% of patients with congenital abnormalities of platelet function have SPD. The inheritance is autosomal recessive in some families but autosomal dominant in others.

δ-SPD is characterized by:
- a bleeding diathesis of variable degree;
- mildly to moderately prolonged skin bleeding time, inversely related to the amount of ADP or serotonin contained in the granules;
- abnormal platelet secretion induced by several platelet agonists;
- impaired platelet aggregation in 75% of cases (only 33% have aggregation tracings typical for a platelet secretion defect); and
- decreased levels of δ-granule constituents: ATP and ADP, serotonin, calcium and pyrophosphate.

Lumiaggregometry, which measures platelet aggregation and secretion simultaneously, may prove a more accurate technique than platelet aggregometry for diagnosing patients with δ-SPD and, more generally, with platelet secretion defects.

Hermansky–Pudlak syndrome (HPS) and Chédiak–Higashi syndrome (CHS) are rare syndromic forms of δ-SPD. HPS is an autosomal recessive disease of subcellular organelles of many tissues involving abnormalities of melanosomes, platelet δ-granules and lysosomes. It is characterized by tyrosinase-positive oculocutaneous albinism, a bleeding diathesis resulting from δ-SPD and ceroid-lipofuscin lysosomal storage disease. HPS can arise from mutations in different genetic loci.

CHS is a lethal disorder (death usually in the first decade of life) with:
- autosomal recessive inheritance;
- variable degrees of oculocutaneous albinism;

• very large peroxidase-positive cytoplasmic granules in a variety of hematopoietic (neutrophils) and nonhematopoietic cells;
• easy bruisability as a result of δ-SPD;
• recurrent infections, associated with neutropenia, impaired chemotaxis and bactericidal activity; and
• abnormal natural killer (NK) cell function.

Two types of hereditary thrombocytopenia may be associated with δ-SPD:
1 Thrombocytopenia and absent radii syndrome (TAR); and
2 Wiskott–Aldrich syndrome.

Abnormalities of the α-granules

Gray platelet syndrome (GPS) derives its name from the gray appearance of the patient's platelets in peripheral blood smears as a consequence of the rarity of platelet granules. The inheritance pattern seems to be autosomal recessive, although in a single family it seemed to be autosomal dominant.

Affected patients have a lifelong history of mucocutaneous bleeding, which may vary from mild to moderate in severity, and prolonged bleeding time. They have mild thrombocytopenia with abnormally large platelets and isolated reduction of the platelet α-granule content. Mild to moderate myelofibrosis has been described in some (hypothetically ascribed to the action of cytokines released by the hypogranular platelets and megakaryocytes in the bone marrow). The basic defect in GPS is probably defective targeting and packaging of endogenously synthesized proteins in α-granules.

The Quebec platelet disorder is an autosomal dominant qualitative platelet abnormality, characterized by:
• severe post-traumatic bleeding complications unresponsive to platelet transfusion;
• abnormal proteolysis of α-granule proteins;
• severe deficiency of platelet factor V;
• deficiency of multimerin;
• reduced to normal platelet counts; and
• markedly decreased platelet aggregation induced by epinephrine.

Multimerin, one of the largest proteins found in the human body, is present in platelet α-granules and in endothelial cell Weibel–Palade bodies. It binds factor V and its activated form, factor Va. Its deficiency in patients with the Quebec platelet disorder is probably responsible for the defect in platelet factor V, which is likely to be degraded by abnormally regulated platelet proteases.

Jacobsen or Paris–Trousseau syndrome is a rare syndrome that is associated with:
• a mild hemorrhagic diathesis;
• congenital thrombocytopenia with normal platelet life span;
• increased number of marrow megakaryocytes (many presenting with signs of abnormal maturation and intramedullary lysis); and
• a deletion of the distal part of one chromosome 11 [del(11)q23.3→qter] has been found in affected patients.

Abnormalities of the α- and δ- granules

α,δ-Storage pool deficiency is characterized by deficiencies of both α- and δ-granules. The clinical picture and the platelet aggregation abnormalities are similar to those of patients with GPS or δ-SPD.

Abnormalities of the signal-transduction pathways

Congenital abnormalities of the arachidonate–thromboxane A_2 pathway, involving the liberation of arachidonic acid from membrane phospholipids, defects of cyclo-oxygenase or thromboxane synthetase, are associated with platelet function defects and mild bleeding. Other congenital abnormalities of the platelet signal-transduction pathways have been described involving:
• G-proteins (Gαq deficiency);
• phosphatidylinositol metabolism (partial selective PLC-β2 isozyme deficiency); or
• defects in pleckstrin phosphorylation and hyper-responsiveness of platelet Gsα.

Abnormalities of membrane phospholipids

Scott syndrome is a rare bleeding disorder associated with the maintenance of the asymmetry of the lipid bilayer in the membranes of blood cells, including platelets leading to reduced thrombin generation and defective wound healing. The cause of the defect is still unclear.

In Stormorken syndrome, resting, unstimulated platelets from patients with this syndrome display a full procoagulant activity. Therefore, this condition represents the exact opposite in terms of platelet membrane function to the Scott syndrome, yet, surprisingly, it is also associated with a bleeding tendency. Platelets from patients with this condition respond normally to all agonists, with the exception of collagen.

Miscellaneous abnormalities of platelet function

Primary secretion defects

The term primary secretion defect was probably used for the first time by Weiss, to indicate all those ill-defined abnormalities of platelet secretion not associated with platelet granule deficiencies. The term was later used to indicate the platelet secretion defects not associated with platelet granule deficiencies and abnormalities of the arachidonate pathway, or all the abnormalities of platelet function associated with defects of signal transduction.

With the progression of our knowledge of platelet pathophysiology, this heterogeneous group, which brings together the majority of patients with congenital disorders of platelet function, will become progressively smaller, losing those patients with better defined biochemical abnormalities responsible for their platelet secretion defect. An example is heterozygous $P2Y_{12}$ deficiency state, which was included in this group of disorders until their biochemical abnormality was identified.

Other platelet abnormalities

Spontaneous platelet aggregation and decreased responses to thrombin are observed in patients with the Montreal platelet syndrome, a rare and poorly characterized congenital thrombocytopenia with large platelets.

Platelet function abnormalities have also been reported in osteogenesis imperfecta, Ehlers–Danlos syndrome, Marfan syndrome, hexokinase deficiency and glucose-6-phosphate deficiency.

Table 9.2 Acquired platelet defects.

Medications affecting platelet function
Uremia
Dysproteinemias
Acute leukemias and myelodysplastic syndromes
Cardiopulmonary bypass
Liver disease
Antiplatelet antibodies
Myeloproliferative disorders
    Essential thrombocythemia
    Polycythemia vera
    Chronic myelogenous leukemia
    Agnogenic myeloid metaplasia

Acquired platelet defects

Platelet function can be impaired in several hematologic and non-hematologic conditions and by medications (Table 9.2).

Uremia

The bleeding time (BT) may be severely prolonged in patients with uremia, but it can be corrected by increasing the hematocrit with red blood cell (RBC) transfusions or with erythropoietin, suggesting that in many instances the defective primary hemostasis in uremia is a consequence of anemia. (It is known that RBCs normally facilitate the platelet interaction with the vessel wall.)

However, correction of the hematocrit fails to correct the BT in some patients, suggesting that other factors impair platelet–vessel wall interaction in this condition. Abnormalities of interaction of adhesive glycoproteins with their platelet receptors, defective platelet activation and platelet procoagulant activity have been described. Both dialyzable and non-dialyzable substances may be responsible.

Myeloproliferative disorders

Functional and biochemical abnormalities of platelets from patients with myeloproliferative disorders include:
• decreased release of arachidonic acid from membrane phospholipids;

- reduced conversion of arachidonic acid to its active metabolites;
- reduced responsiveness to TxA_2;
- deficiency of platelet granules;
- deficiency of the α_2/β_1 integrin; and
- decreased number of α_2-adrenergic receptors.

Other factors, in addition to platelet functional defects, contribute to the bleeding diathesis of these patients, including increased whole blood viscosity and thrombocytosis.

Cardiopulmonary bypass

Cardiopulmonary bypass causes transient thrombocytopenia and platelet function defects, which contribute to the increased bleeding risk of these patients. Platelet function defects associated with extracorporeal circulation include:
- defective aggregation;
- platelet granule deficiencies;
- abnormal interaction with VWF; and
- generation of platelet-derived microparticles.

These abnormalities result from platelet activation and fragmentation, hypothermia, contact with the blood–air interface and exposure to traces of platelet agonists such as thrombin, ADP and plasmin.

Medications

Many drugs affect platelet function (Table 9.3), sometimes causing a prolongation of the BT. In some instances, the inhibition of platelet function is the target of the drug, as in the case of antiplatelet agents that are given to reduce the risk of cardiovascular or cerebrovascular accidents. In other cases, the induced abnormalities of platelet function are to be considered side-effects of the drug, which are in most instances without obvious clinical consequences.

Liver disease

Chronic liver disease is associated with a prolongation of the BT disproportionate to the degree of thrombocytopenia that usually complicates this condition. Whether the described defects are caused by intrinsic or extrinsic abnormalities of the platelets is unclear.

Table 9.3 Drugs affecting platelet function.

Non-steroidal anti-inflammatory drugs
Aspirin, indomethacin, ibuprofen, sulindac, naproxen, phenylbutazone

Thienopyridines
Ticlopidine, clopidogrel, thromboxane A_2 receptor

Gp IIb/IIIa antagonists
Abciximab, eptifibatide, tirofiban

Drugs that increase the platelet cAMP or cGMP levels
Prostacyclin, iloprost, dipyridamole, theophylline, nitric oxide, nitric oxide donors

Anticoagulants and fibrinolytic agents
Heparin, streptokinase, tPA, urokinase

Cardiovascular drugs
Nitroglycerin, isosorbide dinitrate, propranolol, frusemide, calcium-channel blockers, quinidine, ACE inhibitors, verapamil, diltiazem

Volume expanders
Dextran, hydroxyethyl starch

Psychotropic drugs, anesthetics
Imipramine, amitriptyline, nortriptyline, chlorpromazine, promethazine, fluphenazine, trifluoperazine, haloperidol, halothane, dibucaine, tetracaine, butacaine, nepercaine, procaine plaquenil

Chemotherapeutic agents
Mitomycin, daunorubicin, BCNU

Miscellaneous drugs
Antihistamines, radiographic contrast agents, clofibrate

ACE, angiotensin-converting enzyme; cGMP: cyclic guanosine 3′,5′-monophosphate CAMP: cyclic adenosine 3′,5′-monophosphate.

Therapy

Platelet transfusions should be used only in severe bleeding episodes, which are usually seen in patients with BSS or, less frequently, Glanzmann thrombasthenia. Recombinant factor VIIa is a good, albeit expensive, alternative to platelet transfusions. Antifibrinolytic agents, such as aprotinin and tranexamic acid, or the vasopressin analog desmopressin (DDAVP) should be used in all other circumstances, because they are relatively cheap, do not cause platelet refractoriness and are not associated with the risk of transmitting blood-borne viral diseases.

Further reading

Balduini CL, Cattaneo M, Fabris F, Gresele P, Iolascon A, Savoia A, for the Italian Gruppo di Studio delle Piastrine. Inherited thrombocytopenias: proposal of a diagnostic algorithm by the Italian Gruppo di Studio delle Piastrine. *Haematologica* 2003;**88**:582–92.

Bennett JS. Acquired platelet function defects. In: Gresele P, Page C, Fuster V, Vermylen J, eds. *Platelets in Thrombotic and Non-Thrombotic Disorders*. Cambridge: Cambridge University Press, 2002.

Cattaneo M. Congenital disorders of platelet secretion. In: Gresele P, Page C, Fuster V, Vermylen J, eds. *Platelets in Thrombotic and Non-Thrombotic Disorders*. Cambridge: Cambridge University Press, 2002.

Cattaneo M, Mannucci PM. Desmopressin. In: Michelson AD, ed. *Platelets*. Orlando, FL: Academic Press, 2003.

Cattaneo M, Lecchi A, Randi AM, McGregor JL, Mannucci PM. Identification of a new congenital defect of platelet function characterized by severe impairment of platelet responses to adenosine diphosphate. *Blood*. 1992;**80**:2787–96.

Cattaneo M. Inherited platelet-based bleeding disorders. *J Thromb Haemost* 2003;**1**:1628–36.

Cattaneo M, Gachet C. ADP receptors and clinical bleeding disorders. *Arterioscler Thromb Vasc Biol* 1999;**19**:2281–5.

Cattaneo M, Mannucci PM. Current status of non-transfusional haemostatic agents: (EHA-4 Educational Book). *Haematologica* 1999;**84**:120–3.

Clemetson KJ, Clemetson JM. Platelet adhesive protein defect disorders. In: Gresele P, Page C, Fuster V, Vermylen J, eds. *Platelets in Thrombotic and Non-Thrombotic Disorders*. Cambridge: Cambridge University Press, 2002.

Murphy S. Platelet storage and transfusion in platelets. In: Gresele P, Page C, Fuster V, Vermylen J, eds. *Platelets in Thrombotic and Non-Thrombotic Disorders*. Cambridge: Cambridge University Press, 2002.

Poon M-C. Factor VIIa. In: Michelson AD, ed. *Platelets*. Orlando, FL: Academic Press, 2003.

Rao AK. Congenital platelet signal transduction defects. In: Gresele P, Page C, Fuster V, Vermylen J, eds. *Platelets in Thrombotic and Non-Thrombotic Disorders*. Cambridge: Cambridge University Press, 2002.

Ruggeri ZM. Structure of von Willebrand factor and its function in platelet adhesion and thrombus formation. *Best Pract Res Clin Haematol* 2001;**14**:257–79.

Chapter 10

Disseminated intravascular coagulation and other microangiopathies

Raj S. Kasthuri and Nigel S. Key

Disseminated intravascular coagulation

Disseminated intravascular coagulation (DIC) is an acquired clinicopathologic syndrome characterized by chaotic activation of the coagulation system, resulting in widespread intravascular deposition of fibrin-rich thrombi. DIC is not itself a disease state, but rather is a secondary manifestation of some other underlying disorder. Depending on the underlying cause and rapidity of the process, the clinical spectrum may range from subclinical laboratory abnormalities to multiorgan failure (MOF), metabolic derangement, hemodynamic instability, widespread bleeding and death.

The following definition of DIC has been proposed by the DIC Scientific and Standardization Committee of the International Society on Thrombosis and Hemostasis (ISTH): "DIC is an acquired syndrome characterized by the intravascular activation of coagulation with loss of localization arising from different causes. It can originate from and cause damage to the microvasculature, which if sufficiently severe, can produce organ dysfunction."

Synonyms for DIC in the medical literature include the defibrination syndrome, consumption coagulopathy, generalized intravascular coagulation, thrombohemorrhagic phenomenon and disseminated intravascular fibrin formation.

Etiology

A broad range of pathological conditions – the most important of which are listed in Table 10.1 – may trigger DIC. Sepsis syndromes are among the most frequently encountered causes. Although the

Table 10.1 Conditions associated with disseminated intravascular coagulation (DIC).

Infection
Sepsis syndromes (Gram-positive and Gram-negative bacteria)
Viral infections (e.g. dengue, Ebola)
Other (e.g. ricketsial, malarial infections)

Trauma/tissue damage
Head injury
Pancreatitis
Fat embolism
Any other serious tissue damage (crush or penetrating injury)

Malignancy
Solid tumors
Acute leukemias (especially AML-M3)
Chronic leukemias (CMML)

Obstetric complications
Abruptio placentae
Amniotic fluid embolism
Eclampsia and pre-eclampsia
Retained dead fetus

Vascular disorders
Giant hemangiomas (Kasabach–Merritt syndrome)
Other vascular malformations
Large aortic aneurysm

Severe allergic/toxic reactions
Toxic shock syndrome
Snake, spider venoms

Severe immunologic reactions
Acute hemolytic transfusion reactions
Heparin-induced thrombocytopenia, type II

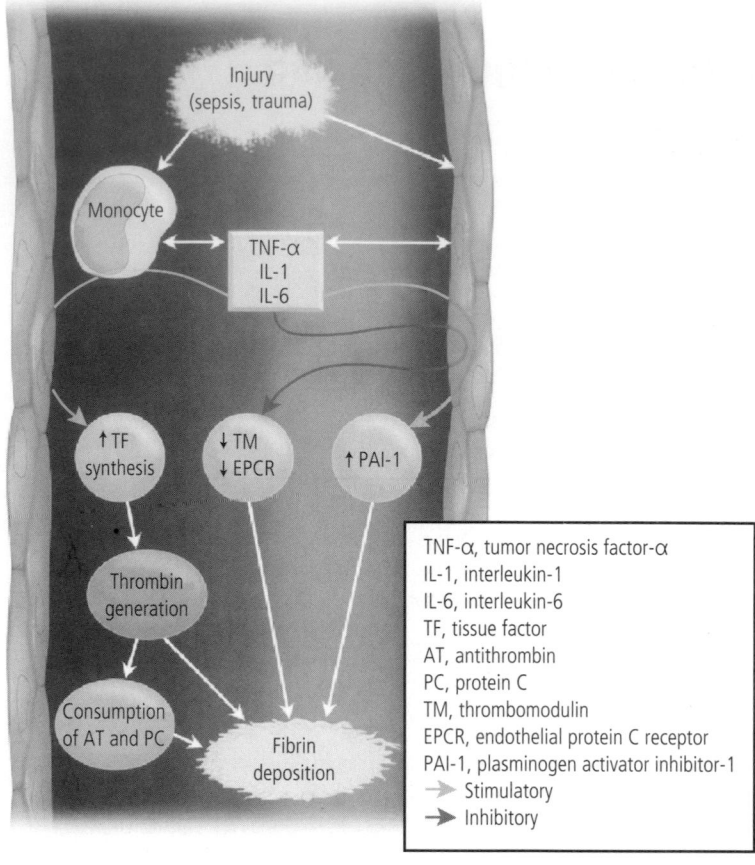

TNF-α, tumor necrosis factor-α
IL-1, interleukin-1
IL-6, interleukin-6
TF, tissue factor
AT, antithrombin
PC, protein C
TM, thrombomodulin
EPCR, endothelial protein C receptor
PAI-1, plasminogen activator inhibitor-1
→ Stimulatory
→ Inhibitory

Figure 10.1 Pathogenesis of disseminated intravascular coagulopathy (DIC).

highest risk is seen with Gram-negative bacterial infections, Gram-positive infections as well as non-bacterial infections can also be associated. Trauma, complications of pregnancy and malignancy are other common causes of DIC in clinical practice.

Pathogenesis

The pathogenesis of DIC involves simultaneous dysregulation of several homeostatic mechanisms. These can be broadly divided into:
- excessive activation of coagulation;
- down-regulation of physiologic anticoagulation pathways; and
- inhibition of fibrinolysis (Fig. 10.1).

Dysfunction of the vascular endothelium, a vast and pervasive organ, is prominent as both a cause and a consequence of these processes. The net result is widespread generation of thrombin and conversion of circulating fibrinogen to insoluble fibrin thrombi, aggravated by the relative inability of the fibrinolytic mechanism to remove intravascular fibrin.

Obstruction of small and medium-sized vessels caused by intravascular fibrin may lead to (multiple) organ dysfunction, especially affecting the kidneys, brain, lung, liver and heart. Obstruction may also lead to simultaneous activation of coagulation with consumption of clotting factors and platelets, aggravated by impaired hepatic production of these factors. Thus, abnormal prolongation of coagulation screening tests, thrombocytopenia and a seemingly paradoxical bleeding tendency may occur in some patients with more advanced forms of DIC.

The passage of erythrocytes through the fibrin meshwork in the microvascular circulation may lead to red cell fragmentation. This microangio-pathic hemolytic anemia (MAHA) is much less common than in the group of disorders known as the "thrombotic microangiopathies," where it is in fact a *sine qua non*.

Activation of coagulation

Although coagulation may be initiated *in vitro* by both the intrinsic (contact) and extrinsic (tissue factor) pathways, only the tissue factor pathway is operative *in vivo*. Unlike most other soluble clotting factors circulating in plasma, tissue factor (TF) is a cell-bound membrane protein. By virtue of its predominant extravascular location, TF is normally present on cells that are relatively inaccessible to blood clotting factors in the absence of vessel injury.

However, the systemic response to infection and injury results in the synthesis and release of pro-inflammatory cytokines such as tumor necrosis factor α (TNF-α), interleukin 1 (IL-1), and IL-6, which may trigger TF synthesis by monocytes and endothelial cells (Fig. 10.1). With other forms of DIC, it is likely that additional stimuli capable of activating and/or propagating coagulation (such as fat, brain lipids, cancer procoagulant protein or amniotic fluid) are released into the circulation.

Decreased physiological anticoagulants

DIC is associated with an acquired deficiency of naturally occurring anticoagulants, particularly antithrombin (III) and protein C. Plasma levels are decreased secondary to consumption and increased enzymatic degradation by activated neutrophils.

Endothelial dysfunction adversely affects the protein C/protein S/thrombomodulin pathway in other ways also. The same pro-inflammatory cytokines that up-regulate TF synthesis simultaneously down-regulate endothelial synthesis of the cofactors thrombomodulin and endothelial cell protein C receptor (EPCR). The end result is decreased conversion of protein C to activated protein C on the endothelial cell surface.

Inhibition of fibrinolytic pathway

The role of the fibrinolytic system is to generate plasmin on fibrin surfaces, in an effort to restore vascular patency via enzymatic digestion of fibrin strands. In many forms of DIC, fibrinolysis is actively suppressed because of elevated levels of plasminogen activator inhibitor type 1 (PAI-1). PAI-1 inhibits the plasminogen activators tissue plasminogen activator and urokinase, preventing the generation of plasmin from plasminogen. Thus, by failing to clear intravascular fibrin thrombi, the inhibition of fibrinolysis by PAI-1 also contributes to the net procoagulant state and end-organ hypoperfusion in DIC.

Clinical manifestations

As predicted from the complex underlying pathophysiological derangements, patients with DIC may suffer simultaneous bleeding and thrombotic manifestations. Clinical features are determined to some extent by the underlying etiology. Thus, while vaso-occlusive manifestations are significantly more prevalent overall, certain subtypes of DIC may be associated with bleeding, usually in the form of microvascular oozing from mucocutaneous surfaces. In obstetric disorders, this may be explained by the hyperacuity of the process leading to rapid consumption of clotting factors and platelets, while in acute promyelocytic leukemia (AML-M3), production of plasminogen activators by leukemic cells may lead to hyperfibrinolytic bleeding.

The most common result of microvascular occlusion is end-organ dysfunction, as for example in sepsis syndromes. This process may lead to renal, cardiac and/or pulmonary failure. Vaso-occlusion may occasionally lead to more clinically overt thrombotic manifestations, such as purpura fulminans in meningococcal or pneumococcal sepsis, which is a clinical syndrome presenting as skin necrosis and digital gangrene (Fig. 10.2). The systemic prothrombotic state may also lead to the development of a localized large vessel arterial or venous thromboembolic event.

It is important to realize that a substantial subset of patients with DIC may suffer only subclinical laboratory abnormalities, with insidious or even absent clinical features.

Diagnosis

The diagnosis of DIC should take into account

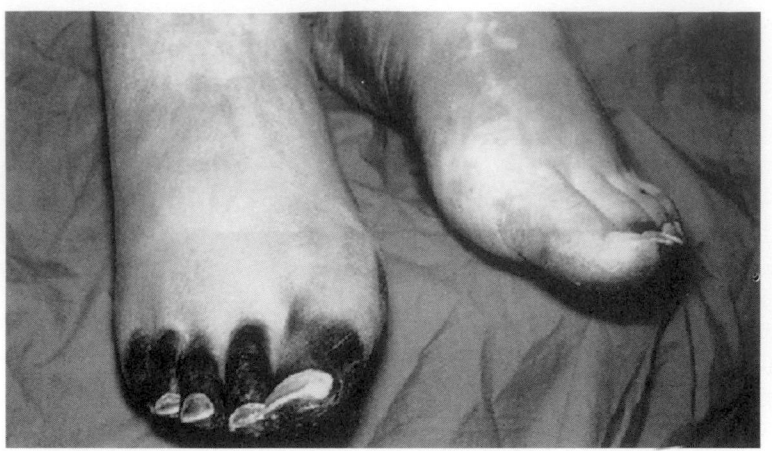

Figure 10.2 Gangrenous feet resulting from pneumococcal infection and DIC. Splenectomy had been performed 11 years earlier. Reprinted from *Blood in Systemic Disease* 1e, Greaves and Makris, 1997, with permission from Elsevier.

both the clinical presentation as well as the laboratory findings. It is important to appreciate that there is no single diagnostic laboratory test for DIC; DIC is always secondary to another underlying pathological condition. A diagnostic scoring algorithm utilizing widely available coagulation tests has been recently proposed (Table 10.2), with a score of 5 or more meeting the definition of "overt" DIC. It should be noted that the term "fibrin-related products" includes:

• Direct assays for the presence of fibrin (e.g. soluble fibrin monomers).
• Indirect assays of fibrin generation (such as D-dimer, fibrin degradation products [FDPs]).

Importantly, the proposed algorithm should be applied only if an underlying disorder known to be associated with DIC (e.g. sepsis, severe trauma) exists. This scoring system is currently undergoing prospective validation by the ISTH subcommittee on DIC.

The design of this scoring system has a pathophysiologic basis, incorporating the concept of "non-overt" (compensated) and "overt" (decompensated) DIC as distinct entities. To some extent, these subsets reflect different points in the continuum, although it is clear that non-overt DIC may be associated with adverse outcomes in critically ill patients independently of progression to overt DIC.

Overt DIC

This may be defined as a state in which the vascular

Table 10.2 Diagnostic scoring system for overt DIC. Do not use this algorithm unless the patient has an underlying disorder that is associated with DIC.

Global coagulation test results	Score (0, 1 or 2 points)
Platelet count	$> 100 \times 10^9/L = 0$ $50 - 100 \times 10^9/L = 1$ $< 50 \times 10^9/L = 2$
Elevated fibrin-related markers (soluble fibrin monomers, D-dimers, fibrin/fibrinogen degradation products)	No increase = 0 Moderate increase = 1 Strong increase = 2
Prolonged prothrombin time (in seconds above upper limit of normal)	$< 3\,s = 0$ $3 - 6\,s = 1$ $> 6\,s = 2$
Fibrinogen level	$> 1.0\,g/L = 0$ $< 1.0\,g/L = 1$
Total score =	

If score ≥ 5, compatible with overt DIC, recommend repeating score daily.
If score < 5, suggestive (not affirmative) for non-overt DIC, repeat scoring in 1–2 days.
Adapted from Taylor FB Jr, Toh CH, Hoots WK, Wada H, Levi M. Towards definition, clinical and laboratory criteria, and a scoring system for disseminated intravascular coagulation. *Thromb Haemost* 2001;**86**:1327–30.

endothelium and blood and its components have lost the ability to compensate and restore homeostasis in response to injury. The result is a progressively decompensating state that is manifest as thrombotic multiorgan dysfunction and/or bleeding.

Table 10.3 Diagnostic scoring system for non-overt DIC. At the present time, although this algorithm with a scoring system has been proposed, interpretations with regards to cut-off scores for diagnosis of non-overt DIC are unclear. At present, trends over time will be more useful than individual single point scores. Adapted from Taylor FB Jr, Toh CH, Hoots WK, Wada H, Levi M. Towards definition, clinical and laboratory criteria, and a scoring system for disseminated intravascular coagulation. *Thromb Haemost* 2001;**86**:1327–30.

Criteria				Score (0, 1 or 2 points)
1 *Risk assessment*				
Is there an underlying disorder that is associated with DIC?				Yes = 2 No = 0
2 *Major criteria*				
Platelet count	$> 100 \times 10^9/L = 0$ $< 100 \times 10^9/L = 1$	+		Rising = −1 Stable = 0 Falling = 1
Prothrombin time (in seconds above upper limit of normal)	$< 3\,s = 0$ $> 3\,s = 1$	+		Falling = −1 Stable = 0 Rising = 1
Soluble fibrin or FDPs	Normal = 0 Raised = 1	+		Falling = −1 Stable = 0 Rising = 1
3 *Specific criteria*				
Antithrombin				Normal = −1 Low = 1
Protein C				Normal = −1 Low = 1
TAT complexes				Normal = −1 High = 1
Total score =				

FDP, fibrin degradation product; TAT, thrombin–antithrombin complex.

Non-overt DIC

This may be defined as a clinical vascular injury state that results in great stress to the hemostatic system, the response to which, for the moment, is sufficient to forestall further rampant inflammatory and hemostatic activation.

The scoring system for the diagnosis of non-overt DIC (Table 10.3) includes, in addition to the above global studies, more specific (but less widely available) tests that are surrogate markers of intravascular thrombin generation (e.g. thrombin–antithrombin (TAT) complexes); indicative of ongoing consumption of coagulation inhibitors (such as antithrombin and protein C levels).

Although perceived as a classic finding, a low plasma fibrinogen level is not a sensitive marker of DIC. In fact, high plasma levels are much more frequently encountered. Fibrinogen levels are probably influenced more by the degree of activation of secondary fibrino(geno)lysis than the degree of consumption during thrombus formation.

Treatment

The development of DIC in patients with sepsis or trauma has been shown to be independently associated with increased morbidity and mortality. Thus, prompt and at times pre-emptive therapy becomes important in these patients.

Managing the underlying disease

The mainstay of treatment in patients with DIC is management of the underlying disease. The reversibility of DIC depends to a large degree on the underlying cause. Delivery of the fetus and placenta may promptly restore homeostasis in patients with obstetric DIC. Eradication of infection with antibiotics and/or surgery may not necessarily have the same rapid effect in sepsis syndromes, possibly because of established widespread endothelial injury.

Supportive care and blood products

Good supportive care in the management of patients with DIC includes adequate hemodynamic support to maintain perfusion and appropriate supportive transfusion of blood products. Given the mechanisms involved in the development of DIC, there is always the theoretical fear of "fueling the fire" with transfused blood cell and plasma products, although the evidence that this occurs in practice is underwhelming. To complicate matters further, there are no consensus guidelines for optimal transfusion management of these patients.

Treatment of patients with DIC who are actively bleeding or at high risk for bleeding should include platelet transfusions, fresh frozen plasma, cryoprecipitate and packed red cells as needed. Patients requiring invasive procedures should be covered peri-procedure with plasma and platelet transfusions as needed. Reasonable transfusion goals in these circumstances are platelet counts $> 50 \times 10^9$/L, fibrinogen > 1.0 g/L, and maintenance of prothrombin time (PT) and activated partial thromboplastin time (APTT) as close to the normal range as possible. There is no role for the prophylactic administration of blood products in patients with DIC. The approach to these patients should be individualized based on their clinical and laboratory manifestations.

Systemic anticoagulation

On the basis of the pathophysiology of DIC, an argument may be made for the use of systemic heparin anticoagulation. While the literature remains divided about this approach, the few available controlled trials have failed to demonstrate a clear benefit. The routine use of heparin in DIC not associated with a clinical thrombotic event is generally discouraged given the demonstrated risk of bleeding complications in these patients. There is some consensus that treatment is indicated for those with a documented thromboembolic event or extensive deposition of fibrin leading to acral ischemia or purpura fulminans. In the case of large vessel thromboembolic events, full therapeutic doses of unfractionated heparin are indicated, whereas in microvascular occlusive syndromes, lower doses (e.g. 500–800 U/h) may be preferable. Low molecular weight heparin has been successfully used as an alternative to unfractionated heparin in some studies. The role of direct thrombin inhibitors (such as hirudin or argatroban) in DIC also remains to be established in controlled trials. Although these agents might theoretically be more effective than heparins, they also carry a higher risk of bleeding.

Antifibrinolytic therapy

Because fibrinolysis is generally down-regulated concomitant with excessive fibrin formation in DIC, treatment with antifibrinolytic agents (such as ε-aminocaproic acid or tranexamic acid) is generally contraindicated. There may be exceptions to the rule, such as patients with acute promyelocytic leukemia who may develop a form of DIC characterized by hyperfibrinolytic bleeding that may result in intracranial hemorrhage. In this instance, prophylactic use of antifibrinolytics has proven effective.

Specific inhibitors of coagulation

In view of the depletion of natural anticoagulants during DIC, it is logical to suppose that replacement therapy using one or more of the missing natural anticoagulants is warranted.

Several preliminary trials with antithrombin, mainly in patients with sepsis, demonstrated some improvement in the duration of DIC and resolution of laboratory abnormalities. However, a significant benefit in mortality could not be demonstrated in a more recent, large, randomized controlled study (the KyberSept Trial). Thus, the merits and risks of antithrombin therapy in patients with DIC remain unclear at this time.

On the other hand, a recent, large, randomized controlled trial (the PROWESS Study) using recombinant activated protein C (Drotrecogin alfa [activated]) to treat patients with sepsis did demonstrate improved survival compared with placebo. This effect was probably mediated not only by an antithrombotic effect, but also by anti-inflammatory and profibrinolytic effects of this agent. However, excess bleeding was seen in patients treated with activated protein C, which inactivates factors Va and VIIIa. Therefore, caution is required in patients with severe thrombocytopenia ($< 30 \times 10^9$/L) or otherwise at high risk of bleeding. The role of activated protein C in the treatment of other forms of DIC has not been adequately evaluated to date.

Thrombotic microangiopathies

The thrombotic microangiopathies are a group of related disorders characterized by widespread microvascular occlusion by platelet-rich aggregates. The accelerated consumption of platelets results in thrombocytopenia. Red cell fragmentation occurs secondary to turbulent blood flow in areas of the microcirculation obstructed by platelet-rich thrombi. Peripheral blood smear examination reveals the presence of fragmented red cells (schistocytes or helmet cells) associated with elevated serum lactate dehydrogenase levels, a condition known as microangiopathic hemolytic anemia (MAHA).

A number of syndromes are included under the rubric of thrombotic microangiopathies (Table 10.4), and a clear distinction between them at the time of presentation may be difficult or impossible. This is especially true of thrombotic thrombocytopenic purpura (TTP) and the hemolytic uremic syndrome (HUS).

The classic clinical pentad in TTP includes:
* thrombocytopenia;
* MAHA;
* renal failure;
* neurologic abnormalities; and
* fever,
but frequently not all features are present.

"Classic" HUS is characterized by:
* MAHA;
* thrombocytopenia; and

Table 10.4 Underlying etiologies of thrombotic microangiopathies.

Thrombotic thrombocytopenic purpura
Familial (ADAMTS-13 deficiency)
Acquired
   Idiopathic
   Drug-related (quinine, ticlopidine)

Hemolytic uremic syndrome
Familial (including factor H deficiency)
Acquired

Secondary thrombotic microangiopathies
Malignancy
Malignant hypertension
Transplantation
   Stem cell transplantation
   Solid organ transplantation
Pregnancy-related
   Pre-eclampsia
   HELLP syndrome
Collagen vascular disease
   Scleroderma renal crisis
   Systemic lupus erythematosus
   Antiphospholipid antibody syndrome

---

* prominent renal failure, following an acute diarrheal illness.

The clinical presentation of many of the secondary thrombotic microangiopathies may also be indistinguishable on initial evaluation. The diagnostic dilemma is further compounded by the urgent requirement for plasma exchange in a subset of these patients (discussed below). Therefore, it is appropriate to utilize the generic diagnosis of "TTP/HUS" in patients presenting with thrombocytopenia and MAHA in the absence of a clinically apparent cause or DIC. Plasma exchange should then be initiated while further evaluation to rule out an alternative diagnosis continues.

Pathophysiology

Although the clinical manifestations of these syndromes show considerable overlap, pathogeneses (where understood) of some of the individual entities may differ considerably.

Thrombotic thrombocytopenic purpura

Unlike the case with DIC, microvascular thrombi are relatively fibrin-poor, but are enriched in von Willebrand factor (VWF) and platelets. Microvascular platelet deposition in TTP is secondary to endothelial secretion of unusually large VWF multimers. Under normal conditions, these unusually large multimers (which are particularly "sticky" for platelets) are prevented from entering the circulation by an enzyme that cleaves VWF.

Predominantly synthesized in the liver, this metalloprotease enzyme is known as ADAMTS-13. A qualitative or quantitative defect of ADAMTS-13 allows the unusually large multimers of VWF to remain anchored to endothelial cells, resulting in widespread platelet adherence, microvascular obstruction and end-organ dysfunction.

Studies have demonstrated that many (but apparently not all) patients with definite TTP have < 5% activity of ADAMTS-13 in their plasma. In the familial form of TTP, affected individuals are usually homozygous or doubly heterozygous for mutations in the gene for ADAMTS-13, located on chromosome 9. In the idiopathic acquired form of TTP, immunoglobulin G (IgG) antibodies against the enzyme may be detectable, suggesting an autoimmune etiology.

More modest reductions in ADAMTS-13 enzyme activity in plasma (5–50%) may be found in liver disease, malignancy, inflammation, pregnancy and in the neonatal period.

Hemolytic uremic syndrome

Microvascular platelet thrombus formation in the classic form of HUS is believed to be toxin-induced. Specifically, prodromal infection of the gastrointestinal tract by verotoxin-producing *Escherichia coli* O157:H7, or certain other serotypes of *E. coli* or *Shigella dysenteriae* is characteristic of this disorder. These toxins, which gain access to blood via the colonic circulation, ultimately target cerebral and glomerular epithelium, mesangial cells and tubular epithelium in the kidneys, and vascular endothelium. In these locations, verotoxins mediate cytokine release, endothelial activation and injury, and direct activation of platelets. The release of platelet adhesogens from damaged endothelium results in microvascular platelet thrombi formation and renal injury.

The small subset of individuals with familial HUS tend to have more severe disease, and a greater risk of recurrence. Some of these patients are deficient in complement factor H which inactivates C3b, a product of the alternate complement pathway. The absence of this regulatory mechanism can lead to autoantibody or immune complex-mediated glomerular injury, with platelet activation, increase in local endothelial procoagulant properties, and ultimately microvascular thrombus formation.

Other thrombotic microangiopathies

Ticlopidine, clopidogrel and (particularly) quinine appear to cause thrombotic microangiopathy through an antibody-mediated mechanism. The pathogenesis of many of the other secondary thrombotic microangiopathies listed in Table 10.4 remains poorly understood.

Differential diagnosis

Faced with a thrombocytopenic patient with MAHA, DIC should be ruled out by review of the history (to rule out an underlying disorder associated with DIC) and by confirmation that screening studies of coagulation such as the PT, APTT and fibrinogen level are normal. The direct antiglobulin (Coombs) test should be negative. Stool cultures are indicated if there has been a preceding diarrheal illness. A careful review of drug exposures, particularly for drugs such as quinine, is essential.

In a pregnant patient – particularly one in the latter stages or in the immediate postpartum period – it may be very difficult to distinguish TTP/HUS (which requires urgent plasma exchange) from preeclampsia with or without the associated HELLP (hemolysis, elevated liver enzymes and low-platelets) syndrome. In general, these syndromes resolve promptly with delivery, whereas TTP/HUS may persist.

The diagnostic utility of a low plasma ADAMTS-13 enzyme activity remains uncertain. The presence of a very low level (< 5%) is probably diagnostic but not necessarily exclusive to TTP, and laboratory demonstration of an inhibitory antibody to the enzyme helps to identify an auto-immune etiology. However, it is also clear that many patients with otherwise clinically indistin-guishable TTP do not have severe ADAMTS-13 deficiency. Therefore, the assay cannot be viewed as the gold standard for diagnosis or for guiding treatment decisions at present.

Clinical manifestations

The distinction between TTP and HUS, when pos-sible, is based on the presence of significant renal failure and preceding history. Thus, in the classic (endemic) form of acquired HUS, which is most common in children less than 5 years of age, a bloody diarrhea resulting from E. coli or S. dysen-teriae is a prodromal hallmark. In the epidemic form of the disease, which may occur after eating infected meat or dairy products, approximately 10–30% of infected individuals develop the full-blown syndrome. The use of antimotility agents after an E. coli infection may increase the risk of HUS. Recurrence of this type of HUS is uncommon.

Patients with familial forms of HUS (the Upshaw–Schulman syndrome) tend to present early in childhood and frequently have a relapsing clinical course that may progress to end-stage renal disease.

Classic TTP occurs much more frequently in adulthood and is associated with neurologic dysfunction, which characteristically manifests as transient focal (e.g. dysphasia) or global (e.g. con-fusion, seizure) symptoms. Neurologic symptoms may be the first sign of relapse in a patient with a previous history of TTP. The risk of recurrence in the idiopathic acquired form of TTP is in the range of 10–30%, with most (but not all) events occur-ring within the first year. Patients with familial forms of TTP may present later in life than those with familial HUS.

The thrombotic microangiopathy related to chemotherapy, cyclosporine, transplantation or total body irradiation tends to occur weeks to months following exposure to these agents.

Treatment

In the era prior to plasma exchange, the mortality rate of TTP approached 100%. Since the institu-tion of plasma exchange, TTP/HUS has become a curable disease. Thus, prompt diagnosis is essen-tial. The diagnostic criteria have therefore become broader and, as already described, all patients with thrombocytopenia and MAHA who do not have another explanation for these findings should be suspected of having TTP/HUS.

Plasma exchange

The most important treatment modality in these patients is plasma exchange, which is superior to plasma infusion. A single plasma volume exchange replacing with fresh frozen or cryosupernatant plasma should be performed daily along with mon-itoring of platelet counts, serum lactate dehydro-genase (LDH) and periodic review of the peripheral smear.

Neurologic symptoms generally resolve rapidly following institution of plasma exchange. Meas-ures of ongoing hemolysis such as the LDH may also improve promptly with therapy, although the anemia may persist and occasionally may require supportive transfusions. The recovery from renal failure may be unpredictable and often slow and incomplete, such that some patients may need prolonged dialysis. The platelet count is the most reliable marker of disease activity on which to base treatment decisions. An improvement reflects reso-lution, whereas worsening of thrombocytopenia at any point in the course of the disease reflects an exacerbation and the need for more aggressive therapy.

In those patients who fail to demonstrate an initial response, more intense therapy such as greater volumes of plasma exchanged once or even twice daily is indicated.

Plasma exchange is most beneficial in patients with TTP/HUS who fall into the "idiopathic acquired," "pregnancy-related," and "drug-related" categories. It is probably ineffective in other forms of thrombotic microangiopathy such as that asso-ciated with stem cell transplantation, which may be more related to the use of cyclosporine A as well as graft-versus-host disease, total body irradiation and cytomegalovirus infection.

In responsive patients, there are no set criteria to guide the optimal duration of treatment. Once the platelet count normalizes, a decision can be made to discontinue plasma exchange. A fall in the platelet count may occur within the first 1–2 weeks, reflecting disease exacerbation, and plasma exchange then needs to be reinstituted. One approach has been to decrease the frequency of plasma exchanges rather than to abruptly discontinue. Ultimately, however, discontinuing plasma exchange is the only way to evaluate if hematological remission has been achieved.

There is still debate as to whether plasma exchange is indicated in patients with postinfectious HUS. The vast majority of disease in young children will resolve with supportive care alone, but plasmapheresis is probably indicated and useful in affected adults.

Immunosuppression

In many centers, glucocorticoids are used as an adjunct to initial plasma exchange, but there are few data to support this practice. Certainly, it is reasonable to consider glucocorticoids in patients who are refractory to plasma exchange. Other immunosuppressive modalities such as vincristine, cyclophosphamide or rituximab, the monoclonal antibody against CD20, have all also been reported to be of value in refractory cases.

Other treatments

In patients with multiple relapses, splenectomy during hematologic remission is a possible option.

In the context of ADAMTS-13 deficiency, episodes of familial TTP have been reversed or prevented by the infusion of fresh frozen or cryosupernatant plasma. These products contain the metalloprotease enzyme and in this subset of congenitally deficient patients plasmapheresis can therefore be avoided.

Patients with TTP/HUS rarely experience bleeding, despite sometimes very significant thrombocytopenia. Routine prophylactic platelet transfusion is contraindicated, because of fears that it may precipitate further vaso-occlusive phenomena. However, it is occasionally necessary to administer platelets to a patient with one of these syndromes who is actively bleeding.

The use of antimicrobial agents in HUS increases the release of Shiga toxin from the organism and could paradoxically increase the risk of HUS.

The sequence of the ADAMTS-13 metalloprotease has now been determined and gene therapy for treatment of patients with familial forms of the disease may become a reality in the future.

Further reading

Bernard GR, Vincent JL, Laterre PF, et al. Efficacy and safety of recombinant human activated protein C for severe sepsis. N Engl J Med 2001;344:699–708.

Dhainault JF, Yan SB, Margolis BD, et al. Drotrecogin alfa (activated) (recombinant human activated protein C) reduces host coagulopathy response in patients with severe sepsis. Thromb Haemost 2003;90:642–53.

George JN. How I treat patients with thrombotic thrombocytopenic purpura–hemolytic uremic syndrome. Blood 2000;6:1223–9.

George JN, Vesely SK, Terrell DR. The Oklahoma thrombotic thrombocytopenic purpura–hemolytic uremic syndrome (TTP/HUS) registry: a community perspective of patients with clinically diagnosed TTP–HUS. Semin Hematol 2004;41:60–7.

Hoots WK. Non-overt disseminated intravascular coagulation: definition and pathophysiological implications. Blood Rev 2002;16(Suppl 1):S3–9.

Levi M, Ten Cate H. Disseminated intravascular coagulation. N Engl J Med 1999;341:586–92.

Okajima K, Sakamoto Y, Uchiba M. Heterogeneity in the incidence and clinical manifestations of disseminated intravascular coagulation: a study of 204 cases. Am J Hematol 2000;65:215–22.

Rock GA, Shumak KH, Buskard NA, et al. Comparison of plasma exchange with plasma infusion in the treatment of thrombotic thrombocytopenic purpura. N Engl J Med 1991;325:393–7.

Taylor FB Jr, Toh CH, Hoots WK, Wada H, Levi M. Towards definition, clinical and laboratory criteria, and a scoring system for disseminated intravascular coagulation. Thromb Haemost 2001;86:1327–30.

Vesely SK, George JN, Lammle B, et al. ADAMTS13 activity in thrombotic thrombocytopenic purpura–hemolytic uremic syndrome: relation to presenting features and clinical outcomes in a prospective cohort of 142 patients. Blood 2003;102:60–8.

Chapter 11
Venous thromboembolism

Lori-Ann Linkins and Clive Kearon

Introduction

Venous thromboembolism (VTE), which includes deep vein thrombosis (DVT) and pulmonary embolism (PE), is a leading cause of morbidity and mortality. This chapter reviews the pathogenesis, prevalence and natural history of VTE as well as providing an overview of the management of VTE. The management of VTE will be discussed in three subsections: diagnosis, treatment and prevention. Venous thromboembolism in pregnancy is addressed as a special category within each section, and in more detail in Chapter 15.

Pathogenesis of venous thromboembolism

Virchow was the first to identify stasis, vessel wall injury and hypercoagulability as the pathogenic triad responsible for thrombosis. This classification of risk factors for VTE remains valuable. A summary of risk factors for VTE is given in Table 11.1.

Venous stasis

The importance of venous stasis as a risk factor for VTE is demonstrated by the fact that most deep vein thrombi associated with stroke affect the paralyzed leg, and most DVT associated with pregnancy affect the left leg, the iliac veins of which are prone to extrinsic compression by the pregnant uterus and the right common iliac artery.

Vessel damage

Venous endothelial damage, as a consequence of accidental injury, manipulation during surgery

Table 11.1 Risk factors for venous thromboembolism (VTE).

Patient factors
Previous VTE*
Age over 40 years
Pregnancy, puerperium
Obesity
Inherited hypercoagulable state

Underlying condition and acquired factors
Malignancy*
Estrogen therapy
Cancer chemotherapy
Paralysis*
Prolonged immobility
Major trauma*
Lower limb injuries*
Heparin-induced thrombocytopenia
Antiphospholipid antibodies
Lower limb orthopedic surgery*
Surgery requiring general anaesthesia > 30 min

Combinations of factors have at least an additive effect on the risk of VTE.
* Common major risk factors for VTE.

(e.g. hip replacement) or iatrogenic injury, is an important risk factor for VTE. Hence, three-quarters of proximal DVTs that complicate hip surgery occur in the operated leg and thrombosis is common with indwelling venous catheters.

Hypercoagulability

A complex balance of naturally occurring coagulation and fibrinolytic factors, and their inhibitors, serve to maintain blood fluidity and hemostasis. Inherited or acquired changes in this balance predispose to thrombosis.

Inherited predisposition to VTE

The most important inherited biochemical disorders that are associated with VTE result from:
• defects in the naturally occurring inhibitors of coagulation: deficiencies of antithrombin, protein C or protein S; and
• resistance to activated protein C caused by factor V Leiden.

The first three of these disorders are rare in the general population (combined prevalence of < 1%), have a combined prevalence of approximately 5% in patients with a first episode of VTE, and are associated with a 10- to 40-fold increase in the risk of VTE. The factor V Leiden mutation is common, occurring in approximately 5% of white people and approximately 20% of patients with a first episode of VTE (i.e. an approximate fourfold increase in VTE risk).

Elevated levels of a number of coagulation factors (I, II, VIII, IX, XI) are associated with thrombosis in a "dose-dependent" manner. It is probable that such elevations are often inherited, with strong evidence for this with factor VIII.

A mutation in the 3′ untranslated region of the prothrombin gene (G20210A), which is associated with an approximately 25% increase in prothrombin levels, occurs in approximately 2% of white people and approximately 5% of those with a first episode of VTE (i.e. an approximate 2.5-fold increase in risk).

Abnormalities of the fibrinolytic system have questionable importance as risk factors for VTE.

Acquired predisposition to VTE

Acquired hypercoagulable states include estrogen therapy, antiphospholipid antibodies (anticardiolipin antibodies and/or lupus anticoagulants), systemic lupus erythematosus, malignancy, combination chemotherapy and surgery. Patients who develop heparin-induced thrombocytopenia also have a very high risk of developing arterial and venous thromboembolism.

Hyperhomocysteinemia, caused by hereditary and acquired factors, is also a risk factor for VTE.

Table 11.2 Natural history of venous thromboembolism (VTE). (Adapted from Kearon C. Diagnosis of pulmonary embolism. *CMAJ* 2003;**168**:183–94.)

- VTE usually starts in the calf veins
- Over 80% of symptomatic DVTs are proximal
- Two-thirds of asymptomatic DVT detected postoperatively by screening venography are confined to the distal (calf) veins
- Approximately 20% of symptomatic isolated calf DVTs subsequently extend to the proximal veins, usually within a week of presentation
- PE usually arises from proximal DVT
- The majority (approximately 70%) of patients with symptomatic proximal DVT have asymptomatic PE (high probability lung scans in approximately 40%), and vice versa
- Only one-quarter of patients with symptomatic PE have symptoms or signs of DVT
- Approximately 50% of untreated symptomatic proximal DVTs are expected to cause symptomatic PE
- Approximately 10% of symptomatic PE are rapidly fatal
- Approximately 30% of untreated symptomatic non-fatal PE will have a fatal recurrence

DVT, deep vein thrombosis; PE, pulmonary embolism.

Prevalence and natural history of venous thromboembolism

VTE is rare before the age of 16 years, likely because the immature coagulation system is resistant to thrombosis. However, the risk of VTE increases exponentially with advancing age (i.e., 1.9-fold per decade), rising from an annual incidence of approximately 30 in 100,000 at 40 years, to 90 in 100,000 at 60 years and 260 in 100,000 at 80 years. Clinically important components of the natural history of VTE are summarized in Table 11.2.

Management of venous thromboembolism

Diagnosis of venous thromboembolism

Objective testing for DVT and PE is essential because clinical assessment alone is unreliable. Failure to diagnose VTE is associated with a high mortality, while inappropriate anticoagulation can lead to serious complications, including fatal hemorrhage.

Diagnosis of deep vein thrombosis

The clinical features of DVT include localized swelling, redness, tenderness and distal edema. However, these features are non-specific and approximately 75% of ambulatory patients with suspected DVT will have another cause for their symptoms. The differential diagnosis for DVT includes:

- cellulitis;
- ruptured Baker cyst;
- muscle tear, muscle cramps, muscle hematoma;
- external venous compression;
- superficial thrombophlebitis; and
- post-thrombotic syndrome (see Plate 5, facing p. 120).

Of the patients who actually have venous thrombosis, approximately 85% have proximal vein thrombosis, while in the remainder thrombosis is confined to the calf.

Objective tests

Venography

This the gold standard for the diagnosis of DVT. Venography has advantages over other tests as it is capable of detecting both proximal vein thrombosis and isolated calf vein thrombosis. However, the disadvantages are that it:

- is invasive, expensive and requires technical expertise;
- exposes patients to the risks associated with contrast media, including the potential for an allergic reaction or renal impairment.

For these reasons, non-invasive tests such as venous ultrasonography and D-dimer testing, alone or in combination with clinical assessment, have largely replaced venography.

A summary of the test results that effectively confirm or exclude deep vein thrombosis are given in Table 11.3.

Although *clinical assessment* cannot unequivocally confirm or exclude DVT, clinical evaluation using empiric assessment or a structured clinical model (Table 11.4) can stratify patients as having a:

- *Low probability of DVT:* with a prevalence of DVT of approximately < 10%.

Table 11.3 Test results that confirm or exclude deep vein thromboisis (DVT). (Adapted from Kearon C *et al.* 1998.)

Diagnostic for first DVT

Venography: Intraluminal filling defect

Venous ultrasound: Non-compressible proximal veins at two or more of the common femoral, popliteal and calf trifurcation sites

Excludes first DVT

Venography: All deep veins seen, and no intraluminal filling defects

D-dimer: Normal test which has a very high sensitivity (i.e. ≥ 98%) and at least a moderate specificity (i.e. ≥ 40%)

Venous ultrasound: Normal

and

(a) Low clinical suspicion for DVT at presentation

or

(b) Normal D-dimer test which has a moderately high sensitivity (i.e. > 85%) and specificity (i.e. ≥ 70%) at presentation

or

(c) Normal serial testing (at 7 days)

Low clinical suspicion for DVT at presentation *and* a normal D-dimer test that has a moderately high sensitivity (i.e. ≥ 85%) and specificity (i.e. ≥ 70%) at presentation

Diagnostic for recurrent DVT

Venography: Intraluminal filling defect

Venous ultrasound:

(a) A new non-compressible common femoral or popliteal vein segment

or

(b) An approximate 4.0 mm increase in diameter of the common femoral or popliteal vein compared to a previous test

Excludes recurrent DVT

Venogram: All deep veins seen and no intraluminal filling defects

Venous ultrasound: Normal or ≤ 1 mm increase in diameter of the common femoral or popliteal veins on venous ultrasound compared to a previous test, *and* remains normal (no progression of venous ultrasound) at 2 and 7 days

D-dimer: Normal test which has a very high sensitivity (i.e. ≥ 98%) and at least a moderate specificity (i.e. ≥ 40%)

- *Moderate probability of DVT:* with a prevalence of DVT of approximately 25%.
- *High probability of DVT:* with a prevalence of DVT of approximately 60%.

Such categorization is useful in guiding the performance and interpretation of objective testing.

Venous Doppler ultrasonography

This is the non-invasive method of choice for diagnosing venous thrombosis. The common femoral

Variables	Points
Active cancer (treatment ongoing or within previous 6 months or palliative)	1
Paralysis, paresis or recent plaster immobilization of the lower extremities	1
Bedridden > 3 days or major surgery within 4 weeks	1
Localized tenderness along the distribution of the deep venous system	1
Entire leg swollen	1
Calf swelling 3 cm > asymptomatic side (measured 10 cm below tibial tuberosity)	1
Pitting edema confined to the symptomatic leg	1
Dilated superficial veins (non-varicose)	1
Alternative diagnosis as likely or more likely than DVT	−2

Total points

Pretest probability calculated as follows:

	Total points
High	> 2
Moderate	1 or 2
Low	< 1

Table 11.4 Model for determining clinical suspicion of deep vein thrombosis (DVT). (From Wells PS, Hirsh J, Anderson DR, *et al.* A simple clinical model for the diagnosis of deep-vein thrombosis combined with impedance plethysmography: potential for an improvement in the diagnosis process. *J Intern Med* 1998;**243**:15–23.)

Note: In patients with symptoms in both legs, the more symptomatic leg is used.

vein, superficial femoral vein, popliteal vein and proximal deep calf veins are imaged in real time and compressed with the transducer probe. Inability to compress the vein fully is diagnostic of venous thrombosis.

Venous ultrasonography is highly accurate for the detection of proximal vein thrombosis with a sensitivity of approximately 97%, specificity of approximately 94% and negative predictive value of approximately 98% in symptomatic patients. Venous ultrasonography is much more difficult to perform and less accurate in the calf (e.g. sensitivity of approximately 70%). For these reasons, and because isolated calf DVT is both uncommon and of limited importance, ultrasonography of the calf veins is often not performed.

If DVT cannot be excluded by a normal proximal venous ultrasound in combination with other results (e.g. low clinical probability or normal D-dimer), a follow-up ultrasound is performed after 1 week to check for extending calf vein thrombosis (approximately 2% of patients). If the second ultrasound is normal, the risk of symptomatic VTE during the next 6 months is less than 2%.

The accuracy of venous ultrasonography is substantially lower if its findings are discordant with the clinical assessment and/or if abnormalities are confined to short segments of the deep veins. These patients should have a venogram because the result of the venogram will differ from the venous ultrasound in approximately 25% of these cases.

D-*dimer analysis of blood*

This measures cross-linked fibrin broken down by plasmin. D-dimer levels are usually elevated with DVT and/or PE. Normal levels can help to exclude VTE, but elevated D-dimer levels are non-specific and have low positive predictive value.

D-dimer assays differ markedly in their diagnostic properties for VTE. A normal result with a very sensitive D-dimer assay (i.e. sensitivity of approximately 98%) excludes VTE on its own, i.e. it has a high negative predictive value (NPV). However, very sensitive D-dimer tests have low specificity (approximately 40%), which limits their utility because of high false-positive rates. In order to exclude DVT and/or PE, a normal result with a less sensitive D-dimer assay (i.e. approximately 85%) needs to be *combined* with either a low clinical probability or another objective test that has a high NPV, but is non-diagnostic on its own (Table 11.3). As less sensitive D-dimer assays are more specific (approximately 70%), they yield fewer false-positive results.

Specificity of D-dimer decreases with aging and with comorbid illness such as cancer. Consequently, D-dimer testing may have limited value as a diagnostic test for VTE in hospitalized patients (more false-positive results) and is unhelpful in the early postoperative period.

Magnetic resonance imaging

A recent small, but rigorous, study suggests that magnetic resonance direct thrombus imaging (MRI) is very accurate for the diagnosis of DVT, including thrombosis in the calf and pelvis, and in asymptomatic or pregnant patients. The technique does not require radiographic contrast and has the potential to differentiate acute from old thrombus.

Diagnosis of recurrent deep vein thrombosis

Persistent abnormalities of the deep veins on ultrasound examination are common following DVT. Therefore, diagnosis of recurrent DVT requires evidence of new clot formation. Tests that can diagnose or exclude recurrent DVT are noted in Table 11.3.

Diagnosis of deep vein thrombosis in pregnancy

Pregnant patients with suspected DVT can generally be managed in the *same way as non-pregnant patients* although, with the exception of serial impedance plethysmography, diagnostic approaches have not been evaluated in this population. Pregnant patients with normal non-invasive tests who have a high clinical suspicion of isolated iliac or calf DVT should be considered for venography (a complete study, or a limited study using abdominal shielding, respectively). Alternatively, normal MRI, a normal D-dimer or normal Doppler ultrasound imaging of the iliac veins are likely to be helpful for excluding DVT.

Diagnosis of pulmonary embolism (see Plate 6, facing p. 120)

The clinical features of PE include:
- pleuritic chest pain;
- shortness of breath;
- syncope;
- hemoptysis; and
- palpitations.

As with DVT, these features are non-specific and objective testing must be performed to confirm or exclude the diagnosis of PE.

Pulmonary angiography

This is the gold standard for the diagnosis of PE (Fig. 11.1). However, it has many of the same limitations as venography. A summary of tests that confirm or exclude PE is given in Table 11.5.

Ventilation–perfusion lung scan

This has been the usual initial investigation in patients with suspected PE. A normal perfusion scan excludes PE, but is only found in a minority of patients (10–40%). Perfusion defects are non-specific; only approximately one-third of patients with perfusion defects have PE. The probability that a perfusion defect is caused by PE increases with size and number, and the presence of a normal ventilation scan ("mismatched" defect). A lung scan with mismatched segmental or larger perfusion defects is termed "high-probability." A single mismatched defect is associated with a prevalence

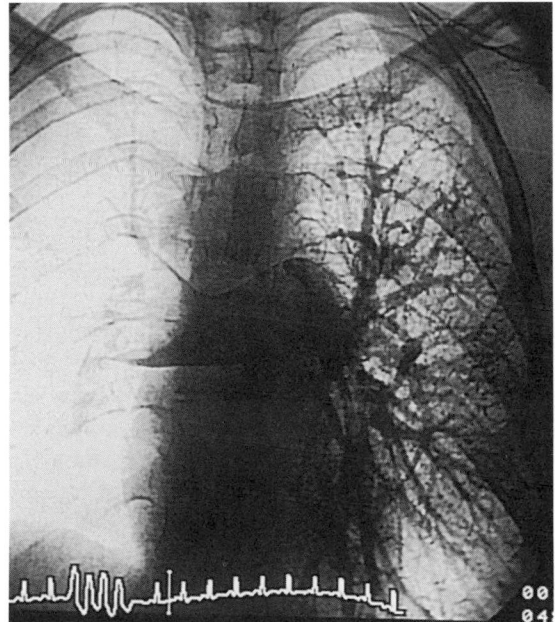

Figure 11.1 Pulmonary angiogram showing massive pulmonary embolism in the right pulmonary artery.

Diagnostic for PE

Pulmonary angiography: Intraluminal filling defect

Helical CT: Intraluminal filling defect in a lobar or main pulmonary artery

Segmental intraluminal filling defect and moderate or high clinical suspicion

Ventilation–perfusion scan: High probability scan and moderate/high clinical suspicion

Diagnostic test positive for DVT: With non-diagnostic ventilation–perfusion scan or helical CT

Excludes PE

Pulmonary angiography: Normal

Ventilation–perfusion scan: Normal

D-dimer: Normal test which has a very high sensitivity (i.e. approximately 98%) and at least a moderate specificity (i.e. approximately 40%)

Helical CT: Normal test *and* normal bilateral leg venous ultrasounds in patients with low or moderate probability for PE

Non-diagnostic ventilation–perfusion scan *and* normal proximal venous ultrasound *and*

(a) Low clinical suspicion for PE

(b) Normal D-dimer test which has at least a moderately high sensitivity (i.e. approximately 85%) and specificity (i.e. approximately 70%)

Low clinical suspicion for PE *and* normal D-dimer, which has at least a moderately high sensitivity (i.e. approximately 85%) and specificity (i.e. approximately 70%)

Table 11.5 Test results which confirm or exclude pulmonary embolism (PE). (Adapted from Kearon C. Diagnosis of pulmonary embolism. *CMAJ* 2003;168:183–94.)

CT, computerized tomography.

of PE of approximately 80%. Three or more mismatched defects are associated with a prevalence of PE of approximtaely 90%. Lung scan findings are highly age-dependent, with a relatively high proportion of normal scans and a low proportion of non-diagnostic scans in younger patients. A high frequency of normal lung scans are also seen in pregnant patients who are investigated for PE.

As with suspected DVT, clinical assessment is useful at categorizing probability of PE (Table 11.6).

Lung scanning combined with clinical assessment
This significantly improves the predictive value. A moderate or high clinical suspicion in a patient with a high probability lung scan is diagnostic (prevalence of PE of approximately 90%); however, a low clinical suspicion with a high probability defect requires further investigation because the prevalence of PE with these findings is only approximately 50%. The prevalence of PE with subsegmental, matched, perfusion defects (low probability scan) and a low clinical suspicion is expected to be less than 10%.

As previously discussed when considering the diagnosis of DVT, a normal D-*dimer result*, alone or in combination with another negative test, can be used to exclude PE (Table 11.5).

Helical (spiral) computerized tomography
Following intravenous injection of radiographic contrast, computerized tomography (CT) can be used to visualize the pulmonary arteries. The main advantage of helical CT over ventilation–perfusion scanning is that fewer examinations are technically inadequate or "non-diagnostic" (i.e. approximately 10% vs. 60%). Helical CT can also identify an alternative diagnosis that may influence clinical management in approximately 25% of patients.

The major disadvantage is that, unlike ventilation–perfusion scanning, a negative result does not exclude PE. Two recent management studies have concluded that a negative helical CT together with negative ultrasound examinations of the proximal deep veins excludes PE in patients with a low or moderate clinical probability. Because PE was found in 5% of the patients who had a high clinical probability (despite negative CT and negative ultrasounds), further testing should be performed in these patients.

Table 11.6 Model for determining clinical suspicion of pulmonary embolism. (From Wells PS, Anderson DR, Rodger M, *et al.* Derivation of a simple clinical model to categorize patients probability of pulmonary embolism: increasing the models utility with the SimpliRED D-dimer. *Thromb Haemost* 2000;83:416–20.)

Variables	Points
Clinical signs and symptoms of deep vein thrombosis (minimum leg swelling and pain with palpation of the deep veins)	3.0
Pulmonary embolism is the most likely diagnosis	3.0
Heart rate > 100 b/min	1.5
Immobilization or surgery in the previous 4 weeks	1.5
Previous deep vein thrombosis/pulmonary embolism	1.5
Hemoptysis	1.0
Malignancy (treatment ongoing or within previous 6 months or palliative)	1.0

Total points

Pretest probability calculated as follows:

	Total points
High	> 6
Moderate	2–6
Low	< 2

Testing for deep vein thrombosis is an indirect way to diagnose pulmonary embolism

Venous ultrasonography of the proximal veins is the usual method, although bilateral ascending venography, or CT or MRI of the legs at the same time as examination of the pulmonary veins, can also be used. Negative tests for DVT do not rule out PE, but they reduce the probability, and suggest that the short-term risk of recurrent PE is low.

Patients with non-diagnostic combinations of non-invasive tests for pulmonary embolism

Patients with non-diagnostic test results for PE at presentation have, on average, a prevalence of PE of approximately 20%.

First management approach

The performance of pulmonary angiography is recommended in those:
- with a high probability ventilation-perfusion scan and low clinical suspicion (consider helical CT scan first, if not already done);
- with subsegmental intraluminal filling defects on helical CT and high clinical suspicion (consider ventilation-perfusion scan first, if not already done);
- with severe symptoms and high post-test probability, but tests are inconclusive;

- with high clinical suspicion, inconclusive helical CT, and serial testing not feasible (e.g. scheduled for surgery, geographic inaccessibility).

Second management approach

While withholding anticoagulants, serial venous ultrasounds are performed to detect evolving proximal DVT, the forerunner of recurrent PE. If serial venous ultrasound for DVT (two additional tests a week apart) is negative, the subsequent risk of confirmed VTE during the next 3 months is less than 1%, which is similar to that after a normal pulmonary angiogram.

As an additional precaution, patients who have had PE and/or DVT excluded should routinely be asked to return for re-evaluation if symptoms of PE and/or DVT persist or recur. A diagnostic algorithm for PE is given in Fig. 11.2.

Diagnosis of pulmonary embolism in pregnancy

Pregnant patients with suspected PE can be managed similarly to non-pregnant patients, with the following modifications:
- Venous ultrasound of the legs can be performed first and lung scanning performed if there is no DVT.
- Patients with unequivocal evidence of DVT can be presumed to have PE.

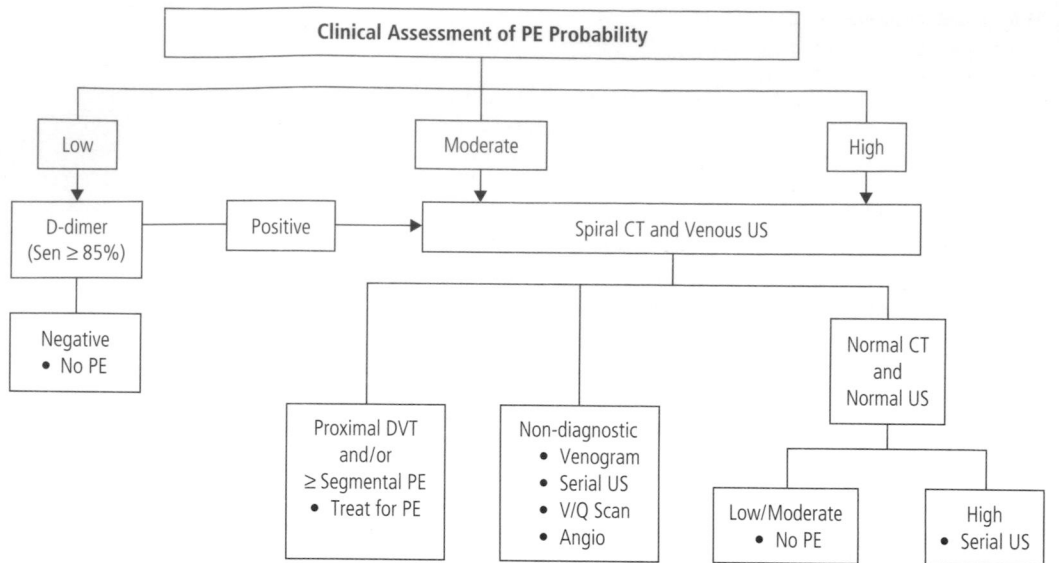

Figure 11.2 Diagnostic algorithm for pulmonary embolism (PE). Choice of additional diagnostic testing depends on clinical presentation and local expertise. CT, computerized tomography; US, ultrasound; V/Q, ventilation–perfusion; angio, pulmonary angiography.

• The amount of radioisotope used for the perfusion scan can be reduced and the duration of scanning extended.

• If pulmonary angiography is performed, the brachial approach with abdominal screening is preferable.

• The use of helical CT in pregnancy is discouraged because of the absence of safety data (if it is necessary, abdominal screening should be used).

These recommendations are based on a belief that the risk of inaccurate diagnosis of suspected PE during pregnancy is greater than the risk of radioactivity to the fetus.

Treatment of venous thromboembolism

Initiation of anticoagulant therapy with heparin

Heparin is a highly sulfated glycosoaminoglycan that produces its anticoagulant effect by binding to antithrombin, markedly accelerating the ability of this naturally occurring anticoagulant to inactivate thrombin, activated factor X (factor Xa) and activated factor IX (factor IXa). At therapeutic concentrations, heparin has a half-life of approximately 60 min. Heparin binds to a number of plasma proteins, a phenomenon that reduces its anticoagulant effect by limiting its accessibility to antithrombin. The concentration of heparin-binding proteins increases during illness, which contributes to the variability in anticoagulant response in patients with thromboembolism. Because of this variability, response to heparin should be monitored with the activated partial thromboplastin time (APTT).

Many trials have established that weight-adjusted low molecular weight heparin (LMWH) is as safe and effective as adjusted-dose unfractionated heparin for the treatment of acute VTE. LMWHs are derived from standard, commercial grade heparin by chemical depolymerization to yield fragments approximately one-third the size of heparin. Depolymerization of heparin results in less binding to heparin-binding proteins and, consequently, improved bioavailability. LMWH therefore has a more predictable anticoagulant response than heparin, which reduces the need for laboratory monitoring. Additional advantages of LMWH are that it can be used to treat patients without hospital admission and need only be injected subcutaneously once daily.

Other potential side-effects of heparin include heparin-induced thrombocytopenia and osteoporosis. These complications occur less frequently in patients receiving LMWH. Patients with heparin-induced thrombocytopenia, with or without associated thrombosis, can be treated with danaparoid, hirudin or argatroban.

Current clinical practice is to treat patients with acute VTE for a minimum of 5 days with heparin in a regimen of at least 30,000 IU/day or 18 IU/kg/h by intravenous infusion (or 33,000 IU/day, by twice daily subcutaneous injection) adjusted to achieve an APTT ratio of 1.5 to 2.5 or with LMWH (at a weight-adjusted dose of either approximately 100 IU/kg every 12 h or approximately 150–200 IU/kg once daily) followed by a course of oral anticoagulant therapy.

Long-term therapy with oral anticoagulants

Vitamin K antagonists (e.g. warfarin) are coumarin compounds that produce their anticoagulant effect through the production of hemostatically defective, vitamin K-dependent coagulant proteins (prothrombin, factor VII, factor IX and factor X). The dose of warfarin must be monitored closely because the anticoagulant response is influenced by multiple over-the-counter and prescription drugs, changes in diet and age of the patient. The international normalized ratio (INR) replaced the prothrombin time (PT) for monitoring oral anticoagulant therapy in the 1970s because, unlike the PT, the INR takes into account differences in the responsiveness of thromboplastins to oral anticoagulants. The target INR for treatment of acute VTE is 2.0–3.0. Nomograms for initiating warfarin are available.

Oral anticoagulants are typically started on day 1 or 2 of treatment of acute VTE and continued for a length of time determined on an individual basis (discussed below). Prolonged high-dose subcutaneous heparin and, subsequently, LMWH (50–75% of acute treatment dose) have also been shown to be effective in treating VTE in the long term.

Duration of anticoagulant therapy

The optimal duration of anticoagulant therapy is determined by both patient- and disease-related factors.

Major transient risk factors

These include VTE that occurs within 3 months of surgery with general anesthesia, plaster cast immobilization of a leg or with hospitalization. The risk of recurrence after stopping anticoagulant therapy is low, approximately 3% in the first year. Three months of anticoagulant therapy is considered adequate.

Minor transient risk factors

These include VTE that occurs within 6 weeks of estrogen therapy, prolonged travel (i.e. > 10 h), pregnancy or less marked leg injuries or immobilization. The risk of recurrence after stopping anticoagulant therapy is expected to be higher than in those patients with a major transient risk factor, but lower than those patients with an unprovoked VTE (e.g. approximately 5% in the first year). Three to 6 months of anticoagulant therapy is considered adequate; the authors' preference is for 6 months.

Unprovoked VTE

The risk of recurrent VTE, after 6 months or more of treatment, when anticoagulant therapy is stopped following an unprovoked VTE is approximately 10% in the first year, and approximately 30% after 5 years. Given the persistent risk of recurrence, and the greater than 90% risk reduction with oral anticoagulants targeted at an INR of approximately 2.5, long-term anticoagulation is the preferred option for patients who have a low risk of bleeding. The rationale for long-term anticoagulation is even stronger for patients with unprovoked PE. As patients with isolated calf DVT have half the risk of recurrence of those with proximal DVT, 6 months of anticoagulant therapy is considered adequate.

Uncontrolled malignancy

Malignancy is associated with a higher than 10%/patient year risk of recurrent VTE after stopping anticoagulant therapy. Those patients at highest risk of recurrence (e.g. patients with progressive or metastatic disease, poor mobility or on-going chemotherapy) should be considered for indefinite anticoagulant therapy. Although vitamin K antagonists can be used, LMWH appears to be the preferred anticoagulant in patients with malignancy, as a recently published study demonstrated that such patients have half the frequency of recurrence if they are treated with LMWH for 6 months instead of oral anticoagulants.

Hypercoagulable states

Patients who have certain hypercoaguable states (anticardiolipin antibodies and/or lupus anticoagulants, homozygous factor V Leiden and likely antithrombin deficiency) have a higher risk of recurrence and may be considered for long-term anticoagulant therapy. Patients heterozygous for factor V Leiden or the G20210A prothrombin gene mutation do not appear to be at increased risk for recurrence.

The implications for duration of treatment of other abnormalities such as elevated levels of clotting factors VIII, IX, XI and homocysteine, and deficiencies of protein C and protein S, are uncertain.

Pulmonary embolism versus deep vein thrombosis

Patients who present with PE appear to have the same risk of recurrent VTE as those who present with proximal DVT. However, patients who initially present with a symptomatic PE are three times more likely to have a PE as their recurrent VTE event (approximately 60%) than patients who initially present with a symptomatic DVT (approximately 20%). Consequently, the case fatality of recurrent VTE in patients who initially presented with a PE is expected to be twofold higher (approximately 10%) after a PE than after an initial DVT (approximately 5%).

A recent clinical trial suggests that patients who present with an unprovoked PE should be considered for long-term anticoagulant therapy. A second episode of VTE does not necessarily indicate a high risk of recurrence or the need for indefinite anticoagulation.

Other potential indicators for increased risk of recurrent VTE

Presence of residual DVT on ultrasound or an elevated D-dimer level after stopping anticoagulant therapy may be associated with an increased risk of recurrent VTE, but it is uncertain if these assessments should influence the duration of therapy.

Risk of bleeding on anticoagulant therapy

The risk of bleeding on anticoagulants differs markedly among patients, depending on the prevalence of risk factors (e.g. advanced age, previous bleeding or stroke, renal failure, anemia, antiplatelet therapy, malignancy, poor anticoagulant control).

A recent meta-analysis in patients who were considered average risk for bleeding and received oral anticoagulant therapy for VTE for 3 months (INR of 2.0–3.0), demonstrated a case fatality of major bleeding of 13.4%. For patients who received anticoagulant therapy for more than 3 months, the case fatality of major bleeding was 9.1%. Therefore the case fatality with an episode of major bleeding appears to be similar to the case fatality of recurrent VTE after an initial PE, and twice that of a recurrence after an initial DVT. Consequently, for a patient to be considered for long-term anticoagulant therapy after a DVT, the patient's estimated risk of recurrence off anticoagulant therapy needs to be greater than the risk of major bleeding on anticoagulant therapy.

New anticoagulants

A variety of new anticoagulants for the prevention and treatment of venous and arterial thromboembolism are under development. Two of these new agents, fondaparinux and ximelagatran, are in advanced stages of clinical testing for treatment of VTE.

Fondaparinux

Fondaparniux is a synthetic analog of the antithrombin-binding pentasaccharide sequence found in heparin and low molecular weight heparin. It produces its anticoagulant effect by binding to antithrombin and enhancing antithrombin's reactivity with factor Xa. It has no direct activity against thrombin. Fondaparinux has excellent bioavailability (100%) after subcutaneous injection and a plasma half-life of approximately 15 h. It is administered subcutaneously once daily. This agent has been shown to be as effective as LMWH in the treatment of DVT and as effective as unfractionated heparin in the treatment of PE.

Ximelagatran

Ximelagatran is the first oral, active, direct thrombin inhibitor. Following absorption, this agent is metabolized to its active form melagatran. Melagatran binds to the active site of thrombin and blocks the enzyme's ability to convert fibrinogen to fibrin. The plasma half-life of melagatran is 4–5 h and it is administered twice daily.

Phase III studies demonstrated that ximelagatran given as monotherapy for 6 months was as effective and safe as LMWH followed by warfarin for 6 months, and that after 6 months of conventional anticoagulant therapy, ximelagatran reduced the risk of recurrent VTE by approximately 85% compared with placebo, without increasing the rate of major bleeding.

Thrombolytic therapy

Systemic thrombolytic therapy accelerates the rate of resolution of DVT and PE at the cost of an approximately fourfold increase in the frequency of major bleeding, and an approximately 10-fold increase in intracranial bleeding. This can be life-saving for PE with hemodynamic compromise (i.e. severe hypotension and/or hypoxia). One trial conducted in patients with submassive PE demonstrated a significant reduction in the combined endpoint of in-hospital death and clinical deterioration requiring escalation of treatment for patients who received thrombolysis in addition to heparin in comparison with patients who received heparin alone. The groups did not differ for all-cause mortality, recurrent PE or major bleeding. Whether thrombolytic therapy decreases the incidence of pulmonary hypertension or recurrences in the long term is yet to be determined. Similarly, thrombo-

lytic therapy may reduce the risk of the post-thrombotic syndrome following DVT, but this does not appear to justify its associated risks. Catheter-based treatments of DVT (i.e. thrombolytic therapy or removal of thrombus) require further evaluation before they can be recommended.

Given the literature to date, the author's practice is to reserve thrombolysis for those patients with hemodynamic compromise secondary to PE. Thrombolysis regimens that are given within 2 h or less, such as 100 mg rt-PA over 2 h, appear preferable.

Major contraindications to thrombolytic therapy include:
- active internal bleeding;
- stroke within the past 3 months; and
- intracranial disease.
  Relative contraindications include:
- major surgery within the past 10 days;
- recent organ biopsy;
- recent puncture of a non-compressible vessel;
- recent gastrointestinal bleeding;
- liver or renal disease;
- severe arterial hypertension; and
- severe diabetic retinopathy.

Surgical treatment

Pulmonary endarterectomy is beneficial in selected patients with thromboembolic pulmonary hypertension. Urgent pulmonary embolectomy is reserved for patients with shock whose blood pressure cannot be maintained despite administration of thrombolytic therapy or those with an absolute contraindication to thrombolytic therapy.

Inferior vena caval filters

A randomized trial demonstrated that a filter, as an adjunct to anticoagulation in patients with proximal DVT, reduced the rate of PE (asymptomatic and symptomatic) from 4.5 to 1.0% during the 12 days following insertion, with a suggestion of fewer fatal episodes (0% vs. 2%). However, after 2 years, patients with a filter had a significantly higher rate of recurrent DVT (21% vs. 12%) and only a non-statistically significant reduction in the frequency of symptomatic PE (3% vs. 6%). This study supports the use of vena caval filters to prevent PE in patients with acute DVT and/or PE who cannot be anticoagulated (i.e. bleeding), but does not support more liberal use of filters. Patients should receive a course of anticoagulation if this subsequently becomes safe.

Treatment of venous thromboembolism during pregnancy

Unfractionated heparin and LMWH do not cross the placenta and are safe for the fetus, whereas oral anticoagulants cross the placenta and can cause fetal bleeding and malformations. Therefore, pregnant women with VTE should be treated with therapeutic doses of subcutaneous heparin (unfractionated heparin or, increasingly, LMWH) throughout pregnancy. The author's practice is to use twice daily LMWH, adjusted to achieve an anti-Xa heparin level of 0.35–0.7 U/ml, 4–6 h after the last injection. Care should be taken to avoid delivery while the mother is therapeutically anticoagulated; one management approach involves stopping subcutaneous heparin 24 h prior to induction of labour and switching to intravenous heparin if there is a high risk of embolism. After delivery, warfarin, which is safe for infants of nursing mothers, should be given (with initial heparin overlap) for 6 weeks and until a minimum of 3 months of treatment has been completed.

Prevention of venous thromboembolism

Venous thromboembolism prophylaxis following surgery

Surgical patients can be stratified according to their risk factors for VTE into low, moderate and high risk categories.

Low risk

This category includes patients under 40 years of age who undergo uncomplicated surgery and have no additional risk factors. The rate of asymptomatic proximal DVT detected by surveillance bilateral venography is 0.4% and the rate of symptomatic PE and fatal PE is 0.2% and less than

0.01%, respectively. Recommended VTE prophylaxis in this group is limited to early mobilization.

Moderate risk

This category includes patients over 40 years of age who undergo prolonged and/or complicated surgery or have additional minor risk factors. The rate of asymptomatic proximal DVT is 5% and the rate of symptomatic PE and fatal PE is 2% and 0.5%, respectively. Recommended VTE prophylaxis in this group includes unfractionated heparin (5000 U/day preoperatively, and 2–3 times daily postoperatively), LMWH (approximately 3000 U/day) or graduated compression stockings alone or in combination with pharmacologic methods.

High risk

This category includes patients who undergo major surgery for malignancy, hip or knee surgery or those who have a history of previous VTE. The rate of asymptomatic proximal DVT is 15% and the rate of symptomatic PE and fatal PE is 5% and 2%, respectively. Recommended VTE prophylaxis in this group includes LMWH (4000 U o.d. with a preoperative start in Europe, or 3000 U b.d. with a postoperative start in North America); warfarin (usually started postoperatively and adjusted to achieve an INR of 2.0–3.0); or fondaparinux (once daily, usually started postoperatively) or intermittent pneumatic compression devices alone or in combination with other methods of prophylaxis. Mechanical methods of prophylaxis should be used in patients who have a moderate or high risk of VTE if anticoagulants are contraindicated (e.g. neurosurgical patients).

Pharmacologic agents for venous thromboembolism prophylaxis in orthopedic surgery

Meta-analyses support the finding that LMWH is more effective than unfractionated heparin following orthopedic surgery and is associated with a similar frequency of bleeding. Warfarin (target INR 2–3 for approximately 7–10 days) is less effective than LMWH at preventing DVT that are detected by venography soon after surgery, but appears to be similarly effective at preventing symptomatic VTE over a 3-month period. An additional 3 or 4 weeks of LMWH after hospital discharge further reduces the frequency of symptomatic VTE after orthopedic surgery (from 3.3% to 1.3%). There is evidence that aspirin reduces the risk of postoperative VTE by one-third. However, as warfarin and LMWH are expected to be more effective (at least a two-thirds reduction in VTE), aspirin alone is not recommended during the initial postoperative period. Fondaparinux has been shown to be more effective than LMWH following major orthopedic surgery; however, fondaparinux may cause marginally more bleeding.

Venous thromboembolism prophylaxis in medical patients

Primary prophylaxis with anticoagulants and/or mechanical methods should be used in hospitalized patients who have a moderate or high risk of VTE. LMWH given for 6–14 days has been shown to reduce the risk of VTE compared with placebo in these patients and the benefit was maintained at 3 months.

Further reading

Agnelli G, Prandoni P, Becattini C, *et al*. Extended oral anticoagulant therapy after a first episode of pulmonary embolism. *Ann Intern Med* 2003;**139**:19–25.

Anderson FA, Spencer FA. Risk factors for venous thromboembolism. *Circulation* 2003;**107**:I9–I16.

Buller HR, Davidson BL, Decousus H, *et al*. Fondaparinux or enoxaparin for the initial treatment of symptomatic deep venous thrombosis: a randomized trial. *Ann Intern Med* 2004;**140**:867–73.

Buller HR, Davidson BL, Decousus H, *et al*. Subcutaneous fondaparinux versus intravenous unfractionated heparin in the initial treatment of pulmonary embolism. *N Engl J Med* 2003;**349**:1695–702.

Decousus H, Leizorovicz A, Parent F, *et al*. A clinical trial of vena caval filters in the prevention of pulmonary embolism in patients with proximal deep-vein thrombosis. *N Engl J Med* 1998;**338**:409–15.

Douketis JD, Kearon C, Bates S, *et al*. Risk of fatal pulmonary embolism in patients with treated venous thromboembolism. *Thromb Haemost* 2002;**88**:407–14.

Fraser DG, Moody AR, Morgan PS, *et al*. Diagnosis of lower-limb deep venous thrombosis: a prospective blinded study of magnetic resonance direct thrombus imaging. *Ann Intern Med* 2002;**136**:89–98.

Geerts WH, Heit JA, Clagett GP, *et al*. Prevention of venous thromboembolism. *Chest* 2001;**119**:132–75S.

Ginsberg JS, Greer I, Hirsh J. Use of antithrombotic agents during pregnancy. *Chest* 2001;**119**:122–31S.

Hirsh J, Dalen JE, Anderson DR, *et al*. Oral anticoagulants: mechanism of action, clinical effectiveness, and optimal therapeutic range. *Chest* 2001;**119**:8–21S.

Hirsh J, Warkentin TE, Shaughnessy SG, *et al*. Heparin and low-molecular-weight heparin: mechanisms of action, pharmacokinetics, dosing, monitoring, efficacy, and safety. *Chest* 2001;**119**:64–94S.

Kearon C. Natural history of venous thromboembolism. *Circulation* 2003;**107**:122–30.

Kearon C, Crowther M, Hirsh J. Management of patients with hereditary hypercoagulable disorders. *Annu Rev Med* 2000;**51**:169–85.

Kearon C, Julian JA, Newman TE, *et al*. Non-invasive diagnosis of deep vein thrombosis. *Ann Intern Med* 1998;**128**:663–77.

Konstantinides S, Geibel A, Heusel G, *et al*. Heparin plus alteplase compared with heparin alone in patients with submissive pulmonary embolism. *N Engl J Med* 2002;**347**:1143–50.

Lee AY, Levine MN, Baker RI, *et al*. Low-molecular-weight heparin versus a coumarin for the prevention of recurrent venous thromboembolism in patients with cancer. *N Engl J Med* 2003;**349**:146–53.

Musset D, Parent F, Meyer G, *et al*. Diagnostic strategy for patients with suspected pulmonary embolism: a prospective multicentre outcome study. *Lancet* 2002;**360**:1914–20.

PEP Trial Collaborative Group. Prevention of pulmonary embolism and deep vein thrombosis with low dose aspirin: Pulmonary Embolism Prevention (PEP) trial. *Lancet* 2000;**355**:1295–302.

Schulman S, Wahlander K, Lundström T, *et al*. Secondary prevention of venous thromboembolism with the oral direct thrombin inhibitor ximelagatran. *N Engl J Med* 2003;**349**:1713–21.

van Strigen MJ, de Monqe W, Schiereck J, *et al*. Single-detector helical computed tomography as the primary diagnostic test in suspected pulmonary embolism: a multicenter clinical management study of 510 patients. *Ann Intern Med* 2003;**138**:307–14.

Warkentin TE, Levine MN, Hirsh J, *et al*. Heparin-induced thrombocytopenia in patients treated with low-molecular-weight heparin or unfractionated heparin. *N Engl J Med* 1995;**332**:1330–5.

Wells PS, Anderson DR, Rodger M, *et al*. Evaluation of D-dimer in the diagnosis of suspected deep-vein thrombosis. *N Engl J Med* 2003;**349**:1227–35.

White RH. The epidemiology of venous thromboembolism. *Circulation* 2003;**107**:14–18.

Chapter 12
Arterial thrombosis

Gordon D.O. Lowe and R. Campbell Tait

Introduction

Arterial thrombosis is a common cause of hospital admission, death and disability in developed countries (and increasingly in developing nations because of global epidemics of smoking, obesity and diabetes). It usually follows spontaneous rupture of an atherosclerotic plaque, and may be:
• clinically silent;
• contribute to atherosclerotic progression resulting in coronary stenosis and stable angina, or lower limb artery stenosis and claudication;
• present as acute ischemia in the heart (acute coronary syndromes – unstable angina, myocardial infarction), brain (transient cerebral ischemic attack or stroke) or limb (acute limb ischemia).

There is now good evidence that patients with acute ischemic syndromes have lower morbidity and mortality if they are promptly diagnosed, admitted as soon as possible to specialist acute units (coronary care, acute stroke or peripheral vascular), undergo risk stratification and receive appropriate treatment. This includes antithrombotic drugs (e.g. aspirin, heparin) and consideration of thrombolysis, thrombectomy, angioplasty or vascular reconstruction in the acute phase; and early, multidisciplinary rehabilitation.

Primary and secondary prevention of arterial thrombosis are everybody's business. All healthcare professionals, including hematologists, should take the opportunity to encourage their patients to adjust their lifestyles (when appropriate); and to consider pharmacologic prevention in all high-risk patients and in all with clinical evidence of arterial disease (Table 12.1).

Hematologists are commonly asked to develop or revise local hospital or area guidelines for investigations in thrombosis, and antithrombotic therapies and their monitoring. In addition, they are often referred patients with arterial thrombosis that is premature, recurrent or which occurs at multiple or unusual sites. Such referrals have increased in recent years, probably because general practitioners and physicians expect that (as with venous thromboembolism) hematologists may define underlying thrombophilias which may require specific management. This review therefore focuses on appropriate hematological investigation of patients with arterial thrombosis, and appropriate antithrombotic therapy in various patient groups.

Evidence in this field is changing rapidly, hence hematologists should keep up-to-date with systematic reviews and evidence-based national guidelines, such as those produced by the British Society for Haematology/British Committee for Standards in Haematology (www.bcshguidelines.com) and the Scottish Intercollegiate Guidelines Network (SIGN; www.sign.ac.uk).

Laboratory investigations

Table 12.2 outlines routine and specialist investigations that are applicable to patients with arterial thrombosis or ischemia.

Routine investigations

Routine hematology investigations include:
• full blood count as a screen for anemia, polycythemia, hyperleukocytic leukaemias and thrombocytosis;
• erythrocyte sedimentation rate (ESR) or plasma

Table 12.1 Summary of lifestyle advice and pharmacologic prevention of cardiovascular disease.

Lifestyle advice

(primary and secondary prevention)

Stop or reduce smoking (cigarette, cigar or pipe)

Take regular exercise (e.g. walk 30 min most days per week)

Lose weight if overweight (BMI over 25 kg/m^2) or obese (BMI over 30 kg/m^2)

Diet: reduce salt and saturated fat; increase fruit, vegetables and fish

Moderate alcohol consumption (less than 16 units/week women, less than 24 units/week men); avoid binge drinking

Pharmacologic

(primary prevention in high-risk patients – annual risk of CHD or stroke ≥ 2%; and secondary prevention in all patients with clinical cardiovascular disease)

Blood pressure reduction (if not achieved by lifestyle advice) to a target of 140/85 mmHg

Beta-blocker following acute myocardial infarction (unless contraindicated)

ACE inhibitor following acute myocardial infarction if LV dysfunction

Cholesterol reduction (usually with a statin at dose of proven efficacy in cardiovascular reduction)

Aspirin (75 mg/day, loading dose 300 mg in acute coronary syndromes or acute ischemic stroke; 300 mg/day following coronary artery bypass grafting)

or

Clopidogrel (75 mg/day) in secondary prevention if aspirin contraindicated or not tolerated

or

Dipyridamole slow-release (200 mg b.d.) in patients with ischemic stroke or TIA, if aspirin contraindicated or not tolerated

Aspirin 75 mg/day *and* clopidogrel 75 mg/day for at least 1 month in acute coronary syndromes or following percutaneous coronary angioplasty ± stenting

Aspirin 75 mg/day *and* dipyridamole 200 mg b.d. in patients with *recurrent* ischemic stroke or TIA despite taking aspirin

Consider oral anticoagulation (usually with warfarin, target INR 2.0–3.0) in patients with atrial fibrillation with previous history of ischemic stroke or other thromboembolic event; or at high risk of thromboembolism (Fig. 12.1). Aspirin (75 mg/day) in other patients with atrial fibrillation, or if balance of benefit over risk of warfarin is uncertain, or if warfarin contraindicated or in patients who elect not to take warfarin

ACE, angiotensin-converting enzyme; BMI, body mass index; INR, international normalized ratio; LV, left ventricle; TIA, transient ischemic attack.

viscosity as a screen for hyperviscosity syndromes and connective tissue disorders and/or vasculitis (e.g. temporal arteritis, systemic lupus erythematosus or polyarteritis nodosa). Hyperviscosity syndromes may be a medical emergency, requiring urgent plasma exchange, plasmapheresis or cytapheresis; vasculitis may require urgent steroid or cytotoxic therapy and biopsy.

Acute elevations in white cell count and platelet counts, ESR or plasma viscosity, and other acute phase reactants such as C-reactive protein and fibrinogen, are common in acute ischemic syndromes; but persistent elevations (e.g. more than 1 month) that are unexplained by complications such as infections, limb necrosis or venous thromboembolism, should raise the suspicion of underlying connective tissue disorder or malignancy.

Routine biochemical investigations should include:

• a lipid profile (specifically low-density lipoprotein [LDL] and high-density lipoprotein [HDL] cholesterol);

• glucose, or another measure of insulin resistance;

• a thyroid screen for evidence of underlying thyrotoxicosis in patients with atrial fibrillation.

Careful control of diabetes and reduction of

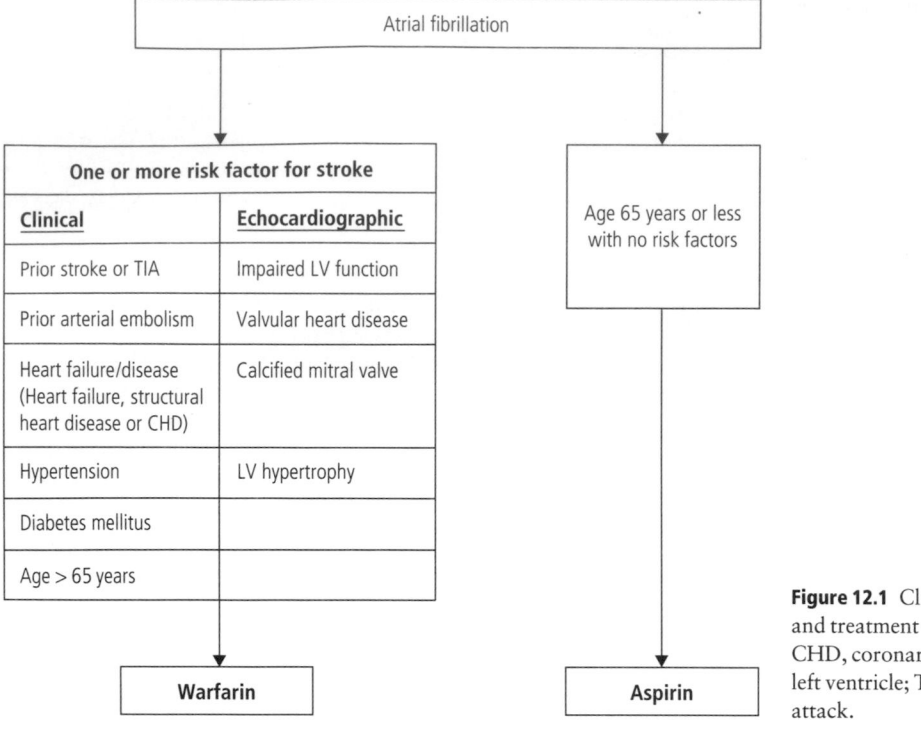

Figure 12.1 Clinical risk stratification and treatment in atrial fibrillation. CHD, coronary heart disease; LV, left ventricle; TIA, transient ischemic attack.

cholesterol have proven value in reduction of both primary and secondary vascular disease in affected individuals.

Specialized investigations

These should be reserved for patients in whom clinical assessment suggests a reasonable expectation of finding a "thrombophilia" which may alter clinical management. Overinvestigation will result in identification of "abnormalities" that are irrelevant to clinical management and a source of confusion and anxiety to patients, family members, carers and healthcare professionals. Table 12.2 summarizes indications for particular tests in adults.

Thrombosis in childhood (apart from that associated with central venous catheters) is uncommon and requires specialist assessment by a pediatric hematologist.

Homocysteine measurement

This is indicated in all patients with premature (e.g.

age under 30 years) arterial thrombosis, to exclude homocysteinuria. In the UK, these assays are more commonly performed in biochemistry rather than hematology laboratories. Blood samples (K_2 edetate) should be kept on ice and centrifuged within 4 h of venepuncture. Such patients may be managed by regional specialists in metabolic medicine.

In recent years, epidemiologic studies have associated high-normal plasma homocysteine levels (and the common underlying MTHFR mutation, suggesting causality) with increased risk of arterial thrombosis (coronary, cerebral and lower limb) as well as venous thrombosis. While vitamin supplementation (vitamin B_{12}, folate, vitamin B_6) reduces plasma homocysteine levels, the first large randomized trial of secondary prevention (after ischemic stroke) was negative for all vascular outcomes. Further trials of vitamin supplementation are in progress.

Meanwhile, the utility of screening for hyperhomocysteinemia in secondary prevention of arterial thrombosis in patients aged over 30 years is unproven. If high homocysteine levels are found,

Table 12.2 Summary of laboratory tests in persons with arterial thromboembolism.

Routine
Full blood count
   anemia (promotes ischemia)
   polycythemia
   hyperleukocytic leukemias
   thrombocytosis
ESR/plasma viscosity
   hyperviscosity syndromes
   vasculitis/connective tissue disorders
Cholesterol
   total cholesterol or LDL : HDL ratio predicts arterial disease

Specialized
Homocysteine
   if arterial thrombosis at age under 30 years
Sickle cell screening
   in persons at ethnic risk
Lupus anticoagulant and anticardiolipin antibodies
   if arterial events at age under 50 years, without prominent clinical
     risk factors
Congenital thrombophilias
   utility unproven
Coagulation factors
   utility unproven
Fibrin D-dimer
   utility unproven
Fibrinolytic factors
   utility unproven
Platelet function studies
   utility unproven (e.g. aspirin resistance)

ESR, erythrocyte sedimentation rate; HDL, high-density lipoprotein; LDL, low-density lipoprotein.

folate supplementation is reasonable because it is cheap and non-toxic (provided vitamin B_{12} levels are normal). It may be that folate supplementation of cereals (as practiced in the USA) or the folate component of a "polypill" (folic acid, aspirin and statin) may be the most clinically effective and cost-effective strategy to reduce cardiovascular risk if homocysteine is shown to have a causal role in arterial (or venous) thrombosis.

Sickle cell screening

This may be appropriate in persons at ethnic risk (almost always non-northern European), although in practice a diagnosis of sickle cell disease (SCD) will usually have been made long before adulthood. Large and small vessel arterial thromboses are responsible for the protean manifestations of SCD. Sickle erythrocytes appear to induce a hypercoagulable state through a variety of mechanisms as assessed by increased platelet activation, thrombin generation and fibrinolysis, and decreased levels of anticoagulant proteins. However, measurement of such parameters has no proven utility in the management of SCD and clinical studies of antiplatelet agents and anticoagulants have yet to show any beneficial effect on the incidence of vaso-occlusive events. Furthermore, it seems likely that the hypercoagulability is a secondary phenomenon to the sickling process – because treatment with hydroxyurea, which increases HbF levels and reduces sickling, is associated with a reduction in measures of hypercoagulability.

Screening for lupus anticoagulant and anticardiolipin antibodies

This is appropriate in all patients with premature (e.g. age under 50 years) cerebral or limb thrombosis or ischemia, and in other indications. Management of the antiphospholipid syndrome is considered in Chapter 14.

Screening for congenital thrombophilias

The factor V Leiden and prothrombin G20210A mutations show modest but statistically significant associations with coronary heart disease (CHD), stroke and peripheral arterial events, especially in younger persons (age under 55 years) and in women. These findings may be relevant to the increases in risk of coronary and stroke events during pregnancy, use of combined oral contraceptives or oral hormone replacement therapy (HRT) (each of which increases resistance to activated protein C).

There is little evidence that other congenital thrombophilias are associated with increased risk of arterial disease and the clinical utility of screening for such abnormalities in patients with arterial thrombosis is at present unproven. Furthermore, there is no evidence that secondary prevention with oral anticoagulants in such patients is more effective than routine antithrombotic prevention with aspirin (Table 12.1).

Ischemic stroke is often associated with a right-to-left cardiac shunt (e.g. patent foramen ovale, atrial septal defect) in younger patients, suggesting the possibility of "paradoxical" cerebral arterial embolism from venous thrombosis. Whether such an event is associated with thrombophilias is unknown; as are the relative benefits and risks of prophylaxis with aspirin, oral anticoagulants or shunt closure.

Coagulation factors

Plasma fibrinogen is associated with CHD, stroke and peripheral arterial events; the risks increase by 30–40% per 1 g/L increase. While there are several plausible biologic mechanisms through which increased circulating fibrinogen levels might promote such risk (atherogenic, thrombogenic, and rheological through increased plasma and blood viscosity), the lack of association of functional genetic polymorphisms with risk of CHD argues against causality. The association of fibrinogen with arterial risk may therefore be coincidental (because of mutual associations with multiple risk factors) or consequential (reverse causality, resulting from effects of atherosclerosis on plasma fibrinogen). The clinical utility of plasma fibrinogen assessment in management of arterial thrombosis is unproven.

Von Willebrand factor (VWF) is weakly associated with risk of CHD; there are few reported studies of functional polymorphisms.

Carriers of hemophilia A (or B), who have plasma levels of factor VIII or factor IX which on average are 50% lower than female non-carriers, have an approximately 35% lower risk of CHD. Together with the 80% lower risk of CHD in male hemophiliacs compared with male non-hemophiliacs, these findings suggest that increasing levels of factor VIII (or factor IX) increase the risks of arterial thrombosis, as well as of venous thrombosis.

The clinical utility of assessment of plasma levels of VWF, factors VIII or IX (or other clotting factors) in management of arterial thrombosis is unproven.

Coagulation activation markers

Plasma fibrin D-dimer levels are associated with increased risks of incident CHD and stroke, including studies of patients with atrial fibrillation. While D-dimer levels might therefore be useful in prediction of stroke in atrial fibrillation, and hence in stratifying choice of antithrombotic therapies, further management studies are required.

Fibrinolytic tests

Circulating levels of tissue plasminogen activator (tPA) antigen, but not of plasminogen activator inhibitor type 1 (PAI-1) are associated with increased risk of CHD in population studies. This association is markedly reduced after adjustment for associated CHD risk factors (obesity and other markers of insulin resistance). The clinical utility of plasma components of the fibrinolytic system in management of arterial thrombosis is unproven.

Platelet function tests

Platelet aggregation studies and measures of platelet activation are not useful in prediction of arterial thrombosis. While there is increasing evidence that aspirin resistance (defined as a laboratory measure of the failure of aspirin to inhibit platelet synthesis of thromboxane A_2, platelet aggregation or the skin bleeding time) is associated with increased risk of recurrent cardiovascular events, further work is required to define the place of such laboratory measures in clinical practice.

In patients with recurrent events despite aspirin, possible empirical approaches are to add a second antiplatelet agent (e.g. adding dipyridamole to aspirin in patients with recurrent ischemic stroke or transient ischemic attack), to increase the dose of aspirin or to change to oral anticoagulant therapy (after considering the increased bleeding risk and the logistical problems of long-term anticoagulant monitoring).

Conclusions

At present, risk stratification for arterial disease

continues to rely on assessment of traditional clinical (smoking, hypertension, obesity) and routine laboratory (cholesterol) risk factors.

The role of thrombophilia screening in patients with arterial disease is unproven, although selected testing for homocysteinuria and antiphospholipid syndrome is indicated in patients with premature arterial thrombosis in the absence of traditional risk factors.

The mainstay of treatment is control, or eradication, of risk factors, coupled with antithrombotic therapy; either an antiplatelet agent, or anticoagulation for patients with atrial fibrillation and additional risk factors (Fig. 12.1).

Further reading

Ataga KI, Orringer EP. Hypercoagulability in sickle cell disease: a curious paradox. *Am J Med* 2003;**115**:721–8.

Danesh J, Wheeler JG, Hirshfield GM, *et al*. C-reactive protein and other circulating markers of inflammation in the prediction of coronary heart disease. *N Engl J Med* 2004;**350**:1387–97.

Danesh J, Whincup P, Walker M, *et al*. Fibrin D-dimer and coronary heart disease: prospective study and meta-analysis. *Circulation* 2001;**103**:2323–7.

Fibrinogen Studies Collaboration. Collaborative meta-analysis of prospective observational studies of plasma fibrinogen and cardiovascular disease. *Eur J Cardiovasc Prevent Rehabil* 2004;**11**:9–17.

Greaves M, Cohen H, Machin SJ, Mackie I, on behalf of the British Committee for Standards in Haematology. Guidelines on the investigation and management of the antiphospholipid syndrome. *Br J Haematol* 2000;**109**:704–15.

Hankey GJ, Eikelboom JW. Aspirin resistance. *BMJ* 2004;**328**:477–9.

Homocysteine Studies Collaboration. Homocysteine and risk of ischemic heart disease and stroke: a meta-analysis. *JAMA* 2002;**288**:2015–22.

Kim RJ, Becker RC. Association between factor V Leiden, prothrombin mutation G20120A, and MTHFR C677T mutations and events of the arterial circulatory system: a meta-analysis of published studies. *Am Heart J* 2003;**146**:948–57.

Klerk M, Verhoef P, Clarke R, Blom HJ, Kok FJ, Schouter EG and the MTHFR Studies Collaboration Group. MTHFR 677C-T polymorphism and risk of coronary heart disease: a meta-analysis. *JAMA* 2002;**288**:2023–31.

Lowe GDO, Danesh J, eds. Classical and emerging risk factors for cardiovascular disease. *Semin Vasc Med* 2002;**2**:229–445.

Lowe GDO, Danesh J, Lewington S, *et al*. Tissue plasminogen activator antigen and coronary heart disease: prospective study and meta-analysis. *Eur Heart J* 2004;**25**:252–9.

Toole JF, Malinow MR, Chambless LE, *et al*. Lowering homocysteine in patients with ischemic stroke to prevent recurrent stroke, myocardial infarction, and death. *JAMA* 2004;**291**:565–75.

Vene N, Mavri A, Kosmelj K, Stegnar M. High D-dimer levels predict cardiovascular events in patients with chronic atrial fibrillation during oral anticoagulant therapy. *Thromb Haemost* 2003;**90**:1163–72.

Wald NJ, Law MR. A strategy to reduce cardiovascular disease by more than 80%. *BMJ* 2003;**326**:1419.

Walker ID, Greaves M, Preston FE, on behalf of the Haemostasis and Thrombosis Task Force, British Committee for Standards in Haematology. Guideline: Investigation and management of heritable thrombophilia. *Br J Haematol* 2001;**114**:512–28.

Wu LA, We LA, Lidar DA, Friesen M *et al*. Patent foramen ovale in cryptogenic stroke: current understanding and management options. *Arch Intern Med* 2004;**164**:950–6.

Chapter 13
Anticoagulation

Gualtiero Palareti and Benilde Cosmi

Introduction

Oral anticoagulants (OACs) have been shown to be effective on the basis of randomized clinical trials in the following conditions:
- primary and secondary prevention of venous thromboembolism;
- prevention of systemic embolism in atrial fibrillation or in patients with tissue or mechanical heart valves;
- prevention of stroke or death in patients with acute myocardial infarction; and
- prevention of acute myocardial infarction in men at high risk.

Properly designed clinical trials are lacking in conditions for which oral anticoagulation is widely accepted:
- prevention of systemic embolism in high-risk patients with mitral stenosis and in patients with systemic embolism of unknown etiology;
- patients with intraventricular thrombosis; and
- patients with dilated cardiomyopathy at high risk of systemic embolism.

For the majority of indications, a moderate anticoagulant effect (international normalized ratio [INR] 2.0–3.0) is effective. No adequate studies have been conducted on the efficacy of oral anticoagulants for the secondary prevention in ischemic cerebrovascular disease, in retinal vein thrombosis or in peripheral arterial disease. In the latter condition, OACs are indicated in patients with venous infrainguinal bypasses at high risk of occlusion.

Contraindications for treatment

A reliable laboratory, an expert physician and a compliant patient are three essential components for appropriate therapy with OACs. Before starting oral anticoagulation, patients should be carefully evaluated for compliance, absolute contraindications and conditions with a higher risk of complications.

OACs cross the placental barrier and can produce both bleeding and a teratogenic effect in the fetus (embryopathy with nasal hypoplasia and stippled epiphyses in the first trimester and central nervous system abnormalities at any time during pregnancy). They could be considered relatively safe after the first trimester up to 36 weeks of gestation. In the last 6 weeks, exposure to OACs could increase the risk of bleeding at the time of delivery. Nursing mothers can be treated with OACs as warfarin does not induce an anticoagulant effect in the breastfed infant.

Major bleeding is an absolute contraindication to OACs for at least 1 month after the event.

Relative medical contraindications to OACs are severe hepatic or renal insufficiency (which increase the risk of bleeding), severe hypertension, severe heart failure, esophageal varices, bleeding diathesis, recent central nervous system (CNS) surgery or trauma, recent hepatic or renal biopsy, active peptic ulcer, bacterial endocarditis, pericarditis, recent CNS hemorrhage, chronic bowel inflammatory disease, menorrhagia, thyrotoxicosis and cerebral aneurisms.

Conditions of non-compliance of the patient such as psychiatric disorders, dementia and chronic alcoholism can also be considered relative contraindications for OACs.

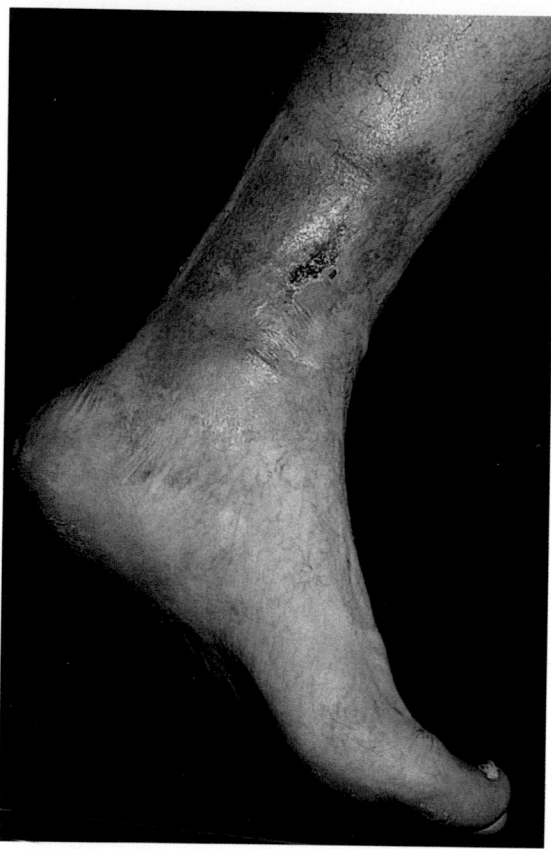

Plate 5 Post-thrombotic sundrome. Although usually the symptoms are confined to itching, mild swelling and pain, when severe there is pigmentation and ulceration over the medial malleolus.

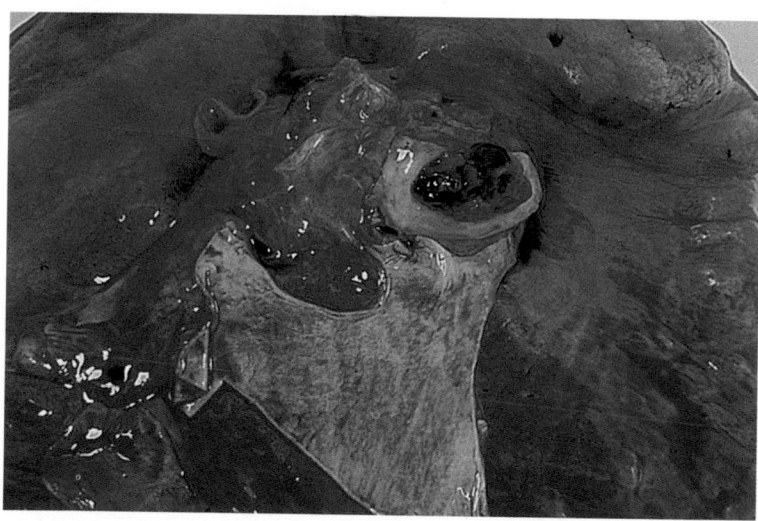

Plate 6 Pulmonary embolus in the pulmonary artery causing sudden death in a young woman who was using the combined contraceptive pill.

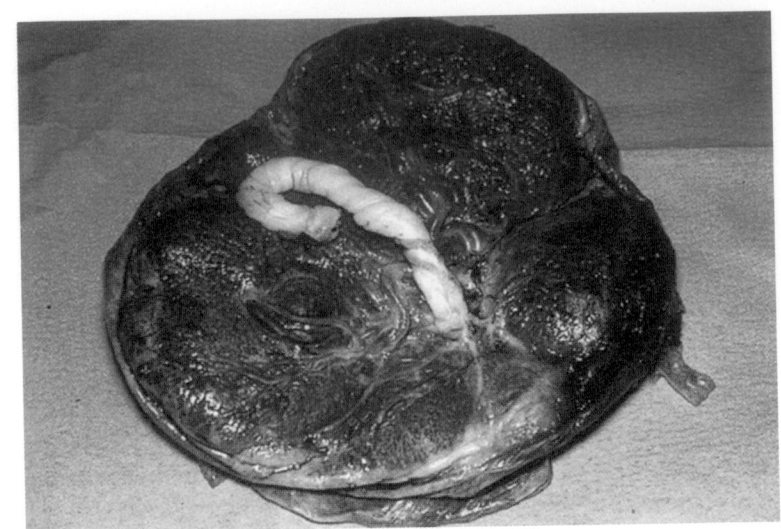

Plate 7 Unusually massive, macroscopic, late pregnancy placental infarction in primary antiphospholipid syndrome. (From Makris and Greaves, *Blood in Systemic Disease*. Reproduced with permission from Churchill Livingstone

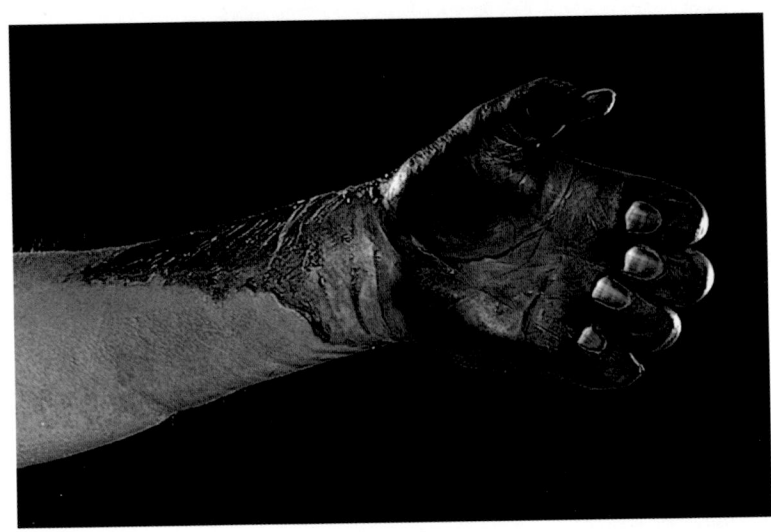

Plate 8 Arterial thrombosis in a patient with malignancy. Reprinted from *Blood in Systemic Disease* 1e, Greaves and Makris, 1997, with permission from Elsevier.

Oral anticoagulant drugs: clinical pharmacology

OACs are 4-hydroxycoumarin compounds, which were developed in the 1940s–1950s and introduced in the treatment of thrombotic disorders in the 1950s. Warfarin, acenocoumarol and phenprocoumon are the compounds currently in clinical use.

They exert their effect by interfering with the vitamin K-dependent hepatic synthesis of coagulation factors II, VII, IX and X as well as the coagulation inhibitors protein C and S. Vitamin K-dependent post-translational γ-carboxylation is critical for coagulation factors to acquire the calcium-mediated ability to bind to negatively charged phospholipid surfaces.

Carboxylation of vitamin K-dependent coagulation factors depends on a carboxylase that requires a reduced form of vitamin K (vitamin KH2), oxygen and carbon dioxide. During this reaction, vitamin KH2 is oxidized to vitamin K epoxide, which is reduced to vitamin K by epoxide reductase and then to vitamin KH2 by vitamin K reductase. OACs inhibit vitamin K epoxide reductase and possibly vitamin K reductase. As a result, intracellular depletion of vitamin KH2 takes place and only partially carboxylated and de-carboxylated proteins are secreted. The antagonizing effect on vitamin K with the resulting production of biologically inactive coagulation factors is the basis for the therapeutic use of OACs.

The effect of OACs is delayed because time is required for the normal coagulation factors to be cleared from plasma and replaced by partially carboxylated or decarboxylated factors. This delay in the onset of OACs effect varies according to the coagulation factor's half-life, which is only 6–7 h for factor VII and 60–72 h for prothrombin.

Animal studies have shown that the reduction of prothrombin and possibly of factor X is more important than the reduction of factor VII and IX for the *in vivo* antithrombotic effect of OACs. As a result, the initial effect of OACs as measured by the prolongation of the prothrombin time

- reflects the reduction of factor VII
- the antithrombotic effect is only observed after the reduction of prothrombin, which requires 60–72 h
- in addition, in the first days of treatment with OACs, a reduction of the levels of protein C and protein S is also observed as the synthesis of these natural anticoagulants is also vitamin K dependent. Protein C half-life is similar to that of factor VII, as a result in the initial phase of Oral Anticoagulant Therapy (OAT) the levels of protein C can be reduced significantly before the onset of the antithrombotic effect of OAT. This can result in warfarin induced skin necrosis (Fig. 13.1).

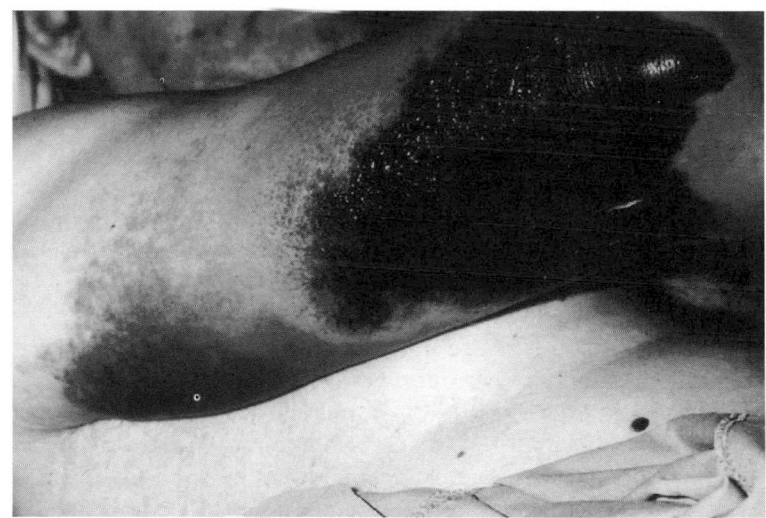

Figure 13.1 Skin necrosis of the elbow in a patient who just started warfarin.

• the delayed onset of the antithrombotic effect of OACs and the potentially prothrombotic effect in the first 24–48 h provide the rationale for overlapping heparin with OACs for 4–5 days until their full antithrombotic effect is obtained.

OAC can be safely started on the first instead of the fifth day of heparin treatment of deep vein thrombosis (DVT). Although in the past unfractionated heparin was the agent primarily used during the overlap, low molecular weight heparin is now the drug of choice (discussed in Chapter 11). Heparin can be safely stopped after a stable therapeutic INR range is reached; i.e. after 2 consecutive days of INR above 2.0.

Initiation of warfarin anticoagulation

Before starting warfarin anticoagulation, it is recommended that the following are performed:
• a baseline INR;
• a full blood and platelet count; and
• assessment of renal function.

Historically, large loading warfarin doses were used at the start of anticoagulation. More recently, this practice has been abandoned as a result of the demonstration that initiating warfarin at a dosage close to that likely required for maintenance therapy not only produces therapeutic anticoagulation in most patients, but is also less risky for complications.

The use of nomograms

There is clear evidence that use of nomograms to guide warfarin initiation is of great help in rapidly and safely achieving therapeutic anticoagulation levels in comparison with a physician-guided warfarin initiation, also resulting in shorter hospital stays for some patients. The use of nomograms may also reduce the need for anticoagulant monitoring in the first days of treatment.

A variety of nomograms for the initial days of warfarin therapy have been devised. Nomogram use requires that baseline INR is normal or near normal (not more than 1.4). A nomogram to start warfarin anticoagulation in children with thrombosis has also been proposed, with an initial dosage

of 0.2 mg/kg. One of the first and most widely adopted nomogram to be used for adult patients was that proposed by Fennerty et al., using 10-mg loading doses. More recently, nomograms suggesting that warfarin be initiated with a 5-mg dose were proposed, with subsequent doses determined by the INR response which can be checked on the third or fourth day.

Advantages of the 5-mg dose

It has been shown that the rate of lowering of prothrombin levels was similar when warfarin was started with either a 5- or 10-mg loading dose. However, the larger loading dose produced a more rapid reduction in protein C levels and a higher frequency in over-anticoagulation (INR > 3.0). A smaller loading dose of warfarin might therefore be less likely to produce a potentially prothrombotic effect in the first 24–48 h of treatment.

Advantages of the 10-mg dose

In contrast to the data suggesting that a low initial warfarin dose is effective and safe, some authors have reported that higher initial doses are better. Patients who receive a 10-mg initial dose of warfarin achieve a therapeutic INR earlier than patients initially treated with 5 mg, and more patients (83%) in the 10-mg group achieve a therapeutic INR by day 5, compared with the 5-mg group (46%). Also, fewer INR assessments are performed in the 10-mg group.

There were no significant differences between the two groups in recurrent events or major bleeding. The authors concluded that 10-mg warfarin initiation nomogram is superior to the 5-mg nomogram because it allows more rapid achievement of a therapeutic INR.

Disadvantages of the 5-mg dose

It has recently been shown that starting anticoagulation with 5 mg warfarin in patients with DVT, entirely treated out of hospital, caused a prolongation of low molecular weight heparin treatment likely caused by a reduced number of INR determinations in outpatients. It has been suggested that either more frequent INR determination should be performed or higher initial dose of warfarin should be adopted in patients younger than 60 years.

Varying dose because of age or diagnosis

Some authors have demonstrated that the initial doses of warfarin should be different according to the age of patients because a reduced dose is required in the elderly.

Patients starting oral anticoagulation after heart valve replacement are more sensitive to warfarin than non-surgical patients, and initial warfarin doses lower than 5 mg are indicated in some.

Guidance during anticoagulation

The effects of OACs are highly variable both within and between individuals. Even though the average daily dose of warfarin is approximately 5 mg, individual patients may require much larger or smaller doses (the daily dose may range between 0.5 and 60 mg).

Furthermore, oral anticoagulants have a narrow therapeutic window, and over- or underdosage can result in over-anticoagulation, with increased risk of hemorrhage, or underanticoagulation, with increased risk of thrombosis, respectively.

The quality of monitoring anticoagulated patients is certainly an important factor influencing the risk of bleeding or thrombotic complications. Guiding warfarin therapy requires some skill and practice. Techniques to reduce the risk of inappropriate warfarin regimens include:
• warfarin regimen nomograms;
• computer-generated warfarin regimens; and
• dedicated anticoagulation clinics.

Several nomograms have been proposed to help warfarin regimens either during the induction phase or during the stabilized phase of anticoagulation. Some nomograms were specifically designed to guide warfarin treatment in some particular types of patients, such as in postorthopedic surgery patients, or in postpartum women.

Evidence is now available that *computer-guided dosing* is effective in helping doctors to prescribe therapeutic regimens, both during long-term maintenance and in the early, highly unstable phase of treatment. The use of computer-guided dosing increases the amount of time spent in the therapeutic range, compared with exclusive management by doctors.

It is a general experience, confirmed by some studies, that the quality of anticoagulation control is higher and the rate of bleeding lower when patients are monitored by *dedicated anticoagulation clinics*. In the dedicated clinic, the specialized training and experience of medical and paramedical staff, proper patient education and the use of computer programs help to ensure optimization of anticoagulant therapy.

Complications of OAC

Bleeding

Bleeding is the most important complication and is a major concern for both physicians and patients, limiting the more widespread use of oral anticoagulation.

The risk of bleeding on OACs in prospective studies has been reported to be:
• 0.1–1.0% patient-years of treatment for fatal episodes;
• 0.5–6.5% for major episodes;
• 6.2–21.8% for minor bleeding.

Differences in the adopted classification of bleeding events and in the composition of the cohorts studied may explain the wide range of bleeding rates reported in clinical studies. Although the criteria for major bleeding were different in different studies, in all studies the most consistent risk factors for major bleeding were:
• intensity of anticoagulation;
• age; and
• the first 90 days of treatment.
An INR ≥ 4.5 increases the risk of hemorrhage sixfold and the risk of major hemorrhage increases by 42% for each one point increase in INR.

The intended intensity, and especially the actually achieved intensity of anticoagulation, is the major determinant of anticoagulation-induced bleeding. In prospective observational studies, such as the Italian ISCOAT study, the following have been shown:

• The lowest rate of bleeding is associated with INR results in the 2.0–2.9 INR range.

• Many bleeding events occur at a very low anticoagulation intensity (< 2.0 INR).

• The increase in bleeding incidence becomes exponential for INR values > 4.5. The risk of bleeding for INR values > 7.0 is 40 times greater than that associated with an INR of 2.0–2.9 and 20 times greater than that when the INR is 3.0–4.4.

• The risk of death in subjects on oral anticoagulation is strongly related to the INR level, with a minimum risk at 2.2 INR.

• High INR values are associated with an excess mortality: for one unit INR increase above 2.5 there is a twofold risk increase.

Intracranial hemorrhage

Intracranial hemorrhage (Fig. 13.2) has a high mortality and morbidity. The rate of intracranial hemorrhage in randomized trials of atrial fibrillation and postmyocardial infarction was 0.3%, while it was 0.5–0.6% in observational studies of patients on OACs for arterial and venous thromboembolic indications. The rate of intracranial bleeding was

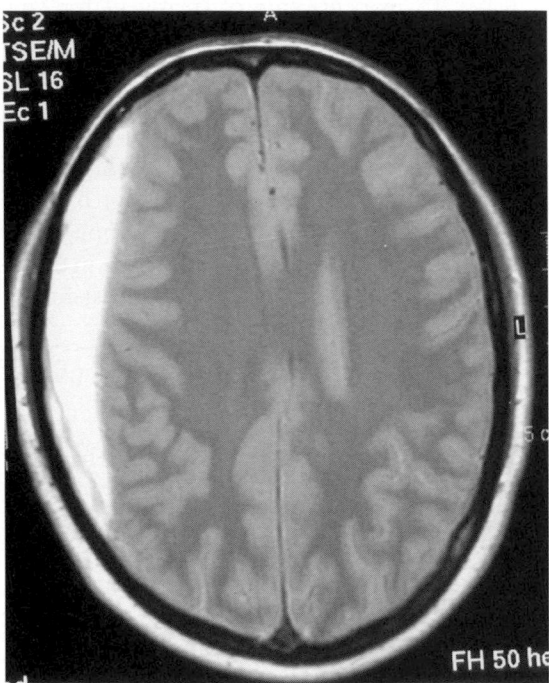

Figure 13.2 Subdural hematoma in a patient on warfarin.

1.15 per 100 patient-years in a meta-analysis evaluating studies in patients taking oral anticoagulant therapy for venous thromboembolism.

Risk factors for intracranial bleeding are:

• Older age.

• Intensity of anticoagulation. The risk increases fourfold for each unit increase in the prothrombin time ratio, and is particularly high for INR > 4.0.

• Ischemic cerebrovascular disease.

• Hypertension.

Various neurologic pathologies such as arterial vasculopathies predispose to intracerebral bleeding. Leukoaraiosis defines a diffuse white matter abnormality seen on computed tomography or magnetic resonance and a dose–response relationship between such abnormality and intracranial hemorrhage has been demonstrated. Amyloid angiopathy increases with age and is associated with asymptomatic microhemorrhages and with spontaneous lobar intracerebral hemorrhage in the elderly. This vasculopathy is a contributing factor to intracranial hemorrhage related to oral anticoagulation.

Extracranial hemorrhage

The rate of major extracranial hemorrhage in randomized trials of patients with atrial fibrillation and postmyocardial infarction was between 0.4 and 1.4% per year. It was 0.9–2.0% per year in observational studies of patients on OACs for arterial and venous thromboembolic indications.

Management of over-anticoagulation and bleeding

Reversal of anticoagulation

Temporary withdrawal of coumarin drug administration

The coumarin drugs have very different half-lives: acenocoumarol has the shortest, phenprocoumon the longest, and warfarin is in between.

Discontinuing coumarin drug intake will result in a slow reversal of anticoagulation, proportional to their half-lives. The majority of over-anticoagulated patients (INR > 4.5) will take 3 days to return to the therapeutic range. For subjects already within the therapeutic range, it will take 3–5 days for the anticoagulation to be completely reversed.

Temporary withdrawal of coumarin administration alone is useful in over-anticoagulated patients, especially if they are treated with acenocoumarol, are at low risk of bleeding and in those anticoagulated patients who are due to undergo elective surgery. This option treatment *cannot* be used alone in patients who are actively bleeding because of the long period necessary for the anticoagulation to be reversed.

Vitamin K administration

Administration of vitamin K (phytonadione) is the recommended mode of reversing the effects of coumarin drugs. However, a patient's response to vitamin K varies, depending on the pretreatment INR value, the route of administration and the dose used. Vitamin K can be administered:
- intravenously;
- orally; or
- subcutaneously.

The intramuscular route is *not* recommended because of irregular, unpredictable absorption and the risk of intramuscular hematoma.

It has been shown that higher doses and longer reversion times are needed with subcutaneous administration when compared with intravenous and oral administration. Vitamin K can be administered intravenously as a slow injection or infused in 5% glucose solution. Intravenous administration can cause anaphylaxis; however, this risk is much lower with the new vitamin K preparation which is stabilized with a mixed micelle vehicle (Konakion® MM) instead of castor oil (Konakion®).

Vitamin K administration in anticoagulated patients is indicated in:
- cases of excessive over-anticoagulation, as recommended by the Seventh Consensus Conference of the American College of Chest Physicians, especially in patients at higher bleeding risk;
- patients who need to undergo invasive procedures that require an INR value < 1.5; and
- cases with active major bleeding.

The oral route

In over-anticoagulated patients oral vitamin K was demonstrated to be much more effective than placebo in correcting excessive INRs. Small amounts of vitamin K given orally can produce a major correction in the INR at 24 h, but the correction is insufficient at 4 h or for cases of major bleeding.

In patients on acenocoumarol, administration of low-dose oral vitamin K offers no advantage to simple omission of a single dose of the drug and may result in an excessive risk of under-anticoagulation.

The intravenous route

Intravenous vitamin K administration leads to an effective reversal of anticoagulation within 6–8 h, and is therefore the **treatment of choice in life-threatening bleeding**. Intravenous vitamin K doses ranging between 0.1 and 3 mg have been shown to effectively reduce very high INR values in the absence of life-threatening bleeding. Higher doses may frequently result in subtherapeutic INR.

Fresh frozen plasma

Administration of fresh frozen plasma (FFP) is intended to correct the deficiency of factors II, VII, IX and X resulting from the effect of coumarin drugs. The recommended FFP dose for warfarin reversal is 15 mL/kg body weight. However, several factors should be considered that **limit the value of FFP** as the best replacement treatment in this indication:
- Large FFP volumes (e.g. approximately 1000 mL for an adult weighing 70 kg) are needed to be given rapidly to replace vitamin K-dependent factors and this may be harmful, especially in patients with compromised cardiovascular conditions.
- FFP may not be virally inactivated and therefore a potential risk of viral infection cannot be excluded.
- The time needed to prepare the plasma, which is stored frozen at −20°C, is usually a cause of delay before transfusion.
- It has been shown that administration of the recommended dose of FFP fails to significantly correct the coumarin-induced coagulopathy, especially for persistently low factor IX levels.

Prothrombin complex concentrates

Concentrates of factors II, VII, IX and X, called prothrombin complex concentrates (PCCs), are available and are highly effective in replacing clotting factors that are deficient in anticoagulated patients. A dose of 30 U/kg is usually effective. The precise optimal dose of PCC remains to be defined but the following have been suggested:

- 25 U/kg for patients with an INR of 2.0–3.9.
- 35 U/kg for an INR of > 4.0.

Potential adverse effects of PCC administration are viral infection and thrombogenicity. Despite all the precautions taken (selection of donors as well as specific viral inactivation procedures), an extremely small risk of viral infection can still persist. Thrombotic events have been reported after PCC transfusion in anticoagulated patients; however, this risk is also small, especially in preparations with added antithrombin and heparin.

The potential risks of PCC indicate that their use should be reserved for patients with major bleeding, especially to those with **intracranial hemorrhage in whom an immediate correction of the coagulopathy is highly recommended.**

Clinical management of over-anticoagulation and bleeding

An unexpected condition of over-anticoagulation is not a rare finding during treatment with OACs. The incidence rate of an INR ≥ 6.0 was found to be as high as 7.8 in 10,000 treatment days in prevalent users and 22.5 in 10,000 treatment days in incident users.

Because it is known that the risk of bleeding increases sharply in association with very high INR values, it is desirable for a patient to spend as little time as possible in a condition of over-anticoagulation. In these cases, the clinical management should be as follows:

- Patients with very high INR values (> 7.0), or with more moderately high INR values but at high risk of bleeding, should receive 1–2 mg vitamin K orally; the INR should be measured the following day and oral vitamin K given again if necessary.
- In patients with an INR of 4.5–6.9, and in those treated with acenocoumarol whatever the INR,

withholding the coumarin drug for 1–2 days followed by a reduction of the weekly dose is usually sufficient.

- All patients with minor bleeding and an INR over the therapeutic range should receive intravenous vitamin K, which will reduce the high INR values within 6–8 h.
- In cases with a major although not life-threatening bleeding, a complete reversal of anticoagulation with intravenous vitamin K is advisable.
- A complete and rapid reversal of anticoagulation is recommended in patients with life-threatening bleeding. PCC infusion will completely correct the coagulopathy within 5–10 min. A dose of 5–10 mg vitamin K should also be administered intravenously.
- Please note the lack of recommendation to use FFP.

Management of patients on oral anticoagulation who require surgery or invasive procedures

There are no universally accepted guidelines for the management of anticoagulated patients requiring surgery or invasive procedures. Clear indications are lacking because of different:

- patients;
- procedures;
- anticoagulant regimens;
- event definition; and
- duration of follow-up;

as well as the absence of randomized clinical trials in this setting.

However, the increasing number of patients undergoing oral anticoagulation demands practical recommendations in spite of the lack of evidence on the efficacy and safety of the recommended procedures.

The general strategy for the management of oral anticoagulation in patients undergoing invasive procedures requires the careful evaluation of three elements:

1 The thromboembolic risk of the individual patient in case of interruption of OAC, in relation to its indications and to the risk of postoperative thromboembolic complications.

2 The bleeding risk of the procedure *per se* and in case anticoagulation is continued.

3 The necessity of alternative anticoagulant drugs (bridging therapy) and their relative efficacy and safety.

The substantial difference between the consequences of major bleeding events and thromboembolic complications should also be taken into account. Permanent disability and death are common after arterial thromboembolism, especially in cases of cerebrovascular events (70–75%), while they are less frequent in cases of venous thromboembolic complications (4–10%) or major postoperative hemorrhage (1–6%).

It is also crucial to consider the attitude of the specialist who performs the procedure, who is generally more concerned about any bleeding resulting from the procedure if oral anticoagulation is continued rather than the risk of thromboembolism if oral anticoagulation is stopped. In the absence of certain indications, a careful evaluation by several specialists is warranted (hematologist, internist, cardiologist, surgeon and anesthesiologist).

There are three possible choices:
1 Continuation of treatment.
2 Temporary discontinuation of therapy without alternative treatment.
3 Temporary discontinuation of therapy with alternative treatment (bridging therapy).

Continuation of oral anticoagulant therapy

In procedures associated with *a low risk of bleeding*, such as traumas of superficial tissues where local hemostatic measures (e.g. pressure, antifibrinolytics, fibrin glue) can be applied, OACs can be continued:
• Punctures and catheterization of superficial veins and arteries (e.g. femoral artery and Seldinger catheter).
• Sternal punctures and bone marrow aspirates.
• Skin biopsies, minor dermatologic surgery, biopsy of mucosa that is easily accessible and explorable (oral cavity, vagina), minor eye surgery.
• Endoscopic examinations without surgery.
• Simple tooth extraction in the absence of infection or surgical incisions. In the latter cases, it is recommended to use local hemostatic agents, suturing of alveolar edges and mouth rinses with a 5% tranexamic acid solution, 4–5 min every 6 h for 5–6 days, combined with antibiotic therapy.

In these cases it is it is advisable to lower the INR to approximately 2 to decrease the hemorrhagic risk without an increase in the thromboembolic risk.

If the expected *risk of bleeding is higher* (e.g. multiple teeth extractions in the presence of infection, closed biopsy, endo-ocular surgery or cataract with retrobulbar anesthetic) and the risk of thromboembolism is not high (in most cases, excluding patients with prosthetic heart valves or cardiac endocavitary thrombosis), OACs can be temporarily reduced, aiming at INR values between 1.5 and 2.

Patients being treated with OAT should be told to avoid, whenever possible, intramuscular injections so to avoid the risk of hematomas (especially if the patient needs many injections).

Temporary discontinuation of oral anticoagulant therapy

This is recommended in cases of trauma to deep tissues not easily accessible to local hemostatic measures:
• major elective surgery, general or specialist;
• explorative cavity punctures (thoracocentesis, paracentesis);
• biopsies of deep tissues (liver, kidney, bone) or mucosa (gastroenteric, respiratory, genital) not accessible; and
• epidural anesthesia.

Preoperative bridging therapy

If the procedure is elective, no immediate reversal of OACs is required and OACs can be discontinued 3–4 days before the procedure (in case of therapeutic INR) as the INR is expected to fall to subtherapeutic values in 3–4 days. The bridging therapy can be commenced 60 h after the last warfarin dose (third morning after last evening dose). The INR should be measured the day before surgery to determine whether it is below 1.5–1.7. If not, 1 mg vitamin K can be given orally and the INR repeated on the day of surgery.

In case of patients at high risk of thromboembolic complications (such as prosthetic heart valves), the goal is to minimize risk by reducing the duration of the bridging therapy to the minimum and by administering bridging therapy for the duration of subtherapeutic INR.

The bridging therapy can be conducted with either unfractionated heparin (subcutaneous or intravenous) when the INR falls below 2.0, bridging therapy can be started with prophylactic unfractionated heparin (5000 units every 8–12 h subcutaneously). Those at very high risk of thromboembolic complications can also be given bridging therapy (previous systemic embolism in atrial fibrillation, prosthetic heart valves, multiple risk factors), adjusted dose heparin (subcutaneous in outpatients or by continuous intravenous infusion in case of hospital admission) can be administered maintaining an APTT value equal to 1.5–2 times the normal value of control.

Bridging therapy can also be administered with low molecular weight heparin:
• subcutaneously as an outpatient in doses recommended for prophylaxis subcutaneously once daily;
• for those at very high risk of thombosis at treatment levels once (150–200 U/kg) or twice (100 U/kg) daily;
• for 2–3 days preoperatively.

Drug administration immediately prior to surgery must be avoided in these cases:
• Subcutaneous unfractionated heparin should be discontinued 12 h before surgery.
• Intravenous heparin should be discontinued 6 h before surgery.
• Low molecular weight heparin should be discontinued no less than 8–10 h at prophylaxis dose or 18 h preoperatively with treatment doses, with an additional 6 h interval in case of planned neuroaxial anesthesia.

In venous thromboembolism, the risk of recurrence is the highest in the first month after the acute event (40%). As a result, invasive procedures should be deferred, if possible, for at least 1 month and preferably 3 months after the acute event. If surgery is necessary within 2 weeks from an acute event, patients should have a vena cava filter inserted preoperatively or intraoperatively.

Postoperative management of anticoagulation

OACs may be resumed only after evaluating each case very carefully as a function of the time needed for tissues to heal and in the absence of bleeding complications.

Intravenous heparin should be resumed after 12 h postoperatively at a rate of no more than 18 U/kg and it has the advantage of rapid elimination if discontinued and of neutralization with protamine. If subcutaneous low molecular weight heparin is preferred, twice daily doses are recommended, started 24 h postoperatively and only after hemostasis has been achieved. In patients with a very high bleeding risk (e.g. after neurosurgery or prostatectomy) heparin is resumed only after clinical evaluation and in general after at least 48–72 h. OACs can be resumed postoperatively as soon as the patients can take solid foods, overlapping with heparin until an INR > 2 is obtained for two consecutive days. In case of emergency surgery, oral anticoagulation must be reversed as soon as possible.

Spinal or epidural anesthesia

Regional anesthesia in association with perioperative prophylaxis or heparin therapy is safe and efficacious with an adequate selection of patient and anesthesiologic technique. There are no controlled studies evaluating the risk of spinal hematoma in the course of therapy or with heparin prophylaxis.

The following can be suggested with intravenous (IV) or subcutaneous (SC) unfractionated heparin:
• Perform the spinal puncture or the positioning of the catheter at least 1 h before starting heparin IV, or more than 4 h after the suspension of the heparin IV and after the administration of the heparin SC.
• Maintain APTT value not more than 1.5 times the control value.
• Remove the catheter only after normalization of the APTT.

Suggestions for the use of low molecular weight heparins:
• to perform spinal puncture or positioning of the catheter 10–12 h after the last dose;
• to remove the catheter at least 10–12 h after the last dose and administer the successive dose, at least 2 h after removal.

In any case it must be remembered·

- Do not administer drugs that interfere with the hemostasis.
- Defer the operation in the presence of hematic spinal tap.
- Constant patient surveillance is essential for the onset of signs or symptoms of medullary compression (sphincteric alterations, progression of paresthesia and limb weakness).
- In the case of spinal hematoma, emergency decompressive laminectomy is mandatory (< 6 h from the onset of the symptoms).

Cataract surgery

With modern techniques, which rely on limited incision of the cornea (non-vascularized tissue), the risk of bleeding from surgery itself is practically null. Possible bleeding complications are linked to the type of anesthesia.

Cases have been reported of retro- and peribulbar hematomas in patients on OACs following retro- and peribulbar anesthesia. Despite the lack of exact data on the incidence of these complications, it should be borne in mind that retro- and peribulbar anesthesia requires normal blood hemostasis and hence discontinuation of OACs, so it should be contraindicated in patients on OACs in whom the thrombotic risk following a suspension of treatment is high. In contrast, cataract surgery can be performed without anticoagulant suspension in all those subjects in whom a topical or general anesthesia can be used.

Evaluating the risk–benefit and cost–benefit ratios of the different options (e.g. surgery without OACs suspension vs. surgery with retrobulbar anesthesia and OACs suspension) should be carried out in each patient on the basis of a general consideration of the risk factors (thrombotic and hemorrhagic).

Further reading

Andrew M, David M, Adams M, *et al.* Venous thromboembolic complications (VTE) in children: first analyses of the Canadian registry of VTE. *Blood* 1994;**83**:1251–7.

Ansell J, Hirsh J, Poller L, *et al.* The pharmacology and management of the vitamin K antagonists. The seventh ACCP Conference on Antithrombotic and Thrombolytic Therapy. *Chest* 2004;**126**:204S–233S.

Chiquette E, Amato MG, Bussey HI. Comparison of an anticoagulation clinic with usual medical care: anticoagulation control, patient outcomes, and health care costs. *Arch Intern Med* 1998;**158**:1641–7.

Crowther MA, Ginsberg JB, Kearon C, *et al.* A randomized trial comparing 5-mg and 10-mg warfarin loading doses. *Arch Intern Med* 1999;**159**:46–8.

Dunn AS, Turpie AG. Perioperative management of patients receiving oral anticoagulants: a systematic review. *Arch Intern Med* 2003;**163**:901–8.

Fennerty A, Dolben J, Thomas P, *et al.* Flexible induction dose regimen for warfarin and prediction of maintenance dose. *British Medical Journal* 1984;**288**:1268–70.

Ginsberg JS, Hirsh J. Use of antithrombotic agents during pregnancy. *Chest* 1998;**114**:S524–30.

Hirsh J, Dalen JE, Anderson DR, *et al.* Oral anticoagulants: mechanism of action, clinical effectiveness, and optimal therapeutic range. *Chest* 2001;**119**:8–21S.

Hylek E. Complications of oral anticoagulant therapy (bleeding and non-bleeding; rates and risk factors. *Semin Vasc Med* 2003;**3**:271–8.

Kearon C. Management of anticoagulation in patients requiring invasive procedures. *Semin Vasc Med* 2003;**3**:285–93.

Kearon C, Hirsh J. Current concepts: management of anticoagulation before and after elective surgery. *N Engl J Med* 1997;**336**:1506–11.

Kovacs MJ, Rodger M, Anderson DR, *et al.* Comparison of 10-mg and 5-mg warfarin initiation nomograms together with low-molecular-weight heparin for outpatient treatment of acute venous thromboembolism: a randomized, double-blind, controlled trial. *Ann Intern Med* 2003;**138**:714–9.

Linkins LA, Choi PT, Douketis JD. Clinical impact of bleeding in patients taking oral anticoagulant therapy for venous thromboembolism: a meta-analysis. *Ann Intern Med* 2003;**139**:893–900.

Makris M, Watson HG. The management of coumarin-induced over-anticoagulation. *Br J Haematol* 2001;**114**:271–80.

Palareti G, Leali N, Coccheri S, *et al.* Bleeding complications of oral anticoagulant treatment: an inception–cohort, prospective collaborative study (ISCOAT). Italian Study on Complications of Oral Anticoagulant Therapy. *Lancet* 1996;**348**:423–8.

Poller L, Shiach CR, MacCallum PK, *et al.* Multicentre randomised study of computerised anticoagulant dosage. *Lancet* 1998;**352**:1505–9.

Chapter 14
Antiphospholipid syndrome

Henry G. Watson

Introduction

The antiphospholipid syndrome (APS) is an acquired prothrombotic or thrombophilic state. An association of antiphospholipid antibodies with a variety of disorders has been made since the first report in patients with systemic lupus erythematosus (SLE) and the clinicopathological criteria for the diagnosis of APS has been agreed internationally. In spite of this, our understanding of the pathogenesis of the condition is limited, particularly with respect to the complications of pregnancy. Also, the laboratory-based diagnosis is a subject of serious concern with disappointing quality assurance data for all tests. In addition, while there are good data to inform on the management of venous thromboembolism, the same is not true for arterial thrombosis. Finally, there are conflicting views on the treatment of women with adverse pregnancy outcome attributable to APS.

Definition of antiphospholipid syndrome

The antiphospholipid syndrome describes a clinicopathologic entity. APS is an acquired prothrombotic state, which probably has an immune-mediated pathogenesis and its diagnosis requires the coexistence of clinical manifestations (thrombosis or adverse pregnancy outcome) with laboratory evidence of antiphospholipid antibodies (Table 14.1).

A variety of other clinical abnormalities, which are frequently observed in association with antiphospholipid antibodies, are not included in the internationally agreed definition of APS. The most common of these are thrombocytopenia and livedo reticularis, which are not uncommonly found in patients who do otherwise fulfill the criteria for APS (Table 14.2). Identification of these other conditions associated should lead to consideration of a diagnosis of APS. It is not clear whether thrombo-

Table 14.1 Diagnostic criteria for antiphospholipid syndrome.

Clinical criteria	Laboratory criteria
Thrombosis Venous, arterial or small vessel thrombosis involving any organ or tissue	IgG or IgM anticardiolipin antibodies at moderate or high titer and/or lupus anticoagulant
Pregnancy Unexplained death of a morphologically normal fetus at or after 10 weeks' gestation Three or more consecutive unexplained abortions before 10 weeks' gestation Severe pre-eclampsia before 34 weeks' gestation	

To fulfill the diagnosis of antiphospholipid syndrome there must be at least one clinical and one laboratory criterion present. The detection of antiphospholipid antibodies must have been performed on two occasions at least 6 weeks apart.

Table 14.2 Some conditions associated with antiphospholipid antibodies but not included in the definition of antiphospholipid syndrome.

Thrombocytopenia
Livedo reticularis
Allograft failure
Transverse myelopathy
Chorea
Multifocal central nervous system syndrome resembling multiple
    sclerosis
Skin necrosis
Pulmonary hypertension
Sensorineural deafness

sis is implicated in the pathogenesis of these conditions and the role of antithrombotic medicines is even less clear.

Clinical features of antiphospholipid syndrome

The main clinical presentation of APS is either with thrombosis or with pregnancy failure. However, the condition is heterogeneous (as are the implicated antibodies) and most individuals do not suffer from all the clinical features of the syndrome. Interestingly, while a combination of venous and arterial thrombotic events may predate the development of a history of pregnancy failure in some women, especially those with SLE, most women who present with adverse pregnancy outcome tend to have this as a sole manifestation.

Thrombosis

Thrombosis may involve both the arterial and the venous systems. The most common presentation is with lower limb deep vein thrombosis, sometimes with clinically significant pulmonary embolus. Other sites for venous thrombosis such as cerebral vein, axillary and subclavian vein, and intrabdominal veins including the portal, hepatic and mesenteric veins are less common but well recognized in APS. Patients tend to be young individuals with unprovoked venous thromboembolism, thrombosis at unusual sites and an absence of a family history of thrombophilia.

Stroke and transient cerebral ischemia are the most common presentations of arterial thrombosis in APS. Myocardial infarction appears rare, although the reason for this is not clear. Embolic thrombus from sterile endocarditis and cardiac valve vegetations are also described.

Microvascular thrombosis is uncommon but is described in the extremely rare "catastrophic antiphospholipid syndrome" that presents with multiorgan failure and which usually progresses unabated in spite of all forms of therapy.

Pregnancy failure

This is now the most common presentation that results in a diagnosis of APS being made. This is in part because of the wish (and pressure) to investigate women who are distressed by this presentation. Recurrent early fetal loss is most commonly seen, although otherwise unexplained fetal death after the first trimester and severe pre-eclampsia before 34 weeks are also recognized features.

The emotive nature of these cases may result in the inappropriate investigation of women with only one or two early abortions, which can result in a chance finding of an innocent antiphospholipid antibody. Having detected antiphospholipid antibodies in these women who do not fulfill the APS criteria, clinicians find it difficult to withhold treatment, resulting in some women spending the whole of subsequent pregnancies on aspirin and heparin, based on very little evidence.

Most proponents of this approach argue that waiting for a third early loss in these women is inappropriate and add that the therapy has so few side-effects that this is not an issue. However, side-effects, although few, are seen and the costs of clinic time and drugs are significant. This practice also converts normal women into patients for the duration of their pregnancy while skewing the perception of benefit for intervention.

Antiphospholipid antibodies

These are a heterogeneous group of antibodies, which are detected because of their capacity to react with phospholipid either in phospholipid-dependent coagulation assays or bound to enzyme-linked immunosorbent assay (ELISA) plates: lupus anticoagulants or anticardiolipin antibodies, respectively.

The earliest descriptions of antiphospholipid antibodies were in individuals with SLE who had false-positive tests for syphilis. Further investigation of these patients indicated that they had circulating antibodies that were capable of binding to the negatively charged phospholipid, cardiolipin. This gave rise to the nomenclature *anticardiolipin antibodies*.

About the same time it was noted that some subjects with SLE had prolonged blood-clotting times in *in vitro* test systems but had no evidence of a bleeding diathesis. The prolonged clotting in phospholipid-dependent tests could not be reversed by addition of normal plasma, indicating the presence of an inhibitor, the so-called *lupus anticoagulant*.

Paradoxically, the presence of the lupus anticoagulant was associated with an increased risk of thrombosis in patients with SLE, and when it became apparent that the presence of either of these antibodies was associated with an increased thrombosis risk the concept of an acquired prothrombotic or thrombophilic state was proposed.

Antiphospholipid antibodies with features of APS may be found either in isolation as a *primary antiphospholipid syndrome* or in association with SLE and other autoimmune conditions such as Sjögren syndrome as a *secondary antiphospholipid syndrome*.

Although they are called antiphospholipid antibodies, it is now clear that the antigenic targets for most of these antibodies are not phospholipid *per se* but instead are proteins that bind to phospholipid. The best known of these is β_2-glycoprotein 1, a circulating protein of unknown function which avidly binds negatively charged phospholipid. Other antigen targets for antiphospholipid antibodies include prothrombin, factor XI, protein C and annexin V, all proteins involved in hemostatic pathways that might be relevant in explaining the thrombotic complications associated with these antibodies. In response to these findings, ELISA assays that have β_2-glycoprotein 1 and prothrombin as antigen are now commercially available.

Despite this knowledge, the pathogenesis of thrombosis and pregnancy failure in APS remains unclear. Laboratory findings combined with the outcome of clinical studies indicate that the processes underlying thrombosis are caused by a prothrombotic state with little evidence that inflammation contributes significantly to the process. No single mechanism has been shown to underlie the prothrombotic tendency and this is perhaps not surprising given the varied sites of thrombosis and the range of target antigens for antiphospholipid antibodies.

Whether antiphospholipid antibodies are indeed directly pathogenic is debated. Laboratory experiments have assessed the effects of antiphospholipid antibodies on many of the processes involved in hemostasis, thrombosis, inflammation and fibrinolysis.

There are data to support that antiphospholipid antibodies may induce tissue factor expression by monocytes, inhibit the function of the natural anticoagulants activated protein C and protein S, induce endothelial cell apoptosis and induce platelet activation by binding via the Fc receptor. All, none or, more likely, a combination of these mechanisms may contribute to the disease process.

The pathogenesis of pregnancy failure in APS is even more difficult to explain. Knowledge of the possible prothrombotic mechanisms has led to the inference that placental ischemia (see Plate 7, facing p. 121) is the main mechanism resulting in pregnancy failure in APS. The evidence from clinical studies suggesting improved outcome in patients treated with antithrombotic medicines such as heparin and aspirin is felt by many to support this hypothesis. However, overt placental ischemia is rare and the observation that the most common manifestation of APS in pregnancy is abortion before 10 weeks (i.e. prior to development of the placental circulation) suggests that other mechanisms must contribute. Antiphospholipid antibodies have been shown to inhibit trophoblastic proliferation and spiral artery invasion *in vitro*. Interestingly, both these effects may be inhibited by heparin, which suggests that at least part of any benefit for heparin may relate to improved implantation.

Recent work has suggested that antiphospholipid antibodies may act by displacing the natural anticoagulant annexin V from endothelial cell surfaces, resulting in a procoagulant state. However, as normal expression of annexin V has been demonstrated in affected pregnancies, the importance of these observations remains unclear.

Diagnosis of antiphospholipid syndrome

APS is a clinicopathologic entity, which depends upon the identification of a clinical diagnosis combined with demonstration of appropriate antiphospholipid antibodies (Table 14.1). Although criteria for diagnosis have been internationally agreed, the diagnosis of APS is still complicated by two main problems:

1 Many antiphospholipid antibodies are non-pathological and are not associated with APS.

2 The standardization of assays for anticardiolipin and lupus anticoagulant is unfortunately very poor.

Transient and non-pathological antiphospholipid antibodies

Both lupus anticoagulants and anticardiolipin antibodies, alone or together, are found in a significant number of normal subjects. Like the finding of a positive direct antiglobulin test in approximately 1 in 10,000 blood donors, the finding is of little consequence to the individual but it does generate further investigation and anxiety in the patient if handled badly. One common source of this type of scenario is in the recruitment of healthy ward and laboratory personnel as normal controls. On some occasions, the antiphospholipid antibody is transient but persistent high-titer anticardiolipin antibodies and strong positive lupus anticoagulants are not uncommon. Some series report the finding of antiphospholipid antibodies, more often anticardiolipin, in up to 5% of normal subjects.

Perhaps the most common cause of transient antiphospholipid antibodies is infection. This is mostly seen seen following viral infection but may complicate bacterial and parasitic infections also. Although these antibodies are not typically associated with significant disease, purpura fulminans resulting from acquired protein S deficiency is a well-documented complication of varicella infec-

Table 14.3 Infections associated with antiphospholipid antibodies.

Viral
Human immunodeficiency virus
Hepatitis C
Varicella

Bacterial
Helicobacter pylori
Syphilis
Leprosy
Leptospirosis

Parasitic
Malaria
Leishmaniasis

tion in children. Some infections such as HIV, hepatitis C, leprosy, syphilis, leptospirosis, leishmaniasis and malaria are associated with persistent antiphospholipid antibodies. These are rarely linked with the development of clinical features of APS (Table 14.3).

The use of certain common drugs is also associated with the development of antiphospholipid antibodies. The association with chlorpromazine is the best documented and although these antibodies are not typically said to be associated with the development of thrombosis it may be that this underlies the recent reported association of psychoactive drugs with an increased risk of venous thromboembolism.

Laboratory assays

Correct diagnosis of APS is ultimately dependent on the availability of accurate diagnostic assays. A vast amount of work has been carried out to try to standardize assays for anticardiolipin and lupus anticoagulant. Although internationally agreed guidelines have been drawn up to address this, the intricacies of the assays and the plethora of non-standardized reagents available make this a difficult area. Summarized below are the key features that require attention in detecting antiphospholipid antibodies.

Lupus anticoagulants

The Scientific and Standardization Committee of the International Society of Thrombosis and Hemostasis recommends that the laboratory diagnosis of lupus anticoagulants (LA) should be carried out on double-centrifuged plasma following a four-step procedure adhering to these principles:

1 Prolongation of a phospholipid-dependent coagulation test.
2 Evidence of inhibitory activity on mixing tests.
3 Evidence of phospholipid dependence.
4 Lack of specificity for any one coagulation factor.

This process allows the detection of inhibitory activity in the plasma and then facilitates differentiation of LA from specific inhibitors of coagulation, which are more rare. As the management of patients with antiphospholipid antibodies often involves antithrombotic medication, while patients with acquired inhibitors of coagulation harbour an often life-threatening bleeding diathesis, differentiation is of paramount importance.

Some laboratories perform LA screening tests such as a dilute prothrombin time and activated partial thromboplastin time (APTT) tests using reagents with a high sensitivity to LA. Others screen requests for clinical detail and perform fewer, more specific tests such as dilute Russell viper venom time (dRVVT) or kaolin clotting time (KCT) to investigate suspected cases.

It is widely agreed that the use of more than one coagulation based test is essential to detect LA. Mixing studies are performed to demonstrate inhibitor activity in test plasma. Errors arising in the mixing procedure relate to the quality of the normal plasma, particularly its platelet content, and to the level of dilution employed. Platelet contamination, even to levels as low as $1000/\mu L$, can result in quenching of the inhibitory effect and therefore to a false-negative result.

Confirmation of the phospholipid dependence of the inhibitor is assessed by adding excess phospholipid to the test system. The rationale for this is that the excess phospholipid neutralizes or bypasses the LA effect. Platelet membrane particles or purer forms of phospholipid may be used for this purpose.

Platelet membrane preparations suffer from significant batch-to-batch variability that does not lend itself to standardization.

Specific coagulation factor assays may help to confirm the nature of an inhibitor. They are probably indicated when there is concern about a bleeding diathesis or when there is discordance in the earlier stages of detecting a LA. Simultaneous reduction of more than one coagulation factor may indicate the presence of a LA.

When using this method to detect a LA, factor assays should be performed at numerous plasma dilutions. Unlike the situation where a specific coagulation factor is present, the apparent coagulation factor activity rises with greater dilution in the presence of a LA; that is, the assay curves are non-parallel. The results from these assays may vary with different reagents.

Anticardiolipin assays

A great deal of effort has gone towards producing new more specific assays to measure anti-β_2-glycoprotein 1 and anti-prothrombin activity in the hope that this would improve diagnostic accuracy. In addition, an international standard for units to measure anticardiolipin antibodies and terminology for the reporting of results has been developed. However, in spite of this, problems in measuring and interpreting anticardiolipin assays persist.

Significant numbers of patients have low-titer anticardiolipin antibodies and in an attempt to address this, the diagnostic criteria state that to fulfill a diagnosis of APS patients must have moderate or high titers of antibody. However, this does not resolve all clinical scenarios. Furthermore, although assay performance has been improved by these changes, inter-assay comparability is still poor and it appears that the new specific assays may be no more sensitive for the diagnosis of APS than standard anticardiolipin and lupus anticoagulant tests.

Quality assurance

Quality assurance is a major issue for laboratories attempting to identify and quantify antiphospholipid antibodies. Although national and international standards and guidelines have been prepared (and are adhered to), recent quality assurance exercises still indicate that there are major problems.

A recent European Concerted Action on Thrombophilia (ECAT) survey indicated that plasma containing a 10 Bethesda unit inhibitor of factor VIII was wrongly identified as a LA in approximately 20% of 128 participating laboratories.

Likewise, a quality assurance exercise report on detection of anticardiolipin antibodies indicated an interlaboratory coefficient of variation of more than 50% in 74% of tests performed, leaving the authors to conclude that in the majority of cases the laboratories could not decide whether a sample was positive or negative.

Management of antiphospholipid syndrome

Thrombosis

The initial management of venous or arterial thrombosis in a patient with APS is, on the whole, no different to the management applied to similar cases without APS. Instead of discussing these in detail it is more relevant to discuss issues that are specific to management of patients with APS. These relate to:

- choice of antithrombotic medication;
- intensity and duration of anticoagulation; and
- monitoring of anticoagulants.

Patients presenting with a first episode of unprovoked deep vein thrombosis or pulmonary embolus have a risk of thrombosis recurrence of approximately 10% per annum, which seems to plateau after 3 years. Based on these data and on considering the risks of life-threatening or fatal hemorrhage on warfarin at 1% and 0.25–0.5%, respectively, most physicians treat these cases with warfarin for 6 months at an international normalized ratio (INR) target of 2.5. In contrast, the reported rates of recurrence of thrombosis in patients with APS is as high as 30–50% per annum and as a result many physicians offer long-term anticoagulation after a first unprovoked event in these cases.

Previous retrospective data suggested that an INR target of 3.5 provided better thromboprophylaxis than a target of 2.5, but recent prospective data from Crowther *et al.* indicate that, certainly for prevention of recurrence of venous thromboembolism, an INR target of 2.5 is optimal.

In all of these cases, the likely benefit and risk to the patient has to be considered and additional risk factors for bleeding on anticoagulants such as increasing age, anemia, previous stroke, history of gastrointestinal bleeding and diabetes mellitus have to be considered.

For patients who present with arterial thrombosis as a manifestation of APS there are differences in approach to management. In the UK, in patients in whom there is no source of cardioembolic stroke such as valvular heart disease or atrial fibrillation, it is usual to offer antiplatelet therapy with aspirin or clopidogrel to patients with ischemic stroke or transient cerebral ischemia. This strategy is probably *not appropriate* for patients with APS. Most patients should be considered for warfarin and, in the absence of good data to indicate a benefit for more intense anticoagulation, should maintain an INR target of 2.5.

The final issue for consideration is of the effect of lupus anticoagulants on monitoring of anticoagulation. Although the use of unfractionated heparin has been largely superseded by low molecular weight heparins, where the former is still used there may be problems monitoring the APTT. Solutions to this are to utilize an APTT reagent that is not sensitive to LA or to use a thrombin time for heparin monitoring. A few lupus anticoagulants produce significant prolongation of the prothrombin time. If this does occur, using a low ISI thromboplastin, which has been locally calibrated prior to use, can usually circumvent it.

Although there is little experience of its use in APS, the oral direct thrombin inhibitor Ximelagatran, which requires no laboratory monitoring of its anticoagulant effect, shows significant promise as an advance in anticoagulant therapy.

Pregnancy failure

Although pregnancy failure is often the only manifestation of disease in patients with primary APS and although the evidence for a prothrombotic state is still not overwhelming, the main focus of therapy over the past 10 years has been to assess the effects of antithrombotic medication. Studies of immunosuppression using prednisolone have shown deleterious effects on pregnancy outcome for both mother and child and studies into the benefit of intravenous immunoglobulin are ongoing. As such, the mainstay of therapy for those women who fulfill the criteria for APS consists of intensive antenatal care combined with aspirin with or without low-dose heparin.

Since 1997, when Rai *et al.* published a significant study of interventions in APS, there has been a trend towards the combined use of low-dose aspirin and heparin in pregnant women with APS. However, two further studies at least challenge the validity of these conclusions:

1 In a randomized study of 98 subjects, the outcomes for aspirin alone were the same as for aspirin and heparin in combination (pregnancy failure rates 28% vs. 22%).

2 A second study reported similar outcomes for patients randomized to supportive care only or to aspirin and supportive care (pregnancy failure rates 15% vs. 20%).

In comparison with these data, the earlier studies, which purported to demonstrate a benefit for combined heparin and aspirin, reported pregnancy failure rates for the aspirin only groups of approximately 60%.

In clinical practice it may be difficult to convince women with a history of pregnancy loss of the validity of treating only those who fulfill the diagnostic criteria and for those who present with an Internet search in hand discouraging heparin may be difficult.

Further reading

Arnout J. Antiphospholipid syndrome: diagnostic aspects of lupus anticoagulants. *Thromb Haemost* 2001;**86**:83–91.

Creagh MD, Malia RG, Cooper SM, Smith AR, Duncan SL, Greaves M. Screening for lupus anticoagulant and anticardiolipin antibodies in women with fetal loss. *J Clin Pathol* 1991;**44**:45–7.

Crowther MA, Ginsberg JS, Julian J, *et al*. A comparison of two intensities of warfarin for the prevention of recurrent thrombosis in patients with the antiphospholipid antibody syndrome. *N Engl J Med* 2003;**349**:1133–8.

Greaves M, Cohen H, Machin SJ, Mackie I. Guidelines on the investigation and management of the antiphospholipid syndrome. *Br J Haematol* 2000;**109**:704–15.

Levine JS, Branch DW, Raunch J. The antiphospholipid syndrome. *N Engl J Med* 2002;**346**:752–63.

Rai R, Cohen H, Dave M, Regan L. Randomized controlled trial of aspirin and aspirin plus heparin in pregnant women with recurrent miscarriage associated with phospholipid antibodies (or antiphospholipid antibodies). *BMJ* 1997;**314**:253–7.

Wilson WA, Gharavi AE, Koike T, *et al*. International consensus statement on preliminary classification criteria for definite antiphospholipid syndrome: report of an international workshop. *Arthritis Rheum* 1999;**42**:1309–11.

Part 3

The clinical interface

Chapter 15
Obstetrics

Isobel D. Walker

Introduction

Thrombosis prevention and management has become the major focus for hematologists with an interest in obstetrics. Normal pregnancy is associated with major changes in all aspects of hemostasis: increasing concentrations of most clotting factors, decreasing levels of some of the natural anticoagulants and reducing fibrinolytic activity so that as pregnancy progresses and during the puerperium the overall balance is shifted towards apparent hypercoagulability. These changes protect the woman from hemorrhage at delivery but increase her risk of thrombosis.

Anticoagulant safety in pregnancy

Coumarins such as warfarin cross the placenta. Maternal coumarin ingestion between 6 and 12 weeks' gestation may result in developmental abnormalities of fetal cartilage and bone. Different series have reported widely varying incidences of warfarin embryopathy but a reasonable estimate of the incidence is approximately 5%. It has been suggested that:
- The risk of warfarin embryopathy is dose-dependent, with an increased risk when the daily warfarin dose exceeds 5 mg.
- Warfarin use later in pregnancy is linked to abnormalities of the fetal central nervous system thought to be the result of repeated cerebral micro-hemorrhages.

In general, coumarins should not be used for the prevention or treatment of venous thromboembolism (VTE) during pregnancy but at present they remain the anticoagulants of choice for the management of pregnant women with mechanical heart valve prostheses. Because of the hemorrhagic risk to both mother and fetus, warfarin should be avoided beyond 36 weeks' gestation.

Neither unfractionated (UF) nor low molecular weight (LMW) heparins nor heparinoids cross the placental barrier. Heparins are devoid of any known teratogenic risk and the fetus is not anticoagulated as a result of maternal heparin use. Systematic reviews suggest that these agents are safe for use in pregnancy. LMW heparins have a number of advantages over UF heparin including better bioavailability with a more predictable dose–response and a longer plasma half-life. The risk of osteoporosis and of heparin-induced thrombocytopenia seems to be lower in patients using LMW heparins than UF heparin. LMW heparins are currently widely used for the prevention and treatment of gestational VTE.

Gestational venous thromboembolism

Venous thromboembolism remains the major cause of maternal mortality and morbidity in the developed world. One large survey recorded an incidence of objectively confirmed VTE of 0.86 in 1000 deliveries. The majority of VTEs occur antenatally. However, when incidences are expressed as events per 1000 years at risk, the risk of deep vein thrombosis (DVT) in the 6 weeks following delivery is approximately threefold higher than the risk of antepartum DVT and the risk of PE about eightfold higher (Table 15.1). Approximately 85% of gestational DVTs are left-sided, compared with only 55% in non-pregnant women. Seventy two percent are ileofemoral. Only 9% are confined to

Table 15.1 Incidence of maternal venous thromboembolism (VTE).

	DVT	PE
Event rate per 1000 deliveries		
Antepartum	0.47	0.10
Postpartum	0.21	0.15
Event rate per 1000 years at risk		
Antepartum (38 weeks)	0.64	0.13
Postpartum (6 weeks)	1.85	1.30

DVT, deep vein thrombosis; PE, pulmonary embolism.

distal calf DVTs. Almost two-thirds of women who have a gestational DVT develop post-thrombotic syndrome.

Thrombophilia and the risk of gestational venous thrombosis

Early studies suggested that, in the absence of anti-coagulant prophylaxis, more than 40% of pregnancies in women with heritable thrombophilia may be complicated by VTE. Because these studies were retrospective reports of events occurring in women from already symptomatic kindred, they were biased and the risk of gestational VTE may have been overestimated. A study of consecutive, unselected women with a history of gestational VTE revealed that:

• For type 1 antithrombin-deficient women, the risk of developing gestational VTE is indeed almost 40% – even in otherwise asymptomatic kindred.

• The incidence of gestational VTE in women with protein C or protein S deficiency is less than that for antithrombin-deficient women.

• The risk of gestational VTE for asymptomatic women heterozygous for factor V (FV) Leiden or for the prothrombin G20210A polymorphism (FII G20210A) is approximately 1 in 300 (Table 15.2).

• The risk is greater in FV Leiden or FII G20210A homozygotes and in women doubly heterozygous for FV Leiden and FII G20210A.

• The contribution of homocysteine levels to the risk of gestational VTE is unclear but the common thermolabile methylene tetrahydrafolate reductase 677 C to T (MTHFR C677T) polymorphism is not associated with an increased risk of gestational thrombosis.

• No formal estimate of the risk of gestational VTE in women with antiphospholipids is available.

Diagnosis of gestational venous thromboembolism

The poor specificity of the clinical diagnosis of DVT and pulmonary embolism (PE) is compounded in pregnancy by the relative frequency of non-thrombotic leg swelling, breathlessness and chest pain in pregnant women.

Objective diagnosis is essential in all women presenting with suspected VTE in pregnancy (in one study of consecutive pregnant patients with clinically suspected DVT, the diagnosis was confirmed on objective testing in less than 10%; in an unpublished study only 2 of 50 pregnant women with clinically suspected PE had the diagnosis confirmed on objective testing). Failure to identify and treat thrombosis places the mother's life at risk. Unnec-

Thrombophilia	Risk of VTE	Estimated OR
Type 1 antithrombin deficiency (quantitative defect)	1 in 4.6 (22.0%)	282
Type 2 antithrombin deficiency (qualitative defect)	1 in 47 (2.10%)	28
Protein C deficiency	1 in 187 (0.50%)	4.4
Factor V Leiden heterozygotes	1 in 401 (0.30%)	3.3
Factor II G20210A heterozygotes	1 in 374 (0.30%)	4.9

Table 15.2 Heritable thrombophilia and risk of gestational VTE.

Based on 93,493 consecutive maternities in two Glasgow hospitals 1985–98.
87 objectively proven VTE; 75 women available for follow-up.

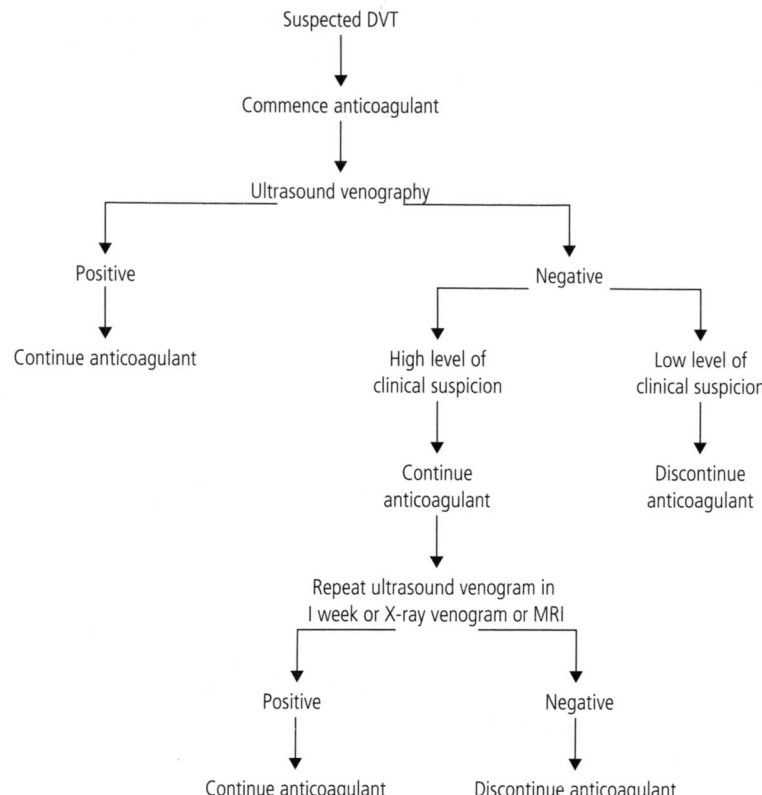

Figure 15.1 Diagnosis of deep vein thrombosis.

essary treatment exposes both the mother and her unborn child to risk.

D-*dimer assays*

These may be unhelpful during pregnancy because normal pregnancy may be associated with elevated D-dimer levels and give many false-positive results; however, a negative result is of value.

Real-time or duplex ultrasound

This is the main diagnostic tool for the confirmation of DVT (Fig. 15.1):
• Patients in whom the presence of a DVT is confirmed should continue anticoagulation.
• Patients with a negative ultrasound and a low level of clinical suspicion do not require continuing anticoagulation.

• Patients with a negative ultrasound but a high pre-test clinical probability of DVT should continue on anticoagulation and have a repeat ultrasound in a week or undergo X-ray venography or magnetic resonance imaging (MRI). If this repeat or extended testing is negative, anticoagulation may be discontinued.

Using V/Q scanning

Patients in whom PE is suspected require a ventilation–perfusion (V/Q) lung scan (Fig. 15.2). Patients with a high or medium probability of PE on V/Q scan should continue anticoagulation. Ultrasound scanning of both legs should be performed in those with a low probability of PE on V/Q scanning. Anticoagulation should be continued in those found to have a DVT.

Women with a low probability V/Q scan, negative bilateral leg ultrasound scans and a low

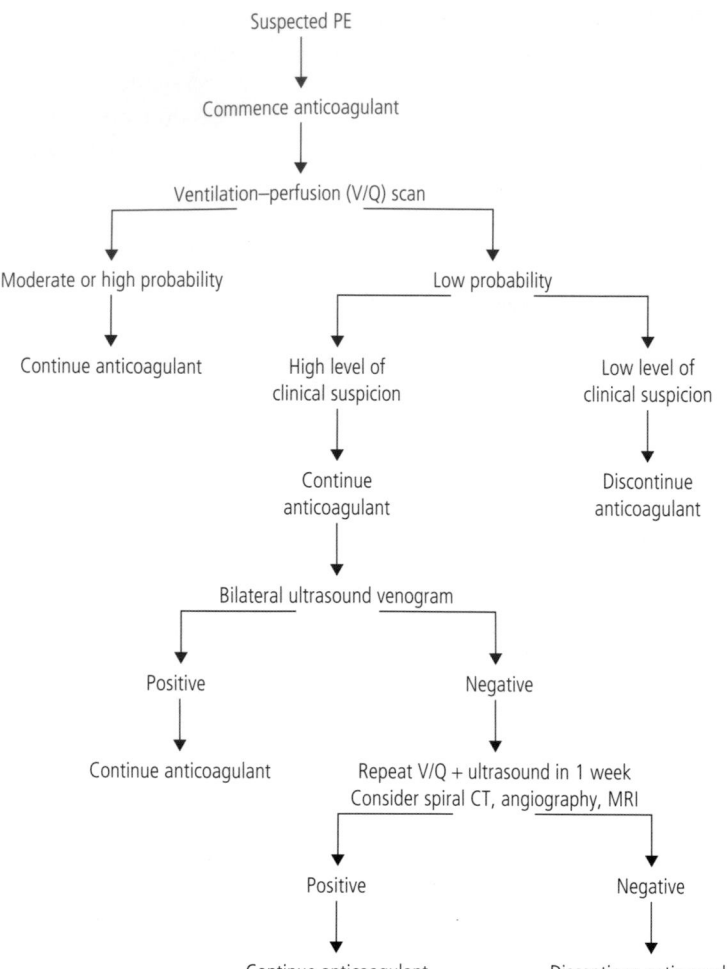

Suspected PE

↓

Commence anticoagulant

↓

Ventilation–perfusion (V/Q) scan

Moderate or high probability   Low probability

Continue anticoagulant

High level of
clinical suspicion   Low level of
clinical suspicion

Continue
anticoagulant   Discontinue
anticoagulant

Bilateral ultrasound venogram

Positive   Negative

Continue anticoagulant   Repeat V/Q + ultrasound in 1 week
Consider spiral CT, angiography, MRI

Positive   Negative

Continue anticoagulant   Discontinue anticoagulant

Figure 15.2 Diagnosis of pulmonary embolism.

pretest clinical probability of PE may discontinue anticoagulation.

In women in whom there is a high pre-test probability of PE but a low probability V/Q scan and negative bilateral leg ultrasound scans, anti-coagulation should continue and the V/Q scan and bilateral leg ultrasounds should be repeated in a week. In these patients and in patients in whom chest X-ray abnormalities make the diagnosis of PE on V/Q scanning difficult, extended investigation including pulmonary angiography, helical computed tomography or MRI should be considered. The radiation doses associated with chest X-ray, V/Q scanning and limited venography are modest and pose a negligible risk to the fetus.

Management of acute venous thromboembolism in pregnancy

In patients presenting with suspected venous thromboembolism

Anticoagulation with UF or LMW heparin should be commenced while awaiting confirmation of the diagnosis – except in the few cases where there is a contraindication to anticoagulation. Some experts suggest continuation of full therapeutic doses of heparin for the remainder of the pregnancy, while others monitor D-dimer levels and if these are low will reduce to prophylactic doses of heparin after 1–2 weeks of therapy. The total duration of anticoagulation should usually be no less than 6 months.

If the thrombotic event occurs very early in pregnancy, anticoagulation should continue for at least 6–12 weeks after delivery. Warfarin can be used after delivery but many women find it more convenient to remain on a LMW heparin for this period. Graduated compression stockings should be used.

Prevention of gestational venous thromboembolism

The common risk factors for gestational VTE are shown in Table 15.3. It has been suggested that, compared with the general obstetric population, women with a history of previous VTE may be at increased risk of a recurrent event in pregnancy. Estimates of the risk of recurrence have varied widely.

In a prospective study of women with a history of a previous objectively confirmed VTE in whom antenatal thromboprophylaxis was withheld, the overall rate of objectively confirmed recurrence during a subsequent pregnancy was 2.4%. There were no recurrent VTEs in women who did not have an identifiable thrombophilia and in whom the previous event was associated with a temporary acquired thrombotic risk factor. The recurrence rate in women who had an identifiable thrombophilia and/or in whom the previous event had occurred apparently spontaneously was 5.9%.

Routine screening of **all** women for thrombophilic defects is **not** justifiable but screening of women who have a history of previous VTE is frequently recommended and many clinicians would also offer thrombophilia screening to women who give a history of proven VTE in a first-degree relative. Patients may be arbitrarily classified as being at highly, moderately or slightly increased risk of gestational VTE (Table 15.4). All women assessed to be at increased risk of gestational VTE should be encouraged to wear graduated compression stockings throughout their pregnancy and puerperium.

High risk of thrombosis

Those with high risk of thrombophilia are:
• Those with type 1 and 2 (reactive site) antithrombin defects, which are associated with a highly increased risk of gestational VTE.
• Patients already committed to long-term anticoagulant prophylaxis for VTE.

These patients merit anticoagulation throughout their entire pregnancy and for at least 6 weeks after delivery. Unfractionated or LMW heparin should be used in doses intermediate between "prophylactic" and full "therapeutic" doses.

Moderate risk of thrombosis

At a moderate risk are:
• Women not on long-term anticoagulation who have a previous history of VTE: spontaneous, gestational, or while using a combined oral contraceptive.
• Women with a previous DVT who have an identifiable thrombophilia (other than antithrombin deficiency) or other persisting thrombosis risk factor.
• Asymptomatic women who give a family history of VTE and who have been found to be heterozygous for protein C deficiency, or homozygous for FV Leiden or FII G20210A, or to have combinations of defects (excluding antithrombin deficiency).

Thromboprophylaxis throughout pregnancy and for 6 weeks following delivery should be considered for these women but, in general, prophylactic doses of a heparin are adequate.

Table 15.3 Common risk factors for gestational VTE.

Obstetric factors
Cesarean section, particularly emergency CS
Extended surgery, e.g. cesarean hysterectomy
Operative vaginal dlivery
Hyperemesis
Pre-eclampsia

Patient factors
Age over 35 years
Obesity; BMI $\geq$ 30 kg/m^2
Dehydration
Immobility > 4 days bed rest
Current infection or other medical illness
Gross varicose veins
Intravenous drug user
Long distance travel
Previous venous thrombosis
Thrombophilia

BMI, body mass index.

Risk	Management of risk group
Highly increased risk	
Antithrombin deficiency (type 1 or 2 reactive site) symptomatic or asymptomatic	Heparin throughout pregnancy in intermediate doses
Women on long-term anticoagulants	Compression stockings throughout pregnancy/puerperium
	Postpartum thromboprophylaxis
Moderately increased risk	
Symptomatic women with any thrombophilia other than antithrombin deficiency and a history of previous VTE	Prophylactic doses of heparin throughout pregnancy
Symptomatic women with a history of previous VTE, spontaneous VTE, gestational VTE, COC-related VTE, persisting thrombotic risk factor	Compression stockings throughout pregnancy/puerperium
Asymptomatic women with a family history of VTE and heterozygous protein C deficient, homozygous FV Leiden or FII G20210A or combined defects	Postpartum thromboprophylaxis
Slightly increased risk	
Asymptomatic women with a family history of VTE and heterozygous protein S deficient or FV Leiden or FII G20210A	Compression stockings throughout pregnancy/puerperium
Women with a history of previous VTE in association with temporary (no longer present) risk factor and no identifiable thrombophilia	Postpartum thromboprophylaxis

Table 15.4 Prevention of gestational VTE.

Low risk of thrombosis

At a slightly increased risk are:
• Asymptomatic women who have been screened for thrombophilia because of a family history of VTE and been found to be heterozygous for protein S deficiency, FV Leiden or FII G20210A may be considered to be at slightly increased risk of VTE.
• Women who have had a previous VTE in association with a temporary and no longer present risk factor and who have no identifiable thrombophilic abnormality may be considered at only slightly increased risk. In these women, the risks associated with antenatal anticoagulation usually outweigh the benefits and, in the majority, antenatal anticoagulation may be avoided but anticoagulant prophylaxis should be offered from delivery until at least 6 weeks' postpartum.

The incidental finding of antiphospholipids in pregnancy should trigger increased clinical surveillance but pharmacologic intervention should be reserved for those women with antiphospholipids who are symptomatic. Women with antiphospholipids and a past history of VTE may usually be considered to be at highly increased risk of recurrent VTE associated with pregnancy.

Management of delivery in women using anticoagulants during pregnancy

Local policies should be decided after discussion with the anesthetists providing the service, bearing in mind the following:
• Epidural or spinal anesthesia is generally safe in women using UF heparin, providing their coagulation screen is normal and their platelet count greater than 80×10^9/L.
• Concern has been raised about a possible increased risk of significant spinal bleeding after neuroaxial block in patients on LMW heparins.
• In spite of considerable debate it remains unclear what period of time should elapse between the last dose of LMW heparin and insertion or removal of

an epidural or spinal catheter, or how long should the time interval be until the next dose. In practice, it may be reasonable to allow at least 12 h to elapse after a prophylactic dose of LMW heparin before inserting an epidural or spinal catheter, but a delay of up to 24 h may be necessary in patients on higher adjusted or full therapeutic doses of LMW heparins.

Thrombophilia and vascular complications of pregnancy

Inadequate or abnormal placental vasculature may result in a number of complications that have potentially serious or even lethal consequences for the mother and her unborn child. These complications include:

- pre-eclampsia;
- placental abruption;
- intrauterine growth retardation; and
- miscarriage and stillbirth.

Recurrent fetal loss (RFL)

This is a well-documented finding in patients with antiphospholipids (APLs). The prevalence of persisting APL positivity among women who have a history of RFL is approximately 15%. In those women with persistent APLs and a history of RFL, the prospective fetal loss rate has been put as high as 90%. However, the detection of positive APL tests in unselected women is not predictive of poor pregnancy outcome.

Testing for the presence of antiphospholipids
After three or more consecutive early pregnancy losses or one unexplained late pregnancy loss, the recommended practice is to test for APLs. It is possible that screening for APLs should be extended to include women who have had two consecutive miscarriages or three or more non-consecutive events. It may also be worthwhile screening women with a history of severe pre-eclampsia or severe placental insufficiency for APLs.

Treatment of RFL resulting from antiphospholipids
Two randomized trials demonstrated improved fetal survival with aspirin plus heparin compared with only aspirin, but a more recent study has suggested that a high success rate can be achieved using low-dose aspirin alone.

The link between heritable thrombophilias and increased fetal loss
A meta-analysis of 31 studies concluded that FV Leiden is significantly associated with early (odds ratio [OR] 2.01) and late (OR 7.83) recurrent fetal loss, and late non-recurrent fetal loss (OR 3.26). FII G20210A is associated with early recurrent (OR 2.56) and late non-recurrent (OR 2.30) fetal loss. Protein S deficiency is associated with recurrent fetal loss (OR 14.72) and late non-recurrent fetal loss (OR 7.39). Protein C and antithrombin deficiencies and MTHFR 677TT are not significantly associated with fetal loss.

Treatment of RFL in heritable thrombophilia
It has been suggested that prophylactic doses of LMW heparin throughout pregnancy may improve pregnancy outcome in women with heritable thrombophilia and a history of RFL but this needs to be tested (in a randomised Clinical trial).

Pre-eclampsia

The weight of evidence currently available would appear to support the conclusion that the more common types of inherited thrombophilia (FV Leiden, FII G20210A and MTHFR 677TT) are not independent risk factors for pre-eclampsia. However, they may characterize a subpopulation of women in whom the risk is elevated or in whom the clinical presentation may be more severe. In particular, there is evidence that carriage of FV Leiden may increase the risk of severe pre-eclampsia in women who are susceptible to this condition.

Venous thrombosis in women using female hormones

Combined oral contraceptives

Since their introduction in the 1960s it has been evident that combined oral contraceptives (COCs) are associated with an increased risk of VTE. While it was originally assumed that the magnitude of this risk was related to the estrogen dose in the COC, more recently the role of the progestogen content has been examined.

Oral contraceptives containing third-generation progestogens (desogestrel or gestodene) are associated with an approximately twofold increase of VTE compared with COCs containing second-generation progestogens (levonorgestrel). COCs cause slight increases in some procoagulant factors and reduce the levels of some natural anticoagulants – in particular antithrombin and protein S. These effects are more marked with third-generation than with second-generation COCs. Although there is a significantly increased risk of VTE for COC users, because these products are used by young women in whom VTE is uncommon, the overall absolute risk of VTE for COC users remains low at approximately 3–4 in 10,000 users/year.

The relative risk of VTE for third-generation COC users is around six- to ninefold that in non-COC users and in a prospective study the absolute risk of VTE associated with third-generation COC use was almost 1 in 1000 new users/year.

FV Leiden heterozygosity increases the risk of VTE associated with COC use. FV Leiden homozygotes using COCs are at even greater thrombotic risk and the interaction between the FV Leiden mutation and COCs is enhanced for users of COCs containing third-generation progestogens. FII G20210A has also been shown to increase the risk of VTE in COC users.

Because of the relative rarity of inherited deficiencies of natural anticoagulants, there is little information about the risk of VTE in women with these defects using COCs. One study noted a significant increase in the risk of venous thrombosis in combined COC users with antithrombin deficiency compared with non-pill using antithrombin-deficient women.

The increased risk of VTE associated with COC use in patients with heritable thrombophilias has led to the suggestion that women should be screened for these defects prior to prescription of a COC. However, it has been estimated that if screening of the adult female population was adopted and advice to avoid COCs given to all women carrying the FV Leiden mutation, more than 2 million women would need to be tested to prevent a single death from COC-related PE each year.

Progestogen-only preparations used to treat menstrual disorders are associated with increased risk of VTE but in the general population progestogen-only pills used for contraception appear **not** to be associated with significantly increased VTE risk.

Hormone replacement therapy

Early studies suggested that hormone replacement therapy (HRT) did not significantly increase the risk of VTE. More recently, however, clear evidence linking HRT use and VTE has been published. The evidence is consistent in demonstrating a relative risk of VTE of the order of 2–4 in women using HRT compared with non-users. As in COC users, the risk of VTE in HRT users seems to be higher near the start of therapy. The risk appears similar irrespective of the type of estrogen used and no significant difference in risk has been observed in users of opposed (with progestogen) versus unopposed estrogen.

The changes in hemostasis associated with HRT use are similar in type and direction to those associated with COC use but lesser in magnitude. Non-oral HRT preparations provoke lesser changes in hemostasis than oral preparations and, theoretically, may be expected to be associated with a lesser relative risk of VTE.

There is limited information about the risk of VTE in users of selective estrogen receptor modulators (SERMs) but in a randomized placebo-controlled trial the relative risk of VTE in users of raloxifene was 3.1 (95% CI 1.5–6.2), suggesting that the risk is similar to that with estrogen-containing HRT. A similarly increased risk of venous thrombosis has been reported in women using tamoxifen for the prevention or treatment of breast cancer.

Ovarian stimulation

VTE is a rare but well-documented complication of pharmacologic ovarian stimulation. The exact prevalence of VTE complications of ovarian stimulation in assisted reproduction protocols is unknown.

Venous thrombosis is usually associated with severe forms of ovarian hyperstimulation syndrome (OHSS) but may occasionally occur in patients who do not display evidence of OHSS. The mechanisms leading to VTE in patients who have undergone ovarian stimulation are not clear but ovarian stimulation has been shown to be associated with increased levels of some coagulation factors and reduced levels of some natural anticoagulants.

Many of the case reports describing VTE in association with OHSS report DVT in subclavian and internal jugular veins and VTE should be suspected in patients who have had ovarian stimulation and who present with neck pain and/or swelling. The reason for localization of VTE in these sites in OHSS patients is not clear. Cases of VTE in ovarian stimulation patients with heritable thrombophilias have been reported.

Efficacy and safety of anticoagulants in pregnant women with prosthetic heart valves

In a review of six published cohort studies and 22 case series, three commonly used approaches to anticoagulation during pregnancy were identified:

1 Oral anticoagulants throughout pregnancy.
2 Replacing oral anticoagulants with UF heparin from weeks 6 to 12.
3 UF heparin throughout pregnancy.

In the first two regimens, heparin was usually substituted for oral anticoagulant close to term.

The incidences of maternal thromboembolic complications and maternal mortality were respectively:
- 3.9% and 1.8% in the group taking oral anticoagulants throughout pregnancy.
- 9.2% and 4.2% in the group taking oral anticoagulants with UF heparin substitution from weeks 6 to 12.
- 33.3% and 15% in the group taking UF heparin throughout pregnancy.

Seventeen of the 25 reported deaths were caused by thrombosis of the prosthesis or related complications and two were a result of hemorrhage. Only a few case reports of LMW heparin use in patients with prosthetic heart valves have been published. Not all have had successful outcomes.

Decisions about the most appropriate anticoagulant regimen during pregnancy for women with mechanical heart valve prostheses must be made on an individual patient basis, after careful counseling, and should be based as far as possible on the relative risks of the various thromboprophylaxis regimens and on whether the patient is perceived to be at high or lower thromboembolic risk.

Women with older type mechanical prostheses (e.g. Starr–Edwards or Bjork–Shiley), women with a prosthesis in the mitral position, women with multiple prosthetic valves and women with atrial fibrillation may be regarded as being at high thromboembolic risk. Women with newer and less thrombogenic valves (e.g. St Jude's or Duromedics), particularly if they are in the aortic position and providing they are in normal sinus rhythm, may be regarded as being at lower thromboembolic risk.

With the information currently available it would be prudent to advise women in the high thromboembolic risk category to use an oral anticoagulant with an INR target of 3.5 throughout pregnancy, although some may choose to substitute adjusted doses of heparin between 6 and 12 weeks' gestation. Warfarin should be avoided close to term and UF or LMW heparin substituted.

On the basis of one report that the risk of fetal complications with warfarin appears to be dose-related, women with mechanical heart valves in the lower thromboembolic risk category may also feel reassured about the relatively low risk to their fetus if they use warfarin throughout pregnancy or with substitution of UF or LMW heparin from weeks 6 to 12 if their daily warfarin requirement does not exceed 5 mg. Women in this category requiring higher daily doses of warfarin may wish to minimize the risk of fetal complication, and be prepared to rely on adjusted doses of UF or LMW heparin, but they must be made aware that there is no good evidence to support the use of these latter regimens.

In general, women with bioprosthetic valves do not require anticoagulation, but anticoagulation may be necessary for other indications.

Further reading

Bates SM, Ginsberg JS. Anticoagulants in pregnancy: fetal effects. *Baillieres Clin Obstetr Gynecol* 1997;**11**:479–88.

Brill-Edwards P, Ginsberg JS, Gent M, *et al.* Safety of withholding heparin in pregnant women with a history of venous thromboembolism. *N Engl J Med* 2000;**343**:1439–44.

Chan WS, Anand S, Ginsberg JS. Anticoagulation of pregnant women with mechanical heart valves: a systematic review of the literature. *Arch Intern Med* 2000;**160**:191–6. [Review, 47 refs.]

Clark P, Brennand J, Conkie JA, McCall F, Greer IA, Walker ID. Activated protein C sensitivity, protein C, protein S and coagulation in normal pregnancy. *Thromb Haemost* 1998;**79**:1166–70.

Greer IA. Thrombosis in pregnancy: maternal and fetal issues. *Lancet* 1999;**353**:1258–65.

McColl MD, Ramsay JE, Tait RC, *et al.* Risk factors for pregnancy associated venous thromboembolism. *Thromb Haemost* 1997;**78**:1183–8.

McColl MD, Ellison J, Reid F, Tait RC, Walker ID, Greer IA. Prothrombin 20210 G → A, MTHFR C677T mutations in women with venous thromboembolism associated with pregnancy. *Br J Obstetr Gynecol* 2000;**107**:565–9.

Morrison ER, Miedzybrodzka ZH, Campbell DM, *et al.* Prothrombotic genotypes are not associated with pre-eclampsia and gestational hypertension: results from a large population-based study and systematic review. *Thromb Haemost* 2002;**87**:779–85.

Rey E, Kahn SR, David M, Shrier I. Thrombophilic disorders and fetal loss: a meta-analysis. *Lancet* 2003;**361**:901–8.

Vandenbroucke JP, Van der Meer FJM, Helmerhorst FM, Rosendaal FR. Factor V Leiden: should we screen oral contraceptive users and pregnant women? *BMJ* 1996;**313**:1127–30.

Vitale N, De Feo M, De Santo LS, Pollice A, Tedesco N, Cotrufo M. Dose-dependent fetal complications of warfarin in pregnant women with mechanical heart valves. *J Am Coll Cardiol* 1999;**33**:1637–41.

Walker ID, Greaves M, Preston FE. Investigation and management of heritable thrombophilia. *Br J Hematol* 2001;**114**:512–28.

Chapter 16
Pediatrics

Mary Bauman and Patricia Massicotte

Introduction

The estimated incidence of symptomatic venous thromboembolism (VTE) in children is significantly less than that in adults. However, advances in tertiary care pediatrics have resulted in rapidly increasing numbers of children requiring anticoagulation therapy; whether for treatment of deep venous thrombosis, or as thromboembolic prophylaxis.

Several mechanisms are likely to contribute to the protective effect of age for VTE:
- A reduced capacity to generate thrombin.
- Increased capacity of α_2-macroglobulin to inhibit thrombin.
- Enhanced antithrombotic potential by the vessel wall.

However, increasing numbers of children are developing VTE as secondary complications to their underlying disorders; 95% of VTEs in children are secondary to serious diseases such as cancer, trauma and/or surgery, congenital heart disease and systemic lupus erythematosus (SLE). Cerebral sinovenous thrombosis (CSVT) is also becoming increasingly diagnosed in children because of the recognition of the associated subtle clinical symptoms and improved cerebrovascular imaging. The etiology of CSVT includes thrombophilia, head and neck infections, and systemic illness.

Infants less than 1 year of age and teenagers are at the greatest risk for VTE. Most children have several risk factors for VTE, with the most common risk factor being the presence of a central venous line (CVL). This can be associated with right atrial thrombosis presenting as cardiac failure, pulmonary embolism (PE), loss of CVL patency and persistent sepsis in the line. The next most frequent manifestation of VTE is non-CVL-associated deep vein thrombosis (DVT) of the lower limb.

The purpose of this chapter is to provide practical guidelines for clinical management of the increasing numbers of pediatric patients presenting with thromboembolic disease.

Clinical symptoms and complications of venous thromboembolism in infants and children

The clinical symptoms and complications of VTE can be classified as acute or long-term.

Acute clinical symptoms

Acute symptoms include:
- loss of CVL patency;
- swelling, pain and discoloration of the related limb;
- swelling of the face and head with superior vena cava syndrome; and
- respiratory compromise in the case of PE.

Long-term complications

Long-term complications include prominent collateral circulation in the skin:
- on the face, back, chest and neck as sequelae of upper venous VTE; and
- on the abdomen, pelvis, groin and legs as sequelae of lower venous thromboembolism.

Post-thrombotic syndrome (PTS) is a serious long-term outcome of VTE consisting of pain, swelling, limb discoloration and ulceration resulting from damage to venous valves in deep vessels. The signs of PTS have been estimated to be present in up to 65% of children post-VTE, but clinically significant PTS occurs in approximately 10–20% of children.

Diagnosis of venous thromboembolism in infants and children

Clinical studies have determined the most sensitive diagnostic methods for diagnosing upper system VTE:
- Ultrasound for jugular venous thrombosis.
- Venography for intrathoracic vessels.

Symptomatic venous thromboembolism of both the upper and lower system

Ultrasound may be used; however, if the clinical suspicion is high for VTE, and the ultrasound is negative, the child should have a venogram of the vessels to rule out VTE.

Central nervous system thrombosis

Magnetic resonance imaging (MRI) is the most sensitive and specific diagnostic method, although computed tomography (CT), is helpful in many patient populations.

There are no studies determining the sensitivity and specificity of diagnostic testing for PE in children. The following radiographic tests may be used to diagnose PE in children: ventilation–perfusion scan, spiral CT, MRI, magnetic resonance verogram (MRV) or, if possible, pulmonary angiogram.

Thrombophilia

The contribution of congenital thrombophilia to childhood thrombosis remains controversial. The need to screen for prothrombotic disorders in children with major illnesses undergoing an invasive procedure or confirmed thrombosis, especially in the presence of clinical risk factors, remains uncertain.

Congenital prothrombotic disorders are relatively rare but include FV Leiden, prothrombin gene G20210A, dysfibrinogenemia, deficiencies of protein C, protein S and antithrombin, increased FVIII. Most children with prothrombin gene mutation do not develop thrombosis until adult life.

Excessive plasma levels of homocysteine resulting from homozygous deficiencies of enzymes such as cystathione β synthase or methylenetetrahydrofolate reductase (MTHFR) may be associated with severe VTE in children. In addition, an association exists between lipoprotein A, antiphospholipid antibody syndrome and VTE in children.

Treatment recommendations in infants and children

Venous or arterial proximal thrombosis

With confirmed symptomatic proximal VTE and asymptomatic proximal VTE in the absence of contraindications (active bleeding, very high risk of bleeding) anticoagulation should be strongly considered. Recommendations for anticoagulants have been largely extrapolated from adult studies with few studies in the pediatric population.

Therapy can be **initiated** with either:
- unfractionated heparin (UFH); or
- low molecular weight heparin (LMWH)

for a minimum of 5–7 days, increased to 10–14 days in extensive DVT or PE.

Following this initial treatment of UFH or LMWH, **continuation** of anticoagulation can take the form of either warfarin or LMWH for the duration of therapy.
- For a DVT secondary to an acquired insult, 3 months of therapy is usually sufficient.
- In cases of idiopathic DVT, at least 6 months should be considered.
- Objective follow-up of the thrombosis is recommended at 3 months.

Central venous line-related thrombosis

There are two aspects to the management of CVL-related VTE:
- Management of the CVL itself (if the CVL is no longer required or not functioning, it should be removed).
- Anticoagulation.

In general, a period (3–5 days) of anticoagulation prior to removal is preferred, especially if there is a known right-to-left shunt. If CVL access is required and the CVL involved is still functioning, then the CVL can remain *in situ*.

For children with a first CVL-related DVT, following the initial 3 months of therapy, prophylactic doses of oral anticoagulants (international normalized ratio [INR] 1.5–1.8) or LMWH (anti-Xa levels of 0.1–0.3) are options until the CVL is removed. However, for recurrent CVL-related VTE, following the initial 3 months of therapy, prophylactic doses of oral anticoagulants (INR 1.5–1.8) or LMWH (anti-FXa levels of 0.1–0.3) should be considered.

Cerebral sinovenous thrombosis

Anticoagulant therapy in children with CSVT is controversial. The diagnosis of CSVT requires either imaging the thrombus within sinovenous channels, or a reduction or obliteration of venous flow within venous sinuses. In the absence of a CNS hemorrhage, anticoagulation is appropriate.

There are three studies in adults using heparin therapy for CSVT showing improved neurologic outcome with therapy. A similar dosage is used as for non-CNS venous thrombosis. Small petechial or localized hemorrhage confined to an area of venous infarction may not be a contraindication to anticoagulation.

Data collected from the Canadian Pediatric Stroke Registry, where 66% of older infants and children were treated using anticoagulant therapy with UFH or LMWH and warfarin, found there were no treatment-related deaths or major hemorrhagic complications. Anticoagulation therapy is given for 3 months if full recanalization is seen on the 3-month monitoring CT venogram or MRV study. If only partial recanalization is seen at 3 months, treatment is extended to 6 months, which is consistent with the treatment approach for adult CSVT.

If no anticoagulants are given (because of significant hemorrhage) repeat MRV or CT venogram should be obtained at 1 week after diagnosis to assess for propagation of the initial thrombosis. Discussion with a hematologist or neurologist

experienced in managing such problems is recommended.

Primary prophylaxis for venous thromboembolism in children

In general, primary prophylaxis for VTE children **cannot be recommended** at this time, because there is no evidence for the efficacy or safety of this approach. However, children having long-term CVLs may benefit from antithrombotic prophylaxis.

Practical guidelines for anticoagulant use in children

Heparin is a descriptive term referring to all heparins including UFH and LMWH. Where possible, avoid intramuscular injections and arterial punctures during anticoagulation therapy. If necessary, appropriate precautions should be taken, including the use of extended periods of external pressure. Avoid concominant antiplatelet drugs. Acetaminophen (paracetamol) or Tylenol is recommended for analgesia. Prior to the initiation of therapy, obtain the patient's weight and blood for hemoglobin, platelets, INR and activated partial thromboplastin time (APTT).

For patients on long-term anticoagulation therapy (longer than 3 months), consider bone densitometry studies at baseline and then every 12 months to assess for possible reduced bone mineral density, which has been described in an uncontrolled study of children on warfarin therapy for more than 1 year, and in adults receiving heparin therapy (there are no data in humans on the effect of LMWH therapy on bone mineral density).

Unfractionated heparin therapy

UFH continues to be a commonly used anticoagulant in pediatric patients as it has a short half-life allowing for quick reversal of anticoagulation by simply discontinuing the infusion, and rapid reversal with the use of protamine sulfate in cases where immediate reversal is required.

As it is supplied in multidose vials in increasing concentrations with similar packaging, extreme caution should be used when dispensing heparin to ensure the correct concentration is being used and to avoid administering an overdose.

Differences in children

The anticoagulant activities of heparin are mediated through antithrombin. Some pediatric patients requiring heparin therapy have very low levels of antithrombin reflecting physiologic, congenital and/or acquired etiologies that may impair the function of therapeutic heparin.

At heparin concentrations in the therapeutic range, the capacity of plasma to generate thrombin is delayed and decreased by 25% in children, compared with adults. Optimal heparin regimens may differ in pediatric patients from adults; however, further studies are needed to delineate this.

A bolus of UFH 75 units/kg should be administered over 10 min, followed by an age-appropriate infusion. Once patients have obtained a therapeutic APTT/anti-Xa level, monitor hemoglobin and platelets daily. A dedicated IV is necessary for UFH infusions and this IV must not be stopped for other medications in order to maintain constant heparin levels.

Maintenance heparin doses are age-dependant. Infants of 28 weeks' gestational age up to 12 months of age require 28 IU/kg/h and children over 12 months of age require 20 IU/kg/h.

Dosing and monitoring

Monitoring of therapy is necessary as a result of the poor bioavailability of UFH. Therapeutic levels need to be achieved and maintained for effective anticoagulant therapy. It has been shown that APTT and anti-Xa levels only correspond in approximately 70% of children and rarely in children less than 12 months of age. In all age groups, if possible, an anti-factor Xa and an APTT should be drawn within 24 h of initiating therapy to ensure that the APTT is accurately reflecting the UFH concentration. In children where the APTT and the anti-factor Xa level do not correspond, then UFH therapy should be monitored using anti-Xa level.

Blood sampling should be performed (APTT or anti-Xa level) 6 h after initiation of therapy and UFH adjusted to maintain an anti-Xa at 0.35–0.7 IU/mL or an APTT that corresponds to the

Table 16.1 Heparin regimen nomogram.

APPT (s)	Anti-Xa (units/mL)	Hold (min)	Rate change	Repeat APTT (h)
< 50	< 0.1	0	Increase 20%	4
50–59	0.1–0.34	0	Increase 10%	4
60–85	0.35–0.70	0	0	24
86–95	0.71–0.89	0	Decrease 10%	4
96–120	0.90–1.20	30	Decrease 10%	4
> 120	> 1.20	60	Decrease 15%	4

therapeutic anti-Xa range. Table 16.1 is an example of a heparin regimen nomogram where the therapeutic APTT is 60–85 s.

Subcutaneous regimens

Therapeutic UFH may be administered subcutaneously. The daily dosage in IU/kg/h is divided into two doses and given subcutaneously every 12 h. Dosage is calculated using the formula:

Patient weight × age dependent unit/kg/hr (i.e. 20/28) × the number of hours of coverage = dose.

Subcutaneous (SC) UFH is monitored using either the APTT or anti-Xa level measured at 6 h after the SC dose. Dosage is adjusted according to the nomogram.

When reversal of anticoagulant therapy for invasive procedures is required, UFH may be used as a "bridge" or substitute anticoagulant in patients who normally receive LMWH or warfarin and are at high risk for thromboembolic disease if these are discontinued preoperatively.

Reversal of unfractionated heparin

If anticoagulation with UFH needs to be discontinued for clinical reasons, termination of the infusion will usually suffice because of the rapid clearance of UFH. If an immediate effect is required, consider administering protamine sulfate. Following IV administration, neutralization occurs within 5 min. The dose of protamine sulfate required to neutralize UFH is based on the dosage of UFH received in the previous 2 h as shown in Table 16.2.

Except for reversal of UFH following cardiopulmonary bypass, the maximum dose of protamine sulfate – regardless of the amount of UFH received

Table 16.2 Reversal of heparin therapy.

Time since end of infusion, or last heparin dose (min)	Protamine per 100 units unfractionated heparin dose (mg) (maximum 50 mg/dose)
< 30	1
30–60	0.5–0.75
61–120	0.375–0.5
> 120	0.25–0.375

– is 50 mg, and should be administered in a concentration of 10 mg/mL at a rate not exceeding 5 mg/min. When administered too quickly protamine sulfate may result in cardiovascular collapse. Patients with known hypersensitivity reactions to fish, and those who have received protamine-containing insulin or previous protamine therapy may be at risk of hypersensitivity reactions to protamine sulfate. An APTT performed 15 min after administration will demonstrate if reversal has been partial or complete.

Heparin-induced thrombocytopenia in children

There have been a number of case reports of pediatric heparin-induced thrombocytopenia (HIT) in the literature, ranging in age from 3 months to 15 years. A high index of suspicion is required to diagnose HIT in children, as many patients in neonatal or pediatric intensive care units who are exposed to heparin have multiple reasons for thrombocytopenia and/or thrombosis.

Platelets should be monitored daily during therapy and if an abrupt drop in platelets by more than 50% from baseline occurs, then a HIT screen should be performed and *all* sources of heparin should be discontinued. Hirudin and argatroban may be used as alternatives to heparin in children with HIT.

Low molecular weight heparin in infants and children

The use of LMWH should be considered in most patients requiring anticoagulation for therapy or prophylaxis. The potential advantages of LMWH for children include:

- The need for minimal monitoring (important in pediatric patients with poor venous access).
- Lack of interference by other drugs or diet, such as exists for warfarin.
- Reduced risk of HIT.
- Probable reduced risk of osteoporosis.

Therapeutic range doses of LMWH are extrapolated from adults and are based on anti-Xa levels, which reflect the pharmacodynamic activity of the LMWH but not accurately its antithrombotic activity. The guidelines for therapeutic LMWH suggest maintaining an anti-Xa level of 0.50–1.0 IU/mL in a sample taken 4–6 h following a subcutaneous injection (for twice daily LMWH administration).

Table 16.3 shows a guideline for initiating and monitoring enoxaparin therapy; modifications for individual clinical circumstances may be necessary. These dosage guidelines apply to enoxaparin only and cannot be directly extrapolated to other LMWHs. The treatment and prophylactic doses of enoxaparin in children are extrapolated from adult clinical trials and a cohort study in children. LMWH is cleared by the kidneys; therefore a blood creatinine level should be measured prior to initiating LMWH therapy. If renal compromise or failure is present, LMWH should be used with caution and frequent anti-Xa levels performed.

Adjust the regimen according to the nomogram in Table 16.4. The therapeutic anti-Xa level for treatment is 0.5–1 IU/mL. This nomogram assumes that there is no bleeding or renal compromise.

Table 16.3 Enoxaparin regimen nomogram: initial dose.

	Age ≤ 2 months	Age ≥ 2 months to 18 years
Initial prophylactic dose	0.75 mg/kg/dose SC q 12 h or 1.5 mg/kg/dose SC once daily	0.5 mg/kg/dose SC q 12 h or 1 mg/kg/dose SC once daily
Initial treatment dose	1.5 mg/kg/dose SC q 12 h	1 mg/kg/dose SC q 12 h
Maximum dose	3 mg/kg/dose SC q 12 h	2 mg/kg/dose SC q 12 h

q, every; SC, subcutaneously.

Table 16.4 Enoxaparin regimen nomogram: dose adjustment.

Anti-Xa level (IU/mL)	Hold next dose?	Change dose?	Next anti-factor Xa level?
< 0.35	No	Increase by 25%	4 h post next morning dose
0.35–0.49	No	Increase by 10%	4 h post next morning dose
0.5–1	No	0	1 × per week at 4 h post morning dose
< 1.20	No	Decrease by 20%	4 h post next morning dose. Hold dose. Do a trough level. If trough < 0.5 at 10 h post dose, administer scheduled dose at 20% of previous dose

Dose adjustments ordered in 0.5-mg increments for doses less than 5 mg and in 1.0-mg increments for doses greater than 5 mg are sufficient to achieve targeted anti-Xa levels.

It is recommended that anti-Xa levels be monitored monthly, and dosage adjustments made accordingly. This is necessary in the pediatric population as children often outgrow their current dosage or, as the medication is cleared by the kidneys, there may be some accumulation over time.

Simplifying administration of heparin therapy in infants and children

LMWH may be administered using an insulin syringe with a short ultrafine needle, where 1 mg of drug (enoxaparin) corresponds to 1 unit. This should reduce measuring error, bleeding, bruising and hematoma formation at the administration site. Similarly, an insulin syringe may be used for all LMWH with accurate calculations for dose measurement.

Subcutaneous therapy may be administered using an Insuflon® catheter (Fig. 16.1). This device is an indwelling subcutaneous vinyl catheter that is inserted into the subcutaneous tissue and may remain in place for 3–7 days. The duration is dependent on assessment of the insertion site prior to each dose. The site must be monitored closely for any bleeding, bruising, leakage and subcutaneous hematoma formation at the site. With presentation of any of these symptoms the Insuflon must be changed prior to administering the next dose. Use of an insulin syringe is also beneficial with the use of Insuflon, again decreasing the occurrence of measuring error and provides easier access to the Insuflon port.

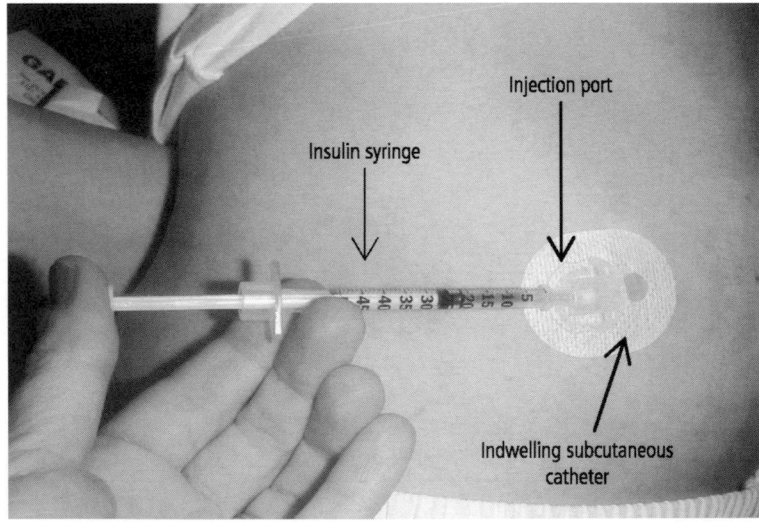

Figure 16.1 Insuflon® catheter *in situ* demonstrating administration of low molecular weight heparin (LMWH) with an insulin syringe.

Reversal of low molecular weight heparin therapy

If anticoagulation with LWMH needs to be terminated for clinical reasons, discontinuation of LMWH injections will usually suffice. If an immediate reversal of effect is required, protamine sulfate reverses 80% of the anti-Xa activity of LMWHs.

Warfarin therapy in infants and children

Currently, therapeutic INR ranges for children are directly extrapolated from recommendations for adult patients because there are no clinical trials that have assessed the optimal INR ranges for children based upon clinical outcomes.

- The target INR for treatment of VTE is 2.5 (range 2.0–3.0).
- The target INR for most children with mechanical valves is 3.0 (range 2.5–3.5).

Difficulties with maintaining these levels, as outlined below, have resulted in the recommendation that warfarin not be used in children less than 12 months of age, except for infants with mechanical heart valves.

Monitoring oral anticoagulant therapy in children is difficult and requires close supervision with frequent dosage adjustments. Reasons contributing to the need for frequent monitoring include diet, medications and primary medical problems.

Breastfed infants are very sensitive to oral anticoagulants because of the low concentrations of vitamin K in breast milk. It is recommended that these children receive daily vitamin K supplements in the form of 50 mL of commercial formula.

In contrast, some children are resistant to oral anticoagulants because of impaired absorption; requirements for total parenteral nutrition (TPN), which is routinely supplemented with vitamin K, and nutrient formulae, which are all supplemented with vitamin K to protect against hemorrhagic disease of the newborn. If possible, supplemental vitamin K should be removed from TPN solutions.

Loading warfarin

The usual loading dose is 0.2 mg/kg as a single daily oral dose, with a maximum of 5 mg (Table 16.5). The loading dose should be reduced to 0.1 mg/kg in patients with liver dysfunction or post-Fontan procedure.

Table 16.5 Warfarin regimen nomogram: loading phase.

Following the initial dose, if your response is:		
INR	1.1–1.4	Repeat initial dose
INR	1.5–2.9	50% of initial dose
INR	> 3.0	Hold until INR < 2.5 then restart at 50% less than the previous dose

Note: These dose reductions are critical to avoid "overshooting" the target range.

Table 16.6 Warfarin regimen nomogram: maintenance phase for target INR 2.5.

INR	*1.1–1.4	Check for compliance, if compliant increase dose by 20%
INR	1.5–1.9	Dose increase by 10%
INR	2.0–3.0	No change
INR	3.1–3.5	Dose decrease by 10%
INR	> 3.5–4.0	Administer one dose at 50% less than maintenance dose. Then restart at 20% less than the maintenance dose
INR	4.1–5.0	Hold × 1 dose then restart at 20% less than maintenance dose
INR	> 5.0	Consider reversal

Note*: In the case of mechanical valves where the target INR is 3.0, the above nomogram may be used by adjusting the INR range up by 0.5. For example, the INR range of 1.1–1.4 would be 1.6–1.9 with a dose adjustment increase of 20%.

Full diet should be tolerated prior to initiating warfarin therapy in children. It is helpful to use LMWH until the child is adequately tolerating feeds, this will result in achieving the maintenance phase safely and efficiently.

Long-term warfarin maintenance dose guidelines

The following dosage guidelines for long-term maintenance of warfarin (Table 16.6) apply primarily to medically stable patients already established on long-term maintenance therapy. Medically unstable patients or those completing the loading protocol may respond differently. Close monitoring with individualized dose adjustment of such patients is essential until they are clearly established on maintenance therapy.

Warfarin reversal

The antidote for warfarin is dependent upon whether urgent or non-urgent reversal is necessary.

• *For non-urgent reversal:* vitamin K$_1$ is administered in a dose of 0.5–2 mg orally, depending upon the patient's size. The administration of vitamin K either subcutaneously or intramuscularly has been shown to be less efficacious than orally, as long as gut absorption is not severely compromised.

• *For urgent reversal* (major bleeding or interventional procedure): prothrombin complex concentrate or fresh frozen plasma (FFP; 20 mL/kg) are administered.

Patients requiring warfarin therapy may be given an ampoule of vitamin K dispensed as 2-mg ampoules to be used orally in the dose recommended above, on the advice of the treating physician if the INR is increased above the therapeutic range. Based on adult recommendations:

• For an INR of 6–10, administer 1.0 mg orally.

• For an INR of > 10, administer 2.0 mg orally. INR must be repeated within 24 h.

Home INR monitors

Whole-blood monitors provide an effective way for monitoring INRs in children on long-term anticoagulant therapy, with needle phobias or poor venous access. The INR is measured using a capillary blood sample. Point-of-care INR monitors (Fig. 16.2) have been evaluated in children and were shown to be acceptable and reliable for use in the outpatient laboratory and in home settings.

Thrombolytic therapy

Systemic thrombolytic therapy is indicated for:

• Arterial occlusions.

• Massive pulmonary embolism.

• Pulmonary embolism not responding to heparin therapy.

• It may also be indicated for acute, extensive DVT and should be limited to situations where there is a risk for loss of life, organ or limb because of thrombosis as there exists a high incidence of hemorrhage.

Contraindications include:

• Acute bleeding.

• Significant potential for local bleeding such as general surgery within the previous 10 days, neurosurgery within the previous 3 weeks, hypertension, AV malformations and severe recent trauma.

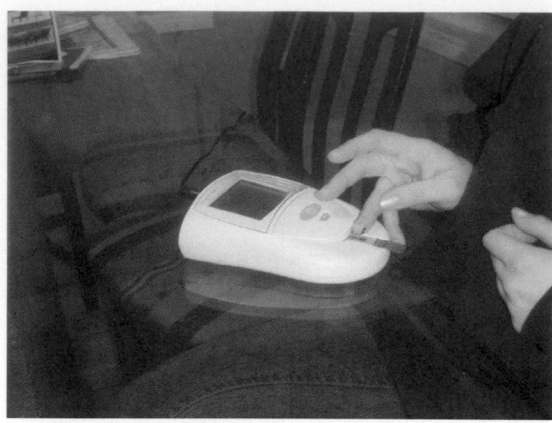

Figure 16.2 A near patient testing instrument for international normalized ratio (INR) measurement. The INR is estimated from a fingerprick drop of blood. Several instruments are available and the one shown is the Coaguchek from Roche Diagnostics.

Alteplase may be administered at 0.1–0.6 mg/kg/h intravenously for 6 h before re-evaluating the thrombus. During alteplase infusion, concurrently administered UFH 10 units/kg/h and precautions to minimize the risk for bleeding should be implemented (such as maintaining fibrinogen > 1.0 g/L, platelets > 100×10^9/L and minimal manipulation of the patient during the infusion).

Vena caval filters

When anticoagulation is contraindicated and the risk of pulmonary embolus is high, placement of a temporary vena caval filter (VCF) may be considered (Fig. 16.3). The VCF serves to mechanically interrupt the inferior vena cava and prevent life-threatening pulmonary emboli. In a retrospective study of the pediatric population where VCFs were placed post DVT or PE, there were no symptomatic recurrent events while the filter was in place. Filters were usually placed through right femoral access and retrieved via right jugular access, with a mean duration of placement of 15 days. Currently, the filters can only be placed in children > 10 kg and with an inferior vena cava (IVC) width (or diameter) of 1 cm because of the size of the filter.

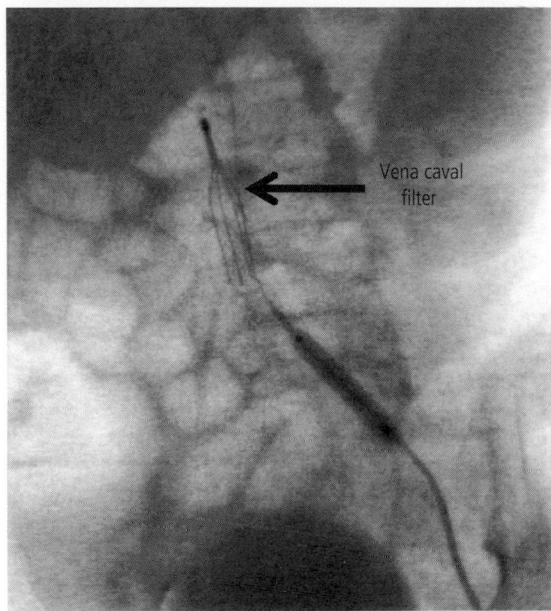

Vena caval
filter

Figure 16.3 Vena caval filter in inferior vena cava.

Clinical pediatric thrombosis assistance

The 1 800 NO CLOTS (1-905-662-5687 outside of North America) telephone consultation service is a 24 h, 7 days-a-week free service provided to healthcare professionals internationally. There are experts in pediatric thrombosis (systemic and CNS) who can provide evidence-based advice concerning the diagnosis, management and long-term outcome of neonates and children with or at risk for thrombosis. The service was set up by Dr Maureen Andrew* in 1991 and remains a testimonial to her dedication, vision and clinical excellence in pediatric thrombosis.

Conclusions

In most children with or at risk for thrombosis, anticoagulation therapy is recommended. Currently, the guidelines for anticoagulation therapy are extrapolated from adult studies. However, unique differences in the hemostatic system compared with adults influences the regimen, monitor-

* Deceased.

ing and response to anticoagulants in children, strongly suggesting that treatment based on adult recommendations may not be safe and/or efficacious. This chapter provides simplified guidelines for the use of anticoagulants in children, based on the evidence that is available in pediatric or adult clinical studies. It is urgent that properly designed clinical studies be completed in children with or at risk for thrombosis, to determine the best and safest method of diagnosis and treatment, and to evaluate the long-term outcome of thrombosis in children.

Further reading

Andrew M, David M, Adams M, *et al*. Venous thromboembolic complications (VTE) in children: first analyses of the Canadian Registry of VTE. *Blood* 1994;**83**:1251–7.

Andrew M, Marzinotto V, Massicotte P, *et al*. Heparin therapy in pediatric patients: a prospective cohort study. *Pediatr Res* 1994;**35**:78–83.

deVeber G, Monagle P, Chan A, *et al*. Prothrombotic disorders in infants and children with cerebral thromboembolism. *Arch Neurol* 1998;**55**:1539–43.

Dix D, Andrew M, Marzinotto V, *et al*. The use of low molecular weight heparin in pediatric patients: a prospective cohort study. *J Pediatr* 2000;**136**:439–45.

Hirsh J, Levine MN. Low molecular weight heparin. *Blood* 1992;**79**:1–17.

Massicotte MP, Dix D, Monagle P, Adams M, Andrew M. Central venous catheter related thrombosis in children: analysis of the Canadian Registry of Venous Thromboembolic Complications. *J Pediatr* 1998;**133**:770–6.

Monagle P, Adams M, Mahoney M, *et al*. Outcome of pediatric thromboembolic disease: a report from the Canadian Childhood Thrombophilia Registry. *Pediatr Res* 2000;**47**:763–6.

Monagle P, Michelson AD, Bovill E, Andrew M. Antithrombotic therapy in children. *Chest* 2001;**119**:344S–370S.

Ranze O, Ranze P, Magnani HN, Greinacher A. Heparin-induced thrombocytopenia in paediatric patients: a review of the literature and a new case treated with danaparoid sodium. *Eur J Pediatr* 1999;**158**:S130–S133.

Schmidt B, Andrew M. Neonatal thrombosis: report of a prospective Canadian and international registry. *Pediatrics* 1995;**96**:939–43.

Williams S, Chait P, Temple M, *et al*. Vena cava filters in children: review of a single centre clinical experience over 7 years. *J Thromb Haemost* 2003;**1**(Suppl 1):OC439.

Chapter 17
Intensive/critical care

Beverley J. Hunt and Sara E. Stuart-Smith

Thrombocytosis

Thrombocytosis is defined as a platelet count of greater than the upper limit of normal. Reactive thrombocytosis is common in Intensive Care Unit (ICU) patients, particularly in association with surgery or trauma, hemorrhage, acute and chronic infection, malignancy, iron deficiency anemia, inflammatory disease and postsplenectomy. The platelet count does not usually exceed $1000 \times 10^9/L$ in reactive thrombocytosis. Differential diagnoses include myeloproliferative disorders such as essential thrombocythemia, chronic idiopathic myelofibrosis and polycythemia vera. If a patient is not actively bleeding, thromboprophylaxis with aspirin 75 mg/day is appropriate.

Thrombocytopenia

Patients with thrombocytopenia may have petechiae, purpura, bruising or frank hemorrhage. A full blood count and blood film will confirm a low platelet count and the presence or absence of other diagnostic features such as red cell fragmentation, platelet morphologic abnormalities or evidence of dysplasia or hematinic deficiency.

Thrombocytopenia may arise because of:
- decreased platelet production;
- increased platelet destruction; and/or
- sequestration in the spleen.

Thrombocytopenia occurs in up to 20% of medical and 35% of surgical admissions to ICU and may be multifactorial. Table 17.1 lists the differential diagnoses of thrombocytopenia in the ICU setting. There is an inverse relationship between severity of sepsis and platelet count.

Platelet clumping

Ethylenediaminetetraacetic acid (EDTA)-dependent antibodies may develop in any patient, which cause platelet clumping *ex vivo*, resulting in pseudothrombocytopenia. If platelet clumping is seen on a blood film, a fresh sample should be taken into an alternative anticoagulant such as citrate.

Patients with sepsis

Immune mechanisms

Although predominately non-immune destruction of platelets occurs in sepsis, immune mechanisms may also contribute, with non-specific platelet-associated antibodies detected in up to 30% of ICU patients. It is thought that immunoglobulin G (IgG) binds to bacterial products on the platelet surface or to an altered platelet surface. A subset of patients with platelet-associated antibodies also has auto-antibodies directed against glycoprotein IIb/IIIa, similar to those implicated in the pathogenesis of immune thrombocytopenic purpura (ITP). Tests for platelet-specific IgG are non-specific and therefore not helpful in the management of septic patients.

Non-immune mechanisms

Bone marrow hemophagocytosis is a common finding in septic thrombocytopenic patients. The marrow is often hypocellular with reduced megakaryocyte numbers.

Consumptive coagulopathy is associated with an elevated prothrombin time or international normalized ratio (INR), activated partial thromboplastin time (APTT), thrombin time, D-dimer and a reduced fibrinogen.

Table 17.1 Differential diagnosis of thrombocytopenia in the Intensive Care Unit (ICU) setting.

Pseudothrombocytopenia
Clotted blood sample
EDTA-dependent antibodies

Drugs
Heparin, including HAT and HITT
IIb/IIIa inhibitors (abciximab, eptifibatide, tirofiban)
ADP receptor antagonists (clopidogrel)
Acute alcohol toxicity

Sepsis
Disseminated intravascular coagulation
Massive blood loss – a dilutional thrombocytopenia

Postcardiopulmonary bypass and intra-aortic balloon pump
Renal dialysis

ITP
Antiphospholipid syndrome

TTP
HUS
Hypersplenism
Hematinic deficiency, particularly acute folate deficiency

Pregnancy-associated thrombocytopenia
Benign gestational thrombocytopenia
Postpartum HUS
HELLP
Pre-eclampsia

Myelodysplastic syndrome
Carcinoma
Post-transfusion purpura
Hereditary thrombocytopenia

ADP, Adenosine diphosphate; EDTA, ethylenediaminetetraacetic acid; HAT, heparin-associated thrombocytopenia; HELLP, hemolysis, elevated liver function tests, low platelets; HITT, heparin-induced thrombocytopenic thrombosis; HUS, hemolytic uremic syndrome; ITP, immune thrombocytopenic purpura; TTP, thrombotic thrombocytopenic purpura.

Other causes of thrombocytopenia should be sought in a critically ill patient. Thrombocytopenia may occur as:
• A complication of heparin treatment. A mild thrombocytopenia of no clinical significance may be seen in the first few days of heparin therapy – heparin-associated thrombocytopenia (HAT).

This should be differentiated from heparin-induced thrombocytopenic thrombosis (HITT; see below).
• Dilutional thrombocytopenia may occur after trauma or complex surgery.
• Acute folate deficiency may be seen in ICU patients.
• Pre-existing disease such as ITP, cancer, hypersplenism and myelodysplastic syndrome may also contribute to a low platelet count.

Thresholds for therapy

The British Society for Haematology guidelines for the prophylactic use of platelets suggest:
• A platelet threshold of 10×10^9/L for platelet transfusion in thrombocytopenic patients without additional risk factors.
• A platelet threshold of 20×10^9/L when there are additional risk factors (sepsis, concurrent antibiotic use or other abnormalities of hemostasis).
• Patients with chronic sustained failure of platelet production, such as myelodysplasia or aplastic anemia, may remain free from serious hemorrhage with platelet counts below $5–10 \times 10^9$/L Long-term prophylactic platelet transfusions may lead to alloimmunization, platelet refractoriness and other complications of transfusion.
• For procedures such as lumbar puncture, epidural anesthesia, gastroscopy and biopsy, insertion of indwelling lines, transbronchial biopsy, liver biopsy and laparotomy, the platelet count should be raised to at least 50×10^9/L.
• For operations on critical sites such as the brain or eyes, recommendations are for a platelet count of greater than $75–100 \times 10^9$/L.

Antiplatelet drugs
Drugs known to have antiplatelet activity should be withdrawn. Any underlying disorder associated with platelet dysfunction, such as uremia, should be treated, and the hematocrit corrected to > 0.30 in those with renal failure. The use of desmopressin (DDAVP) should be considered.

Massive transfusion
In massive blood loss, the platelet count is preserved until relatively late. A platelet count of approximately 50×10^9/L is expected when red

cell concentrates equivalent to two blood volumes have been transfused. The platelet count should be maintained above 50×10^9/L in patients with acute bleeding. A higher target of 100×10^9/L is recommended for those with multiple trauma or central nervous system (CNS) injury.

Disseminated intravascular coagulopathy

Platelet transfusions are indicated in acute disseminated intravascular coagulopathy (DIC) when there is bleeding associated with thrombocytopenia. Management of the underlying disorder and coagulation factor replacement are also required. Frequent full blood count and coagulation screening tests should be carried out, and the platelet count maintained above 50×10^9/L. Platelet transfusions should not be given simply to correct a low platelet count in chronic DIC in the absence of bleeding.

Immune thrombocytopenic purpura

In patients with immune thrombocytopenic purpura (ITP), platelet transfusions are reserved for patients with life-threatening gastrointestinal, genitourinary or CNS bleeding or other bleeding associated with severe thrombocytopenia. In ITP the residual platelets tend to be young and have good hemostatic effect, so patients tend not to bleed unless their platelet count is very low. Platelet transfusions may not produce an incremental rise in patients with ITP because of the effect of the platelet antibodies on the donor platelets. IV methylprednisolone and IVIg can be given to produce platelet increments.

Post-transfusion purpura

Post-transfusion purpura (PTP) is caused by the presence of a platelet specific allo-antibody (usually antihuman platelet antigen-1a [HPA-1a]) in the recipient that reacts with donor platelets destroying them and also the recipient's own platelets. High-dose IVIg (2 g/kg given over 2 or 5 days) is used in the treatment of PTP, with responses in approximately 85% of patients. Large doses of platelet transfusions may be required to control severe bleeding before there is a response to IVIg. There is no evidence that HPA-1a-negative platelets are more effective than those from random donors.

Thrombotic thrombocytopenic purpura

Thrombotic thrombocytopenic purpura (TTP) is a clinical diagnosis characterized by:

- thrombocytopenia;
- microangiopathic hemolytic anemia;
- fluctuating neurologic signs; and
- renal impairment and fever.

Excessive platelet aggregation results in platelet microvascular thrombi, which particularly affect the cerebral circulation. This is mediated by ultra-large von Willebrand factor (VWF) multimers resulting from a deficiency of VWF cleaving protease (VWF-CP), ADAMTS-13. Deficiency of VWF-CP activity may be congenital, resulting from absence of the enzyme, or acquired because of the presence of an autoantibody to VWF-CP. Cirrhosis, acute inflammation, DIC and malignancy have all been associated with reduced VWF-CP activity but do not cause TTP.

TTP is characterized by red cell fragmentation and severe thrombocytopenia.

Red cell fragments may be absent from the peripheral blood in the first 24–48 h following clinical presentation.

Coagulation profiles are usually normal, but secondary DIC resulting from prolonged tissue ischemia is an ominous prognostic indicator.

Renal or skin biopsy performed after recovery of the thrombocytopenia may allow retrospective diagnosis. There is a prominent arteriolar and capillary thrombosis with thrombi largely composed of platelets, which stain strongly for VWF. This contrasts with hemolytic uremic syndrome (HUS) where the primary histologic changes are glomerular and arteriolar fibrin thrombi and subendothelial widening of the glomerular capillary wall.

Factors that may precipitate TTP include (Table 17.2):

- drugs;
- autoimmune disease;
- malignancy; and
- infection.

In some series, up to 14% of TTP episodes have been associated with HIV infection, with the greatest risk at CD4 counts of less than 250×10^9/L. *E. coli* O157 : H7 is more closely linked with HUS but there have been cases with typical TTP features. Recent studies have shown that up to

Table 17.2 Thrombotic thrombocytopenic purpura (TTP) precipitating factors.

Drugs
Oral contraceptives
Ticlopidine
Cyclosporine
Mitomycin C

Infection
HIV
E. coli O157:H7

Autoimmune disease
Systemic lupus erythematosus

Malignancy
Pregnancy
Post bone marrow transplantation

30% of patients with the clinical syndrome of TTP do not have VWF-CP.

Laboratory tests

There is no widely available diagnostic test for TTP. VWF-CP activity can be measured in specialist centers.

A panel of investigations required in a suspected case of TTP includes:
- FBC and film (see Plate 4, facing p. 25);
- Reticulocyte count;
- Clotting screen including fibrinogen and D-dimers;
- Urea and electrolytes;
- Liver function tests;
- Lactate dehydrogenase;
- Urinalysis;
- Direct antiglobulin test;
- HIV and hepatitis serology.

Treatment of thrombotic thrombocytopenic purpura

Treatment should be commenced if a patient presents with neurologic signs and a microangiopathic hemolytic anemia as well as thrombocytopenia, in the absence of any other identifiable cause.

Prior to the advent of plasma exchange, mortality rates were in excess of 90%. With prompt plasma exchange, the mortality has fallen to 10–30%. Thirty-five percent do not have neurologic involvement at presentation, but a reduced level of consciousness has been identified as a poor prognostic indicator, with an overall survival of 54%. The average number of plasma exchange procedures required for remission was 15.8 (range 3–36) in one series.

Plasma exchange

Single volume daily plasma exchange should be commenced within 24 h of presentation. Plasma exchanges using cryosupernatant may be more efficacious than using fresh frozen plasma (FFP). Daily plasma exchange should continue for a minimum of 2 days after complete remission.

In the presence of refractory disease, an alternative plasma product lacking high molecular weight VWF multimeric forms, such as cryosupernatant or solvent detergent plasma should be used for plasma exchange. Intensification of plasma exchange should be considered in life-threatening cases.

Steroids and aspirin

Patients should receive adjuvant corticosteroid therapy with pulsed methylprednisolone 1 g IV daily for 3 days. Low-dose aspirin (75 mg/day) should be commenced on platelet recovery (platelet counts over 50×10^9/L).

Supplementary therapy

Red cell transfusion should be administered according to clinical need. Folate supplementation is required in all patients. Platelet transfusions are contraindicated in TTP unless there is life-threatening hemorrhage. Hepatitis vaccination is recommended.

Immunosuppression

In refractory TTP, advice should be sought from a specialist in this field. Vincristine 1 mg repeated every 3–4 days or intensive immunosuppression using either cyclosporine or cyclophosphamide is indicated in severe refractory or recurrent TTP. Protein A column immunoabsorption may be considered. Relapse is common. Urgent self-referral is advised if a patient develops symptoms suggestive of relapse. Splenectomy may reduce the risk of relapse.

Hemolytic uremic syndrome

Hemolytic uremic syndrome (HUS) is character-ized by:
- a microangiopathic hemolytic anemia;
- thrombocytopenia; and
- renal failure.

There may be associated multiorgan disease including enterocolitis, neurologic complications, and liver, pancreatic and cardiac dysfunction.

The epidemic form (D$^+$) is associated with:
- a prodromal illness;
- bloody diarrhoea; and
- verotoxin enterococcal (VTEC) infection.
  Other courses may be:
- infection e.g. HIV, cytomegalovirus (CMV) or bacterial infection.

Secondary causes of HUS include:
- post solid-organ or bone marrow transplantation;
- drug exposure (pentostatin, cyclosporine, mito-mycin C, heroin and quinine);
- malignancy;
- pregnancy; and
- familial complement factor H deficiency or other complement defects.

Laboratory investigations

Early stool culture is essential for the diagnosis of VTEC-associated HUS. Other investigations are as for TTP.

Treatment of hemolytic uremic syndrome

Management involves meticulous fluid and elec-trolyte balance and blood pressure control, with renal dialysis as required. Antimotility drugs and antibiotic treatment a*dversely* affect the outcome and should be avoided. At present there is no con-clusive evidence that either FFP or plasma exchange improves outcome. Adjuvant treatment with anti-platelet agents, anticoagulation, fibrinolytics or IVIg is not recommended.

HELLP syndrome

HELLP syndrome (hemolysis, elevated liver func-tion tests, low platelets) is diagnosed by:

- the presence of hemolysis;
- elevated liver function tests;
- thrombocytopenia.

It occurs in up to 10% of women with severe pre-eclampsia. Severe thrombocytopenia and abnormal liver function tests can occur in the absence of significant hypertension or proteinuria. Exacerbations may occur postpartum and there is a recurrence risk of approximately 3% in sub-sequent pregnancies. HELLP occasionally presents postpartum, usually within 48 h, but rarely as late as 6 days after delivery.

Common presenting symptoms include:
- nausea;
- malaise;
- epigastric or right upper quadrant abdominal pain; and
- edema.

A neonatal mortality of 10–20% is attributed to placental ischemia. The maternal death rate is less than 1%. Delivery is the treatment of choice and is usually followed by complete recovery within 24–48 h.

The differential diagnosis of pregnancy-associated thrombotic microangiopathy is shown in Table 17.3. Fever rarely occurs in HELLP and may be a useful distinguishing feature. Revision of a diagnosis of pre-eclampsia must be made when a microangiopathy fails to resolve postpartum. There are no diagnostic assays. The differentiation of the thrombotic microangiopathies is based on history, physical examination and routine labora-tory studies.

Sepsis and the systemic inflammatory response syndrome

Sepsis constitutes the systemic inflammatory res-ponse to infection. It is the host response rather than the nature of the pathogen that is the major determinant of patient outcome.

The systemic inflammatory response synd-rome (SIRS) is manifested by two or more of the following:
- temperature > 38°C or < 36°C;
- heart rate > 90 b/min;
- respiratory rate > 20 breaths/minute or $Paco_2$ < 4.3 kPa;

Table 17.3 Differential diagnosis of pregnancy associated thrombotic microangiopathy.

Diagnosis	Classic TTP	Postpartum HUS	HELLP	Pre-eclampsia
Time of onset	Usually < 24 weeks	Postpartum	Usually > 34 weeks	Usually > 34 weeks
Histopathology of lesions	Widespread platelet thrombi	Thrombi in renal glomeruli only	Hepatocyte necrosis and fibrin deposition in periportal sinusoids	Glomerular endothelial hypertrophy and occlusion of placental vessels
Hemolysis	+++	++	++	+
Thrombocytopenia	+++	++	++	++
Coagulopathy	–	–	+/–	+/–
CNS symptoms	+++	+/–	+/–	+/–
Liver disease	+/–	++	+	+
Renal disease	+/–	+++	+	+
Hypertension	Rare	+/–	+/–	+++
Effect on fetus	Placental infarct can lead to IUGR and mortality	None, if maternal disease is controlled	Associated with placental ischemia and increased neonatal mortality	IUGR, occasional mortality
Effect on delivery	None	None	Recovery, but may worsen transiently	Recovery, but may worsen transiently
Management	Early plasma exchange	Supportive care +/– plasma exchange	Supportive, consider plasma exchange if persists	Supportive +/– plasma exchange

CNS, central nervous system; HELLP, hemolysis, elevated liver function tests, low platelets syndrome; HUS, hemolytic uremic syndrome; IUGR, intrauterine growth retardation; TTP, thrombotic thrombocytopenic purpura.

- white cell count $> 12 \times 10^9/\text{L}$, $< 4 \times 10^9/\text{L}$ or > 10% immature forms.

Sepsis is defined as **SIRS resulting from** documented **infection**. Severe sepsis is associated with:
- organ dysfunction;
- hypoperfusion or hypotension, which may include lactic acidosis;
- oliguria;
- an altered mental state; and
- a mortality rate of 30–50%.

Septic shock is defined as **severe sepsis with hypotension** (systolic BP < 90 mmHg or a reduction of > 40 mmHg from baseline) in the absence of other causes for hypertension or inotropic or vasopressor treatment and despite adequate fluid resuscitation.

Coagulation is activated in most patients with severe sepsis as evidenced by:
- elevated D-dimers;
- decreased protein C and antithrombin levels are also common;
- activation of coagulation may lead to depletion of circulating clotting factors with secondary DIC.

Treatment of SIRS

Activated protein C

Recombinant human activated protein C (drotrecogin alfa, activated) is licensed for adjunctive treatment of severe sepsis with multiorgan failure. It has anti-inflammatory, antithrombotic and fibrinolytic properties.

When given as a continuous intravenous infusion, recombinant human activated protein C decreases absolute mortality of severely septic patients by 6.1%, resulting in a 19.4% relative reduction in mortality. The absolute reduction in mortality increases to 13% if the population treated is restricted to patients with an APACHE II (acute physiology and chronic ill health evaluation) score greater than 24.

The most frequent and serious side-effect is bleeding. Severe bleeds increased from 2% in patients given placebo to 3.5% in patients receiving drotrecogin alfa. The risk of bleeding was only increased during the drug infusion time, and returned to placebo levels within 24 h of stopping

System	Description	Score
Respiratory system	< 400 +/– respiratory support	1
Pao$_2$/Fio$_2$ in mmHg	< 300 +/– respiratory support	2
	< 200 and respiratory support	3
	< 100 and respiratory support	4
Cardiovascular system	MAP < 70 mmHg	1
Vasopressors in gamma/kg/min	Dopamine ≤ 5 or dobutamine	2
	Dope > 5 or epi-/norepinephrine ≤ 0.1	3
	Dopamine > 15 or epi-/norepinephrine > 0.1	4
Liver	20–32	1
Bilirubin µmol/L	33–101	2
	102–204	3
	> 204	4
Renal	100–170	1
Creatinine in µmol/L or	171–299	2
urine output in mL/day	300–440 or < 500	3
	> 440 or < 200	4
Coagulation	101–150	1
Platelets × 10^9/L	51–100	2
	21–50	3
	< 20	4
Glasgow Coma Score	13–14	1
	10–12	2
	6–9	3
	< 6	4

Table 17.4 The sequential organ failure assessment (SOFA) score.

the infusion. Patients with a platelet count of < 30 × 10^9/L were excluded from the trials. It has been suggested that such patients could be transfused with platelets and then given activated protein C.

Sequential organ failure assessment score

Sequential organ failure assessment (SOFA) is a scoring system to evaluate the severity of critically ill patients in the ICU. A severity score is needed in clinical research studies to standardize reports, improve the understanding of the course of disease and to allow evaluation of new treatments. Estimates of morbidity serve as a reliable indicator of intensive care performance, allowing comparison between medical centers, cost–benefit analyses and evaluation of new therapeutic or management modalities.

The SOFA score has been designed to report morbidity and to quantify objectively the degree of dysfunction or failure of each organ daily in critically ill patients (Table 17.4).

Heparin-induced thrombocytopenic thrombosis

Heparin-induced thrombocytopenic thrombosis (HITT) is a transient drug-induced autoimmune prothrombotic disorder initiated by heparin. Heparin exposure can induce the formation of pathogenic IgG antibodies that cause platelet activation by recognizing complexes of platelet factor 4 (PF4) and heparin on platelet surfaces. Platelet activation results in thrombocytopenia and thrombin generation, with an increased risk of venous and arterial thrombosis.

HITT antibodies are directed against multiple neoepitope sites. Only a minority of PF4/heparin-reactive HITT sera activate platelets *in vitro*. Some

HITT-IgG recognize PF4 bound to solid phase even in the absence of heparin. PF4 antibodies usually decline to undetectable levels within a few weeks or months of an episode of HITT and there is no anamnestic response.

The frequency of HITT varies widely depending on the type of heparin used and the patient group:
• Unfractionated heparin (UFH) is associated with a higher incidence of HITT than fractionated heparin.
• Surgical patients have a higher frequency of HITT than either medical or obstetric patients with the same heparin exposure.
• Postoperative orthopedic patients receiving UFH have the highest HITT frequency (5%) and require more intense platelet count monitoring than pregnant women receiving LMWH, who have an almost negligible risk.

Laboratory diagnosis

HITT antibodies are detected using either:
• commercially available PF4-dependent antigen immunoassays; or
• functional assays of platelet activation and aggregation.

Clinically insignificant HITT antibodies are common in patients who have received heparin 5–100 days earlier. Functional assays of platelet activation are technically demanding, time consuming and not available in some centers. Testing should be performed when HITT is clinically suspected. Washed platelet activation assays and antigen assays have similar high sensitivity in this context. Standard platelet aggregometry is less sensitive. Diagnostic specificity is greater with washed platelet activation assays than with enzyme immunoassays (EIAs) as EIAs are likely to detect clinically insignificant antibodies.

The diagnosis of HITT should be based on clinical abnormalities (thrombocytopenia with or without thrombosis) as well as a positive test for HITT antibodies as outlined in Table 17.5.

Isolated HITT is the occurrence of thrombocytopenia without thrombosis. Retrospective cohort studies indicate that 25–50% of these patients develop clinically overt thrombosis after stopping heparin, usually within the first week. Subclinical

Table 17.5 Heparin-induced HIT diagnosis based on clinical and laboratory abnormalities.

Clinical	Laboratory
Thrombocytopenia (fall of > 50%) with or without any of the following	A PAA using washed platelets
A Venous thrombosis	Serotonin release assay
Coumarin-induced limb necrosis	Heparin-induced platelet activation test
Deep vein thrombosis	Microparticles by flow cytometry
Pulmonary embolus	B PGA using citrated platelet-rich plasma
Cerebral venous thrombosis	C Antigen assay
Adrenal haemorrhagic infarction	PF4/heparin-EIA
B Arterial thrombosis	PF4/polyvinyl sulphonate-EIA
Lower limb thrombosis	PF4-dependent EIA detecting HIT IgG
Cerebrovascular accident	Fluid phase EIA
Myocardial infarction	Particle gel immunoassay
Other	
C Skin lesions	
Skin lesion at heparin injection site	
Skin necrosis	
Erythematous plaques	
D Acute systemic reaction to heparin	
E Hypofibrinogenemia secondary to DIC	

DIC, Disseminated intravascular coagulopathy; EIA, enzyme immunoassay; PAA, platelet activation assay; PGA, platelet aggregation therapy.

thrombosis was found in eight of 16 patients who underwent routine lower limb duplex ultrasonography for isolated HITT. Early heparin cessation alone does not reduce the risk of thrombosis in patients with isolated HITT, alternative anticoagulation is required.

Approximately 25% of HITT patients receiving a heparin bolus develop signs or symptoms such as fever, chills, respiratory distress or hypertension. Transient global amnesia and cardiorespiratory arrest have also been reported. Of HITT patients, 5–15% go on to develop decompensated DIC.

Treatment of HITT

Thombocytopenia does not usually develop until day 5–10 of heparin treatment and reaches a median nadir of 55×10^9/L. The platelet count falls below 150×10^9/L in approximately 90% of HITT cases. Hemorrhage and platelet counts below 10×10^9/L suggest an alternative cause such as post-transfusion purpura. Patients who have received heparin within the last 100 days may have a fall in platelet count within 1 day of re-exposure to heparin.

Heparin should be stopped immediately, and not repeated, in those who develop thrombocytopenia or a 50% reduction of platelet count. As HITT is strongly associated with thrombosis (odds ratio 12–40), an alternative anticoagulant such as lepirudin or danaparoid should be commenced. Prophylactic platelet transfusions are relatively contraindicated. Therapeutic doses of anticoagulants are recommended even in the absence of thrombosis. Lepirudin (Refludan®), a recombinant hirudin, is licensed for anticoagulation in HITT patients.

Lepirudin

The dose is adjusted according to the APTT and is 400 μg/kg initially by slow intravenous injection, followed by a continuous intravenous infusion of 150 μg/kg/h (max. 16.5 mg/h), adjusted to maintain the APTT between 1.5 and 2.5 times baseline. The APTT should be measured 4 h after the start of treatment or after the infusion rate is altered, and then at least once daily.

As lepirudin is renally excreted, the initial dose should be reduced by 50%, and subsequent doses by 50–85% in patients with mild renal impairment. Although some sources advise that lepirudin should be avoided in severe renal failure, it has been used in severe renal failure or hemodialysis at a dosage of 0.005–0.01 mg/kg/h without initial bolus, with subsequent dosage adjustment according to the APTT.

Danaparoid sodium (Orgaran®)

Danaparoid is a heparinoid that may be used in HITT patients providing there is no evidence of cross-reactivity.

Danaparoid does not cross the placenta but is renally metabolised. It is given by intravenous injection in a regimen of 2500 U (1250 U if body weight less than 55 kg, 3750 U if over 90 kg), followed by an intravenous infusion of 400 IU/h for 2 h, then 300 IU/h for 2 h, then 200 IU/h for 5 days. Anti-Xa target range is between 0.5 and 0.8 anti-Xa IU/mL and should be monitored in those with renal impairment or a body weight of over 90 kg. Danaparoid given by subcutaneous injection has 100% bioavailability. The 24 h intravenous dose can be divided into two or three daily injections.

Argatroban

This is an alternative anticoagulant for use in HITT patients. It is a direct thrombin inhibitor, has hepatobiliary excretion and increases the INR. The dosage is 2 μg/kg/min, without an initial bolus. An APTT target range of 1.5–3.0 times baseline is required. The dosage must be reduced in liver failure. As argatroban increases the INR, a higher than ususal therapeutic target INR during warfarin cotherapy should be used.

Other potential alternative anticoagulants include bivalirudin and novel anti-Xa drugs such as fondaparinux. There is a 5–20% frequency of new thrombosis despite treatment of HITT patients with an alternative anticoagulant.

Thromboembolic disease including massive pulmonary embolus

Venous thromboembolism (VTE) is an important cause of morbidity and mortality in ICU patients. Among patients who died in ICU, PE was reported in between 7% and 27% of postmortem examinations. The mortality rate for PE is less than 8% when the condition is recognized and treated, but approximately 30% when untreated.

Massive PE has a mortality of 18–33% and may present with shock, dyspnoea and confusion. Although pulmonary angiography is regarded as the gold standard in PE diagnosis, in recent years it has been largely replaced by less invasive methods such as echocardiography, magnetic resonance angiography, spiral computerized tomography and ventilation–perfusion lung scanning. As echocardiography can be rapidly performed at the bedside, it is increasingly the modality of choice for confirming massive PE.

Treatment of pulmonary embolus

Heparin

Low molecular weight heparin is equal or superior in efficacy to UFH for the treatment of deep vein thrombosis (DVT) and PE. Thrombolytic therapy should be considered in patients with massive PE, hemodynamic instability or right heart dysfunction. Thrombolytic therapy can help prevent secondary chronic thromboembolic pulmonary hypertension. At 7 years follow-up, pulmonary artery pressure and pulmonary vascular resistance were lower in patients receiving thrombolysis compared with those treated with anticoagulation alone. An inferior vena cava (IVC) filter can be placed in patients with an absolute contraindication to anticoagulation who remain at risk of PE.

Thrombolysis

The streptokinase/urokinase PE thrombolysis trials showed that thrombolytic therapy successfully decreases pulmonary artery pressures acutely with improvements in the lung scan and arteriogram at 12 and 24 h. There was no overall decrease in mortality in those receiving thrombolysis compared with those receiving heparin therapy.

Contraindications to thrombolysis include active internal bleeding, a stroke within 2 months, and an intracranial process such as neoplasm or abscess. Relative contraindications include surgery or organ biopsy within 10 days, uncontrolled hypertension and pregnancy.

The dosage of alteplase is 10 mg IV injection over 1–2 min followed by an IV infusion of 90 mg over 2 h (max. 1.5 mg/kg in patients less than 65 kg). The dosage of streptokinase is 250,000 units by IV infusion over 30 min, then 100,000 units every hour for up to 12–72 h according to clinical condition, with monitoring of clotting parameters. A simplified algorithm for alteplase consisting of 0.6 mg/kg over 15 min has been used successfully in many centers, with equivalence to the standard regimen demonstrated in two prospective randomized studies.

Hemorrhagic complications are higher in patients with a recent invasive procedure such as pulmonary angiogram or placement of an IVC filter. There is a reported incidence of intracranial hemorrhage of approximately 2%, with higher rates in the elderly and those with poorly controlled hypertension. The major hemorrhage rate ranges from 11% to 20%.

Surgical embolectomy

Surgical intervention should be considered for patients whose condition worsens despite intensive medical treatment. A randomized study of embolectomy versus medical therapy is unavailable. Thrombolytic treatment fails in 15–20% of patients. The mortality after surgical embolectomy is approximately 30–40%, with a higher mortality in those with a longer duration of hemodynamic instability, a requirement for cardiopulmonary resuscitation and intubation, high doses of catecholamines, metabolic and respiratory acidosis, and poor urine output. Early diagnosis and treatment leads to improved outcomes.

Thromboprophylaxis in the ICU

VTE is an important cause of morbidity and mortality in ICU patients. Most ICU patients have multiple risk factors including advanced age, serious medical illness, recent surgical procedure or trauma, sepsis, heart failure, mechanical ventilation, malignancy, paralysis, pregnancy or puerperium and indwelling central venous lines. DVT rates

Bleeding risk	Thrombosis risk	Prophylaxis
Low	Moderate	LDH 5000 IU sc b.d. or LMWH at prophylactic doses
Low	High	LMWH in thromboprophylactic doses
High	Moderate	Graduated compression stockings or intermittent pneumatic compression, and LMWH*
High	High	Graduated compression stockings or intermittent pneumatic compression, and LMWH*

Table 17.6 Suggested venous thromboembolism (VTE) prophylaxis in critically ill patients. (Adapted from Geerts W, Selby R. 2003.)

b.d., twice daily; LDH, low-dose heparin; LMWH, low molecular weight heparin; sc, subcutaneous.
* when bleeding risk decreases.

in ICU patients not receiving prophylaxis vary between 13% and 31% in four prospective studies.

With few exceptions, thromboprophylaxis should be used in all ICU patients. Decisions regarding the initiation and method of prophylaxis should be based on the balance of bleeding and thrombotic risk. Patients with a high risk of bleeding should be given mechanical prophylaxis with either graduated antiembolic stockings alone or stockings combined with intermittent pneumatic compression devices until bleeding risk decreases and prophylaxis with heparin can be commenced.

Combined pharmacologic and mechanical methods of prophylaxis may provide enhanced protection, but have not been rigorously tested in the ICU setting. Prophylaxis should be reviewed daily and altered as necessitated by the patient's clinical status. Prophylaxis should not be interrupted for procedures or surgery unless there is a particularly high bleeding risk. Procedures such as insertion or removal of epidural catheters should be planned to coincide with the nadir of anticoagulant effect. Table 17.6 outlines recommendations for prophylaxis in critically ill patients.

Special situations

Renal failure (thrombosis of vascular access, LMWH, uremia)

For continuous hemofiltration, UFH or LMWH is used. Occasionally, antithrombin replacement is indicated in patients undergoing continuous hemofiltration, or other extracorporal circulation procedures, if there are low plasma antithrombin levels. Treatment aims to normalize antithrombin levels.

Patients with sepsis and VTE treated with LMWH, and those with hereditary antithrombin deficiency, may benefit from antithrombin concentrates if the plasma antithrombin level is below 60% of normal.

Renal transplantation and thrombophilia

Some renal transplant recipients have an increased risk of thromboembolism. The hypercoagulability of these patients persists throughout life, but is most marked in the first 6 months after transplantation. In a large series published by the European Dialysis and Transplantation Association in 1983, 4.4% of deaths occurring in renal transplant recipients were secondary to PE.

The hypercoagulable state appears to be multifactorial, with proposed contributing factors including:
• the procoagulant side-effects of certain immunosuppressive agents;
• an increased prevalence of antiphospholipid antibodies;
• hyperhomocysteinemia;
• altered levels of hemostatic factors secondary to nephrotic syndrome;
• post-transplant erythrocytosis; and
• acute CMV infection.

The risk factors outlined in Table 17.7 should be sought in renal transplant patients. Prophylactic measures will be required in high-risk patients.

Immunosuppressive agents

Several immunosuppressive agents have been implicated in post-transplant venous thromboembolic disease:

Table 17.7 Possible additional risk factors for venous thromboembolic disease in renal transplant recipients.

Immunosuppressive agents
Cyclosporine
Corticosteroids
Muromonab-CD3 (OKT3)
Sirolimus
Mycophenolate mofetil

Antiphospholipid antibodies
Elevated homocysteine levels
Nephrotic syndrome
Pretransplant continuous ambulatory peritoneal dialysis
Post-transplant erythrocytosis
Acute CMV infection

CMV, cytomegalovirus.

- *Cyclosporine:* data concerning the thromboembolic complications associated with cyclosporine therapy are contradictory. Although cyclosporine has procoagulant effects *in vivo*, large clinical trials have failed to support a significant difference in thromboembolic events.
- *Corticosteroids:* the thrombotic effects of corticosteroids have been well described and include enhanced endothelial synthesis of VWF, impaired fibrinolysis resulting from suppression of tissue plasminogen activity and increased plasminogen activator inhibitor type 1 synthesis. Long-term steroid treatment results in a hypercoagulable hypofibrinolytic state.
- *Muromonab-CD3 (OKT3):* an IgG2a murine monoclonal antibody that targets the CD3–T-cell receptor complex. It has been used in the prophylaxis and treatment of acute graft rejection but has been largely replaced by newer antirejection drugs. Treatment with OKT3 results in complement activation, cytokine release, coagulation activation and an increased incidence of intragraft thrombosis, particularly when given in combination with steroids.
- *Sirolimus:* an immunosuppressive agent and potent *in vitro* enhancer of platelet aggregation and secretion. In April 2002, the US Food and Drug Administration warned of an increased incidence of hepatic artery thrombosis among liver transplant recipients treated with sirolimus in com-

bination with either cyclosporine or tacrolimus. The situation has not been fully explored by clinical trials in renal transplant patients.
- *Mycophenolate mofetil (MMF):* associated with *in vivo* platelet aggregation in normal subjects and uremic patients. However, this complication appears to be localized and related only to intravenous administration of MMF, with phlebitis and thrombosis in 4% of renal transplant recipients.

Antiphospholipid antibodies

The prevalence of antiphospholipid antibodies in renal transplant recipients has been reported to be as high as 28%. The incidence of post-transplant thrombosis is significantly higher in antiphospholipid positive patients than in negative patients (26% and 8.5%, respectively). Renal artery thrombosis necessitating transplant nephrectomy has been reported, and was recurrent in a second renal transplant in two antiphospholipid antibody-positive renal transplant recipients. These patients require adequate peritransplant anticoagulation.

Homocysteinemia

Stable renal transplant recipients have an excess prevalence of hyperhomocysteinemia, occurring in up to 70% of 207 patients in one series. The main determinant of serum homocysteine concentration was the level of renal function. Patients with hyperhomocysteinemia should be offered treatment dose folic acid.

Nephrotic syndrome or peritoneal dialysis

Nephrotic syndrome contributes to an increased thromboembolic risk by causing elevated levels of some coagulation factors (fibrinogen, factors V, VIII and XIII) and decreased levels of some anticoagulant proteins (antithrombin and protein S), as well as being associated with thrombocytosis, platelet hypercoagulability and hypofibrinolysis.

A hypercoagulable state resulting from transperitoneal protein loss has been reported in patients undergoing continuous ambulatory peritoneal dialysis. These patients have higher levels of factors VII, IX, X and fibrinogen. Transplanted peritoneal dialysis patients are more likely to suffer allograft thrombosis than patients treated with hemodialysis prior to transplantation.

Erythrocytosis

Erythrocytosis is defined as a hematocrit > 52% in men and > 49% in women. The incidence of post-transplant erythrocytosis in renal graft recipients is 8–22%. Long duration of dialysis, acquired cystic disease, polycystic kidney disease, graft artery stenosis, graft hydronephrosis, diabetes, smoking and hypertension may contribute to its development. The incidence of thromboembolic complications is increased. Angiotensin-converting enzyme inhibitors or angiotensin II receptor agonists may be used to reduce the hematocrit. Repeated phlebotomy is used in non-responders.

Cytomegalovirus infection

The CMV virus has a tropism for endothelial cells and can be found in venous or arterial walls. It has been suggested that CMV infection causes increased endothelial cell activation and thus a procoagulant state. In one series, seven of 13 renal transplant recipients who presented with a thromboembolic event had a simultaneous CMV infection. All were non-hospitalized ambulatory patients.

Jehovah's Witnesses

Jehovah's Witnesses (JWs) do not accept transfusion of blood or its major components, based on the belief that to be transfused with blood is equivalent to eating it and therefore prohibited by scripture. Until 2000, any JW known to be transfused with a prohibited blood product was expelled from the society and ostracized by other JWs. Since 2000, any JW who "wilfully and without regret" accepts blood transfusion is no longer expelled but instead "revokes his own membership by his own actions." Doctors should consider the possibility that individual JW patients have interpreted this change as allowing them to accept transfusion under certain circumstances. This will require clarification in a one-to-one consultation in absolute medical confidentiality.

The Association of Anesthetists of Great Britain and Ireland (AAGBI) advise that although it is unlawful to give blood to a patient who has refused it, "for unconscious patients, the doctor will be expected to perform to the best of his/her ability, and this may include giving blood." This would only apply when JW status is unclear and/or relatives or associates cannot produce an Advance Directive document.

Before dismissing the use of blood products there must be a certainty that the patient is a committed JW, has independently and freely decided to refuse transfusion and has thought this decision through to the point of death at the time of making an Advance Directive (living will) or additional consent to surgery.

A copy of the Advance Directive should be placed in the patient's notes and the contents respected. If life-threatening bleeding occurs and time allows, a doctor of consultant status should discuss with the patient, or relative, the implications of withholding blood, and a clear, signed entry should be written in the patient's notes.

The 2000 Watch Tower directive stated that "primary components" of blood must be refused, but that "when it comes to fractions of the primary components, each Christian must conscientiously decide for himself."

Every JW should decide which products are acceptable to him/her during the consent process. All available blood products should be discussed as interpretations of a "fraction of the primary component" may hypothetically include products such as leukocyte-depleted red cells and platelets, IVIg, fibrinogen concentrates and solvent detergent treated FFP.

Most JW patients refuse autologous predonation because blood is separated from the body in storage. Normovolemic hemodilution and some forms of intraoperative cell salvage and hemodialysis may be acceptable because the extracorporeal blood remains in contact with the circulation. Hematological parameters should be optimized preoperatively. Meticulous surgical hemostasis, minimal access surgery and systemic pre- and perioperative administration of antifibrinolytic agents (tranexamic acid or aprotinin) or DDAVP should be considered. The use of topical hemostatic plasma fractionation products such as fibrin glue may be acceptable to some.

JW patients accept crystalloids and synthetic colloids including dextran, hydroxyethylstarch and gelatins (e.g. Gelofusine®) for circulatory support. Most requiring plasma exchange will refuse human albumin but may accept hexastarch or protein A immunoabsorption as alternatives.

Recombinant blood products are acceptable to many JWs. Epoetin beta (NeoRecormon®) contains a trace of albumin, whereas Epoetin alfa does not contain albumin and so is more widely accepted. Epoetin alfa (Eprex®) is licensed for the treatment of moderate anemia (hemoglobin concentration 10–13 g/100 mL) before elective orthopedic surgery in adults with expected moderate blood loss, to reduce exposure to allogeneic transfusion. It is given by subcutaneous injection (max. 1 mL per injection site), 600 units/kg every week for 3 weeks before surgery and on the day of surgery *or* 300 units/kg/day for 15 days starting 10 days before surgery.

Supplementation with folic acid and oral iron, or intravenous folinic acid and iron, should be considered particularly if the patient is maintained on erythropoietin. Frequency and amount of blood sampling should be minimized.

Granulocyte colony-stimulating factor (G-CSF) is acceptable treatment for neutropenia. Recombinant activated factor VII (rFVIIa, NovoSeven®) is licensed for the treatment of bleeding episodes in hemophiliacs with inhibitors, and has been used to treat bleeding in platelet disorders as well as those without a pre-existing hemostatic disorder.

Recombinant factor VIII and XI, particularly second-generation products containing no albumin, facilitate therapy of hemophilia A and B in JW patients. DDAVP is a synthetic product suitable for use in mild hemophilia A and type 1 von Willibrand disease (VWD) and uremia. Some patients with rare hemorrhagic disorders that currently require plasma-derived therapeutic products (e.g. type 2 or 3 VWD) will accept a purified fractionated product.

Some JW will regard their peripheral blood and bone marrow stem cell as a permissible fraction and consent to collection by leukapheresis or marrow aspiration. Specific treatment of the JW with other hematologic disorders is beyond the scope of this chapter. There should be an open, full and confidential discussion of all available options.

Further reading

Aird W. *Endothelial–Platelet Interplay in Sepsis*. American Society of Hematology, 2003.

Bevan, D. Haematological care of the Jehovah's Witness patient. *Br J Haematol* 2002;**119**:25–37.

Dempfle C-E. Coagulopathy of sepsis. *Thromb Haemost* 2004;**91**:213–24.

Geerts W, Selby R. Prevention of venous thromboembolism in the ICU. *Chest* 2003;**125**:357–63S.

Guidelines for the use of platelet transfusions. *Br J Haematol* 2003;**22**:10–23.

Guidelines on the diagnosis and management of the thrombotic microangiopathic haemolytic anaemias. *Br J Haematol* 2003;**120**:556–73.

Kazory A, Ducloux D. Acquired hypercoagulable state in renal transplant recipients. *Thromb Haemost* 2004;**91**(41):646–54.

Le Conte P, Huchet L, Trewick D. Efficacy of alteplase thrombolysis for ED treatment of pulmonary embolism with shock. *Am J Emerg Med* 2003;**21**:438–40.

Olin JW. Pulmonary embolism. *Rev Cardiovasc Med* 2002;**3**(S2):S68–S75.

Tayama E, Onchida M, Treshima H. Treatment of acute massive/submassive pulmonary embolism. *Circ J* 2002;**66**:479–83.

Warkentin TE. *Heparin-induced Thrombocytopenia and Thrombosis*. American Society of Hematology, 2003.

Warkentin TE. Heparin-induced thrombocytopenia: pathogenesis and management. *Br J Haematol* 2003;**121**:535–55.

Chapter 18
Cardiothoracic surgery

Denise O'Shaughnessy and Steven von Kier

Introduction

The importance for surgeons of understanding the normal hemostatic mechanisms cannot be overemphasized. Hemostasis is a mechanism to protect the integrity of the vascular system after tissue injury and the fluidity of the blood is finely balanced between the procoagulants and the natural anticoagulants. Excessive bleeding can be a result of surgical causes, but more often is caused by a derangement of hemostasis, and cardiothoracic surgery is a prime example.

As the incidence of heart disease continues to rise, the consequent demand for coronary artery bypass surgery also increases: with 400,000 in the USA, over 100,000 in Europe and 30,000 in UK per annum. Most of these procedures, together with major heart surgery on congenital defects and valvular heart disease, are performed on beating hearts supported by cardiopulmonary bypass (CPB).

Cardiopulmonary bypass

CPB pumps blood anticoagulated by large doses of heparin (3 mg/kg, approximately 30,000 units), because of the large area of contact of the artifical surfaces of the circuit, through an extracorporeal circuit with an oxygenator. Blood is drained from the right atrium and returned to the aorta, creating a bloodless field for the cardiothoracic surgeon. The patient's clotting is measured by the activated clotting time (ACT) or activated anti-factor X (anti-Xa) levels and residual heparin is reversed by protamine at the end of surgery.

This process:
- activates fibrinolysis;
- disturbs platelet function; and
- often reduces the platelet count.

Reduction in volume of the CPB circuit and improvements in operative techniques, together with cell salvage and the use of antifibrinolytic drugs, have reduced the need for transfusion. Recent "near patient" coagulation testing devices have enabled much of this progress and include the thromboelastogram (TEG®) and platelet function analyzer (PFA-100®).

Bleeding is usually manifest postoperatively, after protamine reversal of heparin, and shed into the mediastinal and pleural drains. There are two main causes of perioperative bleeding:

1 Surgical, due to failure to secure hemostasis at the operative site
2 Non-surgical, due to failure of hemostatic pathways and principally due to
   (a) The procedure itself, in this case ~CPB (the circuit and its effect on hemostasis).
   (b) Incomplete reversal of heparin by protamine.
   (c) Antiplatelet drugs (Aspirin, Clopidrogel, IIb-IIIa inhibitors).
   (d) A pre-existing bleeding disorder (e.g. hemophilia, von Willebrand disease).
   (e) Oral anticoagulation that has not been reversed completely.

Critical rates of blood loss are 500 mL in the first hour, 800 mL at 2 h, 900 mL at 3 h, 1000 mL at 4 h and 1200 mL by 5 h.

The cardiopulmonary bypass circuit

Bigelow showed in dogs that circulatory arrest

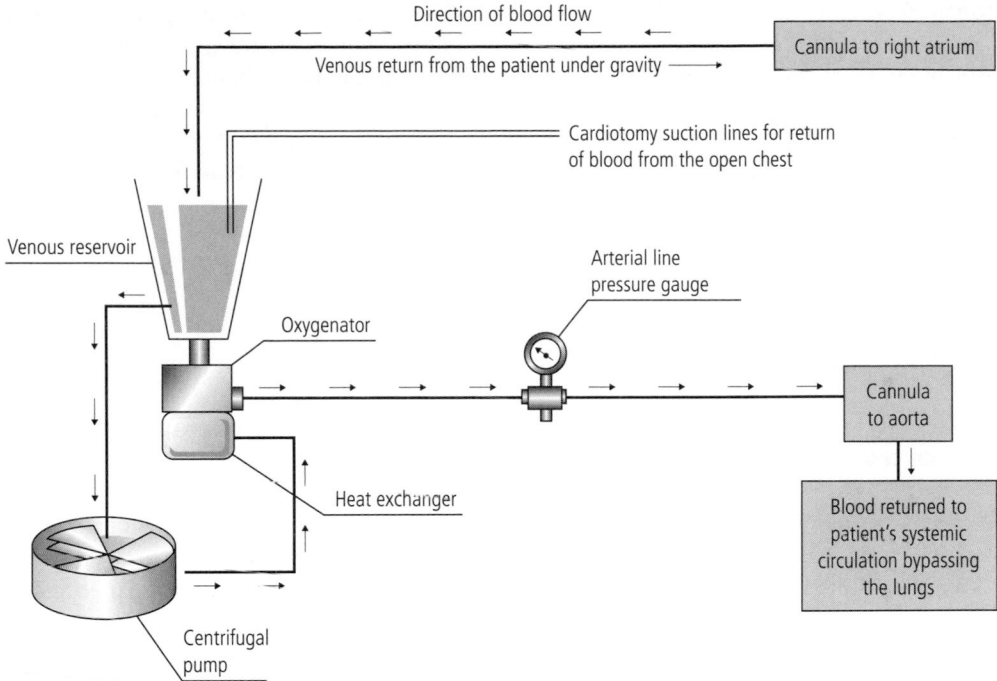

Direction of blood flow

Cannula to right atrium

Venous return from the patient under gravity

Cardiotomy suction lines for return of blood from the open chest

Venous reservoir

Oxygenator

Arterial line pressure gauge

Heat exchanger

Cannula to aorta

Blood returned to patient's systemic circulation bypassing the lungs

Centrifugal pump

Figure 18.1 Cardiopulmonary bypass circuit.

(CA) was possible allowing simple operations without circulatory support, but only for 15 min. Originally invented by Gibbon in the 1930s, the pump oxygenator only worked successfully in the 1950s. Even then, only one in four cases survived and 14–25 L of fresh blood prime was required. At the same time, Lillehei connected a patient to a volunteer donor (parent). He drained the blood from the superior vena cava (SVC) of the patient, and pumped this blood into the femoral vein of the donor. Blood was then returned from the femoral artery of the donor to the carotid artery of the patient. Forty-five patients (mostly children) had operations. The 63% survival, despite no reliable ventilators, blood gas or electrolyte analysis, pacemakers or defibrillators was remarkable. However, this was not a long-term solution.

The Gibbon Mayo pump in 1955 had bubble oxgenators, high flow total cardiopulmonary support, but still required 10–14 units fresh blood prime. Adapations over the next 60 years have reduced adult prime volumes to 1.5–2.5 L crystalloid and pediatric prime volumes to 400–1000 mL

prime including some blood (depending on the size of the child), such that on bypass the hematocrit will not fall below 20% (Fig. 18.1).

Hemostasis in cardiopulmonary bypass

Hemostasis is a dynamic and extremely complex process, involving many interactive factors including coagulation and fibrinolytic proteins, activators, inhibitors and cellular elements (e.g. platelet cytoskeleton, cytoplasmic granules and cell surfaces) as described in Chapter 1.

In order to measure any degree of hemostatic imbalance, we need the ability to measure the net product of the interactions, which is the three-dimensional clot matrix. Once the coagulation cascade is activated, thrombin is formed. Thrombin will cleave soluble fibrinogen into fibrin monomers, which polymerize to form protofibril strands and then undergo linear extension, branching and lateral association, leading to the formation of a three-dimensional matrix of fibrin. This matrix is given rigidity by the anchoring platelet network,

173

thus allowing resistance to shear. Platelet glyco-protein receptors (Gp IIb/IIIa) bind the polymer-ized fibrin network to the actin cytoskeleton of the platelet. Actin is a muscle protein that has the ability to transmit contractility force, which is the major contributor to clot strength.

It follows that in order to treat failures of the hemostatic system adequately we would need to evaluate and target this interaction of platelet and fibrin in order to assess the basic principles of func-tional hemostasis: activation, kinetics, contribu-tion and stability of clotting.

Conventional tests of coagulation

Until recently, hemostatic component therapies were guided by the results of conventional laboratory-based testing (see Chapter 2). These tests, which include the prothrombin time (PT), activated par-tial thromboplastin time (APTT), platelet count and fibrinogen concentrations have been shown to be unrelated to both postoperative bleeding and the need for blood and component therapies.

Inappropriateness of component transfusion

The national blood service for England issues approximately 2.2 million units of blood per year, of which 10% are used in cardiac surgical units. There is a wide unexplained variation in the trans-fusion practice between different cardiac surgical units despite the risk to the patient of contract-ing blood-borne or other infections or having a perioperative adverse event such as myocardial infarction.

This was noticed first by Goodenough *et al.* (1991), who showed that approximately 50% of platelet and 30% fresh frozen plasma (FFP) trans-fusions were inappropriate in a survey of patients undergoing routine heart surgery. (Inappropriate use definition was based upon the American Association of Blood Banks published guidelines for transfusion practice.) Seven years later, Stover *et al.* (1998) showed that little improvement had been made in relation to inappropriate ordering and administration of component products.

In a third study BCSH guidelines for the use of FFP Cryoprecipitate and Cryosupernatant, con-ducted as a national benchmarking audit of blood and component use in primary myocardial revas-cularization in the UK (National Blood Service and Royal Brompton and Harefield NHS Trust), it was shown that a high degree of transfusion practice variability still existed and it confirmed that the majority of platelet and FFP transfusions were inappropriate (as defined by national and interna-tional guidelines).

The need for near patient testing

A number of possibilities exist to explain this poor compliance and wastage of resources. The most obvious to the clinician is the delay between receiving test results when the patient has already developed serious bleeding.

It would seem logical that to improve perform-ance and to reduce inappropriate exposure to component products, near patient testing (NPT) is available, which is able to indicate an abnormal coagulation profile prior to the development of a clinically significant coagulopathy.

Early attempts at near patient testing

A number of suggestions and attempts have been made to develop point-of-care tests to fulfill these requirements. Early attempts at such devices included the use of machines to produce dedicated heparin–protamine response curves. Providing an individual solution for a specific patient was shown to be of benefit to reduce both bleeding and the requirement for red cells in patients undergoing heart surgery.

The potential failing in the concept of using a simple coagulation monitor as the only point-of-care test is shown in Fig. 18.2.

Standard laboratory tests (see Chapter 2)

PT and APTT

These use activators to initiate either intrinsic or extrinsic pathways of coagulation. The end-

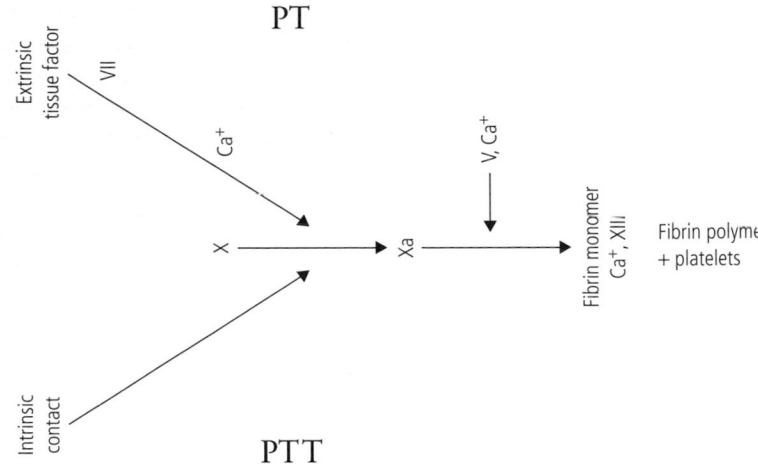

Figure 18.2 Standard laboratory tests. APTT, Activated partial thromboplastin time; PT, prothrombin time.

point for these tests, whether performed in citrated plasma in the laboratory or whole blood in a point-of-care test, is the establishment of fibrin strands.

Activated clotting time

In the ACT test, fresh whole blood is added to a tube containing an activator such as kaolin. It is the test for measuring high doses of heparin (when on bypass). It cannot be used in cases of heparin resistance and is likely to be inaccurate if the patient has an inhibitor (e.g. lupus anticoagulant).

Anti-Xa

Heparin binds to and enhances the activity of antithrombin (AT). Plasma containing heparin is incubated with AT and an excess of factor Xa. It is used primarily to monitor low molecular weight heparin (LMWH), which is not detectable by the APTT clotting test. It is a more accurate test for monitoring unfractionated heparin (UFH) and is the test of choice if there is a lupus anticoagulant present, or heparin resistance. There are NPT devices to measure anti-Xa available but, currently, these are used only in the USA. When monitoring LMWH, testing should be performed 2–3 h after the injection.

Desired levels of Anti-Xa

Prophylaxis LMWH	**Therapy LMWH**
0.2–0.4 IU/mL	0.4–1.0 IU/mL

CPB (large dose UFH)
5–8 IU/mL

None of these standard laboratory tests attempt to go further in order to evaluate the kinetics, strength or relative contribution (platelet to fibrin) of the clot and whether it remains stable over time.

Platelet count

Normal platelet numbers and function are required for normal hemostasis. A platelet count in patients undergoing surgery gives little information to the clinician. A normal platelet count gives no indication as to the functional capacity of the platelet and therefore is of limited value within the decision-making process, especially as many patients who undergo CPB already present as, or become, thrombocytopenic.

Non-standard laboratory tests

Thrombelastography

The thrombelastograph® uses its ability to measure the viscoelastic properties of blood to target hemostatic imbalance. It uses a simple premise, that the end result of the process of hemostasis is to create a single product (i.e. the clot) and that the physical properties of the clot (kinetics, strength and stability) will determine whether the patient will have normal hemostasis, hemorrhage or develop thrombosis.

The concept of coagulation analysis using the thromboelastograph was first described in Germany by Professor Hartert in the 1940s. At this time the device had two components: the mechanism for measuring clot formation and a mirror–galvanometer recording onto light-sensitive paper. The permanent record of activity was developed on this photographic paper and was available some hours, or days, later.

This somewhat slow, if highly innovative method, no longer takes this amount of time to produce data upon which the clinician can base treatment options. However, the principle of enabling a trace that identifies a number of variables related to functional disturbances in the hemostatic system is still key to thrombelastographic analysis.

Coagulation analysis: definitions of coagulation parameters using the thrombelastograph®

R = reaction time

Time from sample placement into the cuvette until the tracing amplitude reaches 2 mm.

This represents the rate of initial fibrin formation and is related functionally to plasma clotting factors of the intrinsic and circulating inhibitor activity (i.e. PT and APTT). Prolongation of the R-value may be a result of coagulation factor deficiencies, anticoagulation (heparin) or severe hypofibrinogenemia. A reduced R-value may be present in hypercoagulability syndromes.

K = clot formation time

Measured from R time to the point where the amplitude of the tracing reaches 20 mm.

The coagulation time represents the time taken for a fixed degree of viscoelasticity to be achieved by the forming clot, as a result of fibrin build-up and cross-linking. It is affected by the activity of the intrinsic clotting factors, fibrinogen and platelets.

Alpha angle (α)

This is a line tangent from the point at which clot formation begins to the peak of the curve. It denotes speed at which solid clot forms. Decreased values may occur with hypofibrinogenemia and thrombocytopenia.

Maximum amplitude/G (MA/G)

This is the greatest amplitude of the TEG® trace and is a reflection of the absolute strength of the fibrin clot. It is a direct function of the maximum dynamic properties of the interaction of fibrin and platelets.

Platelet abnormalities, whether qualitative or quantitative, substantially disturb the MA. There is a significant, albeit complex, relationship between the MA of the TEG® trace and the platelet count. A significant relationship with the MA value and the aggregation responses to collagen and adenosine diphosphate (ADP) has also been reported.

Clot lysis

This can be expressed in a number of ways. Normal clot will retract with time and thus a narrowing of the MA can be expected. The clot lysis index (CLI) (normal range > 85%) is derived as $A_{60}/MA \times 100\%$. This index has been superseded with computer-based data acquisition and handling to give the LY30, the percentage reduction in maximum amplitude at 30 min. Both measures reflect an abnormal decrease in amplitude as a function of time and reflect loss of clot integrity as a result of lysis.

A stylized thrombelastography trace is shown in Fig. 18.3 together with the clotting profile originally outlined in Fig. 18.2. It is easy to recognize that thromboelastography can provide information on clot kinetics, strength and stability, which are not available with conventional laboratory-based testing.

A unique attribute of thrombelastography is its ability to define previously unrecognized changes in certain clinical scenarios. It can be observed that the trace develops more vigorously and produces a more stable and strong clot in certain clinical conditions.

Hypercoaguability

Increased alpha angle and MA associated with a

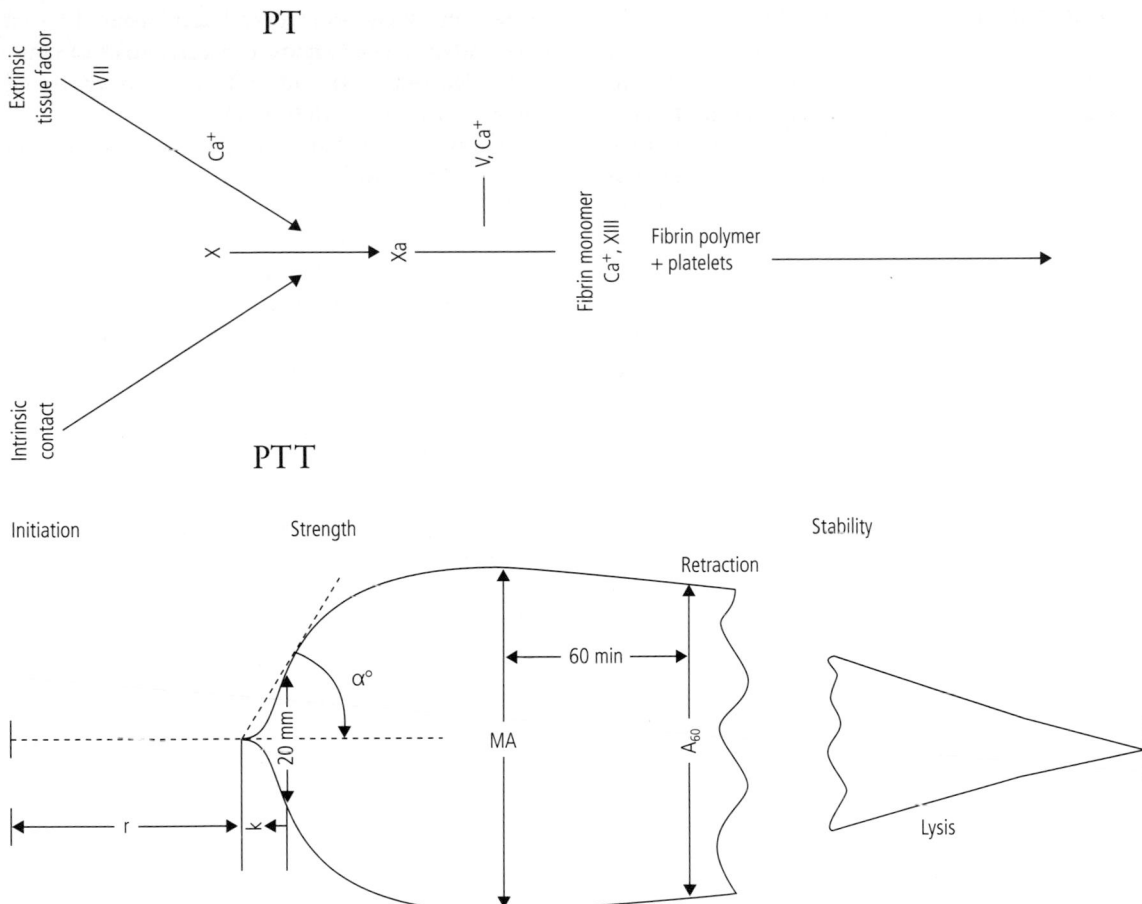

Figure 18.3 The thromboelastogram with the clotting profile from Fig. 18.2.

shorter R-value can be defined as hypercoagulability. This is an increasing focus of attention in many fields, largely because of the recognition of genetic determinants of increased likelihood of developing a thrombotic disease process such as stroke, coronary artery or deep vein thrombosis.

The advent of inhibitor and activator reagents

A now common development of thromboelastography is to use commercially available activator and inhibitor reagent technology to define specific parts of the coagulation system.

Heparinase
This enzyme is known to convert unfractionated heparin to a relatively inactive form. It therefore allows the use of thromboelastography in a patient who is fully heparinized, such as on CPB.

Abcximicab
When this monoclonal antibody to Gp IIb/IIIa receptor on the platelet surface is added to the system, it inhibits the platelet component (80%) of the clot strength shown in the MA, revealing the functional fibrinogen element of the clot (normally 20%).

Tissue factor
An equivalent to the PT is performed by the addition of tissue factor.

Kaolin
The effects of contact activation (equivalent to APTT) are assessed using either celite or kaolin.

Adensine diphosphate and arachidonic acid

As more pharmacologic interventions using platelet inhibitor agents are becoming evident, thromboelastography technology has addressed the issue by using reagent technology to assess the impact of such interventions. On writing this chapter, two new assays have been developed using ADP and arachidonic acid agonists, generating modified MA values which measure the degree of inhibition caused by these antiplatelet agents.

Thromboelastography-based transfusion algorithms

Some centers such as Mount Sinai (New York), Southampton (UK) and Harefield Hospital (UK) have incorporated the TEG® system into their transfusion algorithms.

The Mount Sinai protocol

The measurements used were partly TEG®-based (celite, with and without heparinase), in conjunction with platelet count and fibrinogen concentration from the laboratory:

- If the R-value in the non-heparinase sample was greater than twice that found in the heparinase sample, then the patient was given supplementary protamine.
- If the platelet count was < 100,000 and the MA was < 45 mm, then platelets were administered.
- FFP was given if the celite activated R-value, 10 min post protamine administration, was > 20 mm.
- Low fibrinogen was treated with cryoprecipitate.
- ε-Aminocoproic acid (amicar) was given in the event of excess lysis.

Using this protocol, they showed significant reductions in the use of hemostatic products compared with the more conventional transfusion protocol.

The Harefield protocol

The concept of a TEG®-derived algorithm was taken a stage further, with measurements taken during the bypass phase in order to predict the need for component products. A study was conducted in 60 patients who were considered to have a higher than average risk of bleeding and thus the need for hemostatic products, but were not given aprotinin or tranexamic acid. They were randomly allocated

to have products ordered and administered based upon either a TEG®-derived decision tree or clinician's discretion after the return of conventional laboratory-based testing results.

Results for the TEG® trace were available, on average, 70–90 min before conventional tests of coagulation, fibrinogen and platelet count. This was considered significant in terms of logistical appropriateness. There was also a 50% reduction in the number of patients given hemostatic products, with a reduction in the use of FFP from a total of 16–5 units in transfused patients. The use of platelet concentrates was reduced, with only one patient receiving a single platelet pool in the TEG® guided group.

Future development in blood and hemostatic component management

It is well-recognized that postoperative bleeding and the subsequent need for reoperation to control bleeding is associated with an increase in morbidity and mortality, particularly in cardiac surgery. Replacement therapy using red cells and plasma-based hemostatic components are themselves contributors to morbidity and mortality.

Clinical indications to reduce exposure

The complex relationship between transfusion, mortality and morbidity is ill-defined. There is emerging evidence that blood transfusion is an independent risk factor for death after cardiac surgery. In addition, platelet transfusion is associated with an increased risk of organ dysfunction or death from uncertain causes. Immunomodulation may have a role, because leukodepletion of blood may reduce mortality in the critically ill adult and neonate. Given the complexity of these issues, it would seem to be prudent to avoid transfusion unless necessary and to use simple, safe, available methods to reduce the chances of patients needing a transfusion during surgery.

Logistical indications to reduce exposure

The current donor pool is known to be decreasing at 6%/year, and may well continue to decrease.

This trend is probably multifactorial; however, the ongoing public debate concerning variant Creutzfeldt–Jakob disease (vCJD) has to be considered a significant contributory element. Some estimates put the possible overall donor reduction at 50% because of the eventual inclusion of a screening test for vCJD. It remains to be seen if this trend is capable of being reversed, even with the advent of increased public relations awareness and legislative measures introduced to lower the acceptable donor age limit. This must be viewed against a projected increase in demand for blood and hemostatic products of approximately 4.9% by 2008.

The true role for TEG® analysis is as a platform for an integrated approach to hemostasis management. Evidence-based medicine dictates that we do not prophylactically treat patients with drugs or expose them to non-proven technology. Therefore, it would make sense to return to the original issue surrounding hemostasis management: that of information. A global assessment of patient hemostasis in the preoperative, perioperative or postoperative phase is required. If such information is available, to allow for targeted analysis and trend management of hemostatic imbalance, then the ability to effectively identify, treat and monitor treatment is enhanced.

Information is the key to this whole process and any technology that fails to provide relevant information because of scientific or logistical failures only serves to further exacerbate an already complex clinical management task.

Methods to reduce blood loss

- Mechanical strategies;
- Pharmacologic strategies;
- Preoperative methods;
- Anesthetic methods.

Pharmacologic methods

Pharmacotherapy remains the mainstay of treatment in trying to minimize blood loss in cardiothoracic surgery. Nothing beats meticulous surgical technique, but some loss is inevitable. Both aprotinin and tranexamic acid are antifibrinolytic agents that have been used widely in this setting to reduce blood loss.

Aprotinin

This is a non-specific serine protease inhibitor (inhibits plasmin at low dose, kallikrien at high dose and inhibits activated protein C and thrombin). In addition to its antifibrinolytic properties, it may have effects on preventing platelet activation by blocking the thrombin activated protease-activated receptor 1 (PAR-1) and appears to affect novel anti-inflammatory targets preventing transmigration of leukocytes.

Efficacy is dose-dependent over a wide range of surgery, with high-dose regimens reducing blood requirements and perioperative bleeding by two-thirds.

As aprotinin is derived from bovine lung there is a risk of allergy, especially with repeated doses, therefore a test dose should always be performed.

Tranexamic acid

Tranexamic acid is a synthetically derived antifibrinolytic agent that has its effects by the prevention of the interaction between plasminogen with fibrin via interaction with lysine residues. It has been shown to be safe, reduces blood loss but not transfusion and is cheaper than aprotinin.

Studies comparing antifibrinolytic agents

Antifibrinolytic therapy has been extensively studied in cardiac surgical patients, with three major meta-analyses favoring their use in terms of reduction of exposure to allogenic blood and in reduction in postoperative blood loss. The Cochrane Collaboration identified seven studies that compared aprotinin to tranexamic acid. This showed a non-significant trend to benefit in the aprotinin group; only one of these trials reported the use of cell salvage.

Recombinant factor VIIa

Factor VIIa (NovoSeven®) is approved for the treatment of hemophilia with inhibitors. In recent years there has been increasing interest in using factor VIIa in major hemorrhage in non-hemophilia patients. Randomized clinical trials are now required to determine the role of this product in cardiothoracic surgery.

Preoperative assessment clinics

The prescribing clinician should anticipate and plan ahead for a situation that may necessitate transfusion and aim to reduce the chance that the patient will actually need to be given blood.

Assessment of patients specific to hemostasis:

1 *Diagnosis of any bleeding disorder:* previously undiagnosed bleeding disorders are common and can lead to greater use of donor blood if not known about prior to surgery. Consider specific questions about bleeding history in standard preoperative assessment.

2 *Assessment of patient's current medication, its potential for increasing bleeding tendency and impact on recovery:* commonly used drugs increase bleeding time (e.g. aspirin, NSAIDs, coumarins).

3 *Identification of problems that may require specialist intervention* (ITP, PTP).

4 *Patient's beliefs* (e.g. Jehovah's Witnesses).

Diagnosis of a bleeding disorder

Although most hemostatic defects in hospitalized patients are acquired, underlying mild hereditary disorders may only manifest in the hospital setting such as mild hemophilia A (deficient factor VIII), mild hemophilia B (deficient factor IX) and mild hemophilia C (deficient factor XI), all of which prolong the APPT. If patients are found to have hemophilia it is essential that a hematologist advises on the best treatment, which can vary from DDAVP preoperatively with an antifibrinolytic postoperatively, to the giving of regular doses of a recombinant replacement factor (and regular measurements of factor levels in blood). The latter may not be available in all hospitals out of hours without prior notice.

Assessment of current medication

Some of the drugs can be stopped prior to surgery, others may need to be continued but the surgical team need to be aware.

Antiplatelet drugs. Clopidogrel causes platelet inhibition via a different mechanism to aspirin, and following coronary stenting the two drugs are increasingly being prescribed together. There is growing evidence that the hemorrhagic risk is increased when the two drugs are taken concurrently. An increasing number of patients take antiplatelet agents. Non-steroidal anti-inflammatory drugs (NSAIDs), dipyridamole, aspirin and clopidogrel are all implicated in increased surgical blood loss. Ideally, these drugs should be stopped prior to surgery, to allow platelet function to return to normal.

The time required off the drug to ensure normal platelet function varies. NSAIDs provide reversible inhibition of cyclooxygenase, and their antiplatelet effects are half-life dependent (usually hours). Aspirin and clopidogrel lead to irreversible inhibition of platelet aggregation for the life span of the platelet (approximately 10 days). These drugs need to be stopped for 7 days to be confident of adequate platelet function. However, due consideration must be given to the risks associated with stopping these drugs in surgical patients.

Many patients are presenting for emergency coronary revascularization having had failed coronary stenting procedures. These patients have usually received aspirin and clopidogrel. Hemorrhage during the subsequent surgery may be a major problem. Use of the new TEG® reagents is very useful here as 15% of patients have normal platelet function despite therapy, and in others the degree of dysfunction is variable.

Clopidogrel is a pro-drug. The active metabolite circulates for approximately 18 h after the last dose, and may permanently inhibit any platelets present during this time (whether endogenous or transfused). Surgery is best delayed for at least 24 h after the last dose of clopidogrel. Surgery in patients who have received clopidogrel in the last 7 days should, where possible, be postponed. If the surgery is a genuine emergency, platelets should be made available for transfusion, and consideration given to using aprotinin. Delaying for 24 h after the last dose of clopidogrel will improve the response to platelet transfusion.

Warfarin. With a patient on oral anticoagulant therapy, it is sufficient to stop warfarin 3 days before surgery and restart the usual maintenance dose on the evening of the surgery. If they have a mechanical heart valve or have had a venous thromboembolism in the past, this period should be covered by heparin. Having stopped warfarin, if the INR preoperation is > 2.5, small amounts of vitamin K (1–2 mg) may be given.

Anesthetic techniques to reduce blood loss

There are some basic techniques that the anesthetist and surgeon can use to reduce blood loss during surgery:

• Positioning of the anesthetized patient so as to minimize any venous congestion in the operating field.

• The use of local vasoconstrictors.

• The sequencing of a multistage procedure (e.g. a coronary artery bypass procedure where the saphenous vein is harvested by one member of the team as another is opening and preparing the chest. The vein harvester needs to close his operation site fully before ascending to assist with the chest).

There are also some specific procedures that may help in reducing blood loss:

• preventing hypertension;

• minimizing the period of hypothermia; and

• controlling hypotension.

Further reading

BCSH guidelines for the use of FFP Cryoprecipitate and Cryosupernatant. *Br J Haematology* 2004;**26**:11–28.

Bevan D. A review of cardiac bypass haemostasis, putting blood through the mill. *Br J Haematol* 1999;**104**:208–19.

Carson JL, Duff A, Berlin JA. Perioperative blood transfusion and postoperative mortality *JAMA* 1998;**279**:199–205.

Goodenough LT, Johnston MFM, Toy PTCY, and the Medicine Academic Award Group. The variability of transfusion practice in coronary artery bypass surgery. *JAMA* 1991;**265**:86–90.

Koh MBC, Hunt BJ. The management of perioperative bleeding. *Blood Rev* 2003;**17**:179–85.

Laupacis A, Fergusson D, for the International study of Perioperative Transfusion (ISPOT). Drugs to minimize postoperative blood loss in cardiac surgery: meta-analysis using perioperative blood transfusion as the outcome. *Anasth Analg* 1997;**85**:1258–67.

McGill N, O'Shaughnessy D, Pickering R, Herbertson M, Gill R. Mechanical methods of reducing blood loss in cardiac surgery: a randomized controlled trial. *BMJ* 2002;**324**:1299.

Shore-Lesserson L, Manspeizer HE, Francis S, Deperio M. Intraoperative thrombelastograph analysis (TEG®) reduces transfusion requirements. *Anesth Analg* 1998:**86**:S104.

Spiess BD. Thrombelastograph analysis and cardiopulmonary bypass. *Semin Thromb Hemost* 1995:**21**:S4.

Stover FP, Stegel IC, Parks R, *et al*. for Institutions of the Multicenter study of Perioperative Ischaemia Research. Variabillity in transfusion practice for coronary artery bypass surgery persists despite national consensus guidelines. *Anaesthesiology* 1998;**88**:327–33.

von Kier S, Royston D. Reduced hemostatic factor transfusion using heparinase-modified thrombelastograph analysis (TEG®) during cardioplumonary bypass. *Anesthesiology* 1998;**89**(3A):A911.

Chapter 19

Hepatology

Raj K. Patel and Roopen Arya

Introduction

The liver has a major role in the maintenance of normal hemostasis. In addition to the synthesis of coagulation factors and hemostatic regulators, it acts as a clearance site for activated coagulation proteins. Because of a considerable hepatic functional reserve, coagulopathy tends not to occur until more than 80% of hepatic function is lost.

Hepatic diseases are associated with a variety of defects affecting both primary and secondary hemostasis (Table 19.1). It is therefore not surprising that advanced hepatic disease is associated with bleeding. Chronic liver disease frequently causes portal hypertension with resultant hypersplenism and thrombocytopenia. This leads to formation of fragile vascular anomalies (varices) which may bleed profusely on a background of hemostatic failure. Not all patients with liver disease have bleeding manifestations but these tend to be unpredictable when they occur. Common clinical manifestations include petechiae, ecchymoses, recurrent epistaxes and gingival bleeding. Invasive procedures such as liver biopsy and ascitic shunts are particularly high risk in chronic liver disease as they may precipitate bleeding in previously stable patients.

Liver disease may be classified into two broad categories:
1 *Acute liver disease* (e.g. fulminant hepatic failure secondary to paracetamol overdose).
2 *Chronic liver disease* (e.g. alcohol-induced cirrhosis, primary biliary cirrhosis).

Most advanced cases of liver disease are associated with at least one and frequently multiple hemostatic defects. Orthotopic liver transplantation corrects hepatic function and coagulopathy long-term but is associated with a substantial perioperative increase in bleeding risk.

Pathophysiology of coagulopathy

Impaired coagulation factor synthesis

The liver is the major synthetic site for:
• Coagulation factors of both intrinsic and extrinsic pathways including factors II, V, VII, VIII, IX, X, XI, XII and fibrinogen.
• Anticoagulant proteins (antithrombin, protein C, protein S).
• Fibrinolytic regulators (plasminogen, α_1-antiplasmin).

Coagulation proteins

Loss of hepatocyte function in disease states leads to a reduction in the levels of most coagulation proteins (except factor VIII) and therefore predisposes to bleeding. Reduced levels of these proteins broadly reflect the extent of liver damage but are poor predictors of bleeding risk in individual patients.

Table 19.1 Hemostatic defects in hepatic disease.

Hemostatic abnormality
Reduced biosynthesis of hepatic coagulation factors
Reduced biosynthesis of anticoagulant and fibrinolytic proteins
Reduced clearance of coagulation proteins and inhibitors
Dysfibrinogenemia
Systemic fibrinolysis
Disseminated intravascular coagulation
Thrombocytopenia
Platelet dysfunction

- In acute liver injury (e.g. following paracetamol overdose).
- Prothrombin time (PT) has been shown to be an accurate predictor of hepatocellular damage, bleeding risk and likelihood of progression to fulminant liver failure.
- Factor V concentration is a particularly sensitive and specific indicator of hepatic synthetic function and plasma levels fall with increasing disease severity.
- Malabsorption of fat-soluble vitamins may lead to low levels of circulating vitamin K-dependent coagulation factors.

Whereas the majority of circulating coagulation factors decrease in liver disease, the reverse is true of factor VIII, von Willebrand factor (VWF) and fibrinogen. Fibrinogen and most of factor VIII are synthesized in hepatocytes whereas VWF is synthesized by platelets and vascular endothelium. Circulating levels of these proteins increase in the acute phase response associated with hepatic disease, although low levels of fibrinogen in late disease may herald the onset of acute liver failure.

The formation of abnormal forms of vitamin K-dependent coagulation factors (e.g. des-γ-carboxyl prothrombin) may be seen in both acute and chronic liver disease. These proteins, raised in the absence of vitamin K (PIVKAs), form as a result of an acquired carboxylation defect, but do not reach high enough concentrations to cause bleeding.

Thrombocytopenia and platelet dysfunction

Mild to moderate thrombocytopenia is common in hepatic disease, affecting up to 30% of all cases of chronic liver disease and 90% of subjects with end-stage disease.

Chronic liver disease is associated with:
- Portal hypertension and congestive splenomegaly. The resultant increase in platelet pooling by splenic sequestration is the principal mechanism by which thrombocytopenia occurs in these patients.
- Increasing portal venous pressures, blood is shunted into the systemic circulation via portosystemic collaterals (varices) from which blood loss may occur, particularly on a background of thrombocytopenia.

- Ineffective production of platelets secondary to a decrease in liver thrombopoietin synthesis has been reported.

Alcohol-associated liver disease may cause thrombocytopenia by a variety of mechanisms:
- Alcohol is directly toxic to megakaryocytes, leading to inhibition of megakaryopoiesis and decreased platelet production.
- Folate deficiency resulting from poor dietary intake or ineffective hepatic metabolism may result in ineffective megakaryopoiesis.
- Alcohol ingestion is itself associated with decreased platelet survival.

In fulminant viral hepatitis, the marked thrombocytopenia often encountered is caused by both suppression of megakaryopoiesis by virus; and increased platelet destruction.

The increase in bleeding time seen in many subjects with severe liver disease is often out of proportion to the associated degree of thrombocytopenia, suggesting the presence of platelet dysfunction. The results of platelet function testing in these patients are inconsistent. Whereas some studies have demonstrated abnormalities in primary and secondary aggregation to adenosine diphosphate (ADP), adrenaline, thrombin and ristocetin, others have failed to show any functional defect.

The cause of platelet dysfunction in liver disease is unclear. There is an increase in levels of circulating platelet-inhibitors including fibrin degradation products. Ethanol or abnormal high-density lipoproteins may contribute to aggregatory abnormalities in some cases. In others, intrinsic platelet abnormalities have been demonstrated including acquired storage pool deficiency (platelet nucleotide deficiency), reduced platelet arachidonic acid and abnormalities of platelet membrane composition and signaling.

Disseminated intravascular coagulation

It is generally accepted that many patients with advanced liver disease have activated coagulation and chronic low-grade disseminated intravascular coagulation (DIC). The diagnosis of DIC in subjects with chronic liver disease is complicated by the fact that many of the laboratory abnormalities present are common to both conditions.

Bleeding or thrombosis is usually present in DIC but is not a frequent finding in patients with liver disease coagulopathy alone. Evidence of increased thrombin generation has been demonstrated in chronic liver disease. These effects are at least partially reversible by heparin and include reduced fibrinogen survival and increased markers of thrombin generation (D-dimer, thrombin–antithrombin complexes, fibrinopeptide A and plasmin–antiplasmin complexes). It may be that liver disease confers a state of increased intravascular coagulation where additional factors such as sepsis or bleeding trigger DIC.

A number of possible causes of chronic DIC in liver disease have been suggested:
• Procoagulant factors released from damaged hepatocytes.
• Release of intestinal endotoxins into the portal circulation.
• Impaired clearance of activated coagulation factors by the damaged failing liver.
• In addition, levels of naturally occurring anticoagulants including antithrombin, protein C, protein S and heparin cofactor II are reduced in proportion to the degree of hepatic dysfunction.

Vitamin K deficiency

Vitamin K is a fat-soluble vitamin required for the production of a variety of coagulation proteins including factors II, VII, IX, X, protein C and protein S. Vitamin K deficiency may occur in liver disease as a result of:
• poor dietary intake;
• destruction of vitamin K_2-producing intestinal bacteria by antibiotic therapy;
• bile salts are required for the absorption of vitamin K in the small intestine so biliary obstruction may therefore lead to vitamin K deficiency; and
• prolonged cholestasis secondary to calculi or neoplasia leads to deficiencies in the vitamin K-dependent coagulation proteins and prolongation of the PT.

Dysfibrinogenemia

One of the earliest coagulation abnormalities seen in chronic liver disease is the production of a dysfibrinogen. This molecule is rich in sialic acid residues and results in abnormal fibrin polymerization. The reduced efficiency in fibrin clot production prolongs both the thrombin time and reptilase time, but has not been shown to contribute to clinical bleeding. Dysfibrinogenemia is most commonly seen in chronic hepatitis and cirrhosis but has also been reported in hepatocellular carcinoma.

Hyperfibrinolysis

Accelerated fibrinolysis is well recognized in hepatic cirrhosis. Forty percent of patients awaiting liver transplant show laboratory evidence of hyperfibrinolysis with short euglobulin lysis times and elevated serum fibrin degradation product concentrations. In addition, low plasminogen levels and elevated fibrinopeptide B, D-dimer and plasmin–α_2-antiplasmin complex concentrations may be demonstrated in subjects with chronic liver disease. Possible mechanisms behind this include decreased hepatic clearance of plasminogen activators (e.g. tissue plasminogen activator; tPA) and a decrease in circulating the fibrinolytic inhibitors plasminogen activator inhibitor type 1 (PAI-1), α_2-antiplasmin and histidine-rich glycoprotein.

Clinical manifestations of liver disease coagulopathy

Hemorrhage

Bleeding is a common manifestation of chronic liver disease (Table 19.2) and is associated with

Table 19.2 Clinical manifestations of liver disease coagulopathy.

Ecchymoses
Purpura
Oozing from venipuncture or intravenous cannula sites
Dental bleeding
Hematuria
Gastrointestinal and variceal hemorrhage
Epistaxis
Postoperative hemorrhage

substantial morbidity and mortality. Patients may present with both:

• *Mucosal bleeding:* resulting from thrombocytopenia and platelet dysfunction leading to failure of primary hemostasis.

• *Soft tissue bleeding:* resulting from the reduction in coagulation proteins with failure of secondary hemostasis.

Once liver disease is diagnosed it is important to remember that laboratory tests of hemostasis are poorly predictive of bleeding events. This is partly because liver disease bleeding is not only caused by defects in primary and secondary hemostasis, but also is frequently associated with anatomical abnormalities such as portosystemic varices on a background of raised portal pressure.

Bleeding episodes may also be triggered by operative procedures in previously stable patients. Some patients with advanced chronic liver disease are identified for the first time prior to elective surgery when a coagulation screen is checked. At least 50% of patients with cirrhosis will have varices secondary to portal hypertension at diagnosis and some will be diagnosed for the first time with liver disease following a variceal bleed.

Hepatic venous thrombosis

Budd–Chiari syndrome (BCS) is associated with a variety of acquired and inherited hypercoagulable states including:

• hereditary thrombophilia;
• antiphospholipid syndrome;
• paroxysmal nocturnal hemoglobinuria; and
• myeloproliferative disorders (polycythemia rubra vera is causative in up to 50%).

Laboratory investigation of hemostasis in liver disease

Clotting screen

The prothrombin time (PT) and activated partial thromboplastin time (APTT) are commonly prolonged in chronic liver disease, reflecting a reduction in coagulation factor production by the failing liver (Table 19.3). Patients with abnormal laboratory tests only require treatment to correct coagulopathy when there is evidence of active bleeding or prior to surgery.

Chronic liver disease

No single coagulation test is predictive of hemorrhage in patients with chronic liver disease:

• Factor VII has a short half-life and levels fall early in subjects with hepatic impairment. An isolated prolongation of the PT may be the only demonstrable laboratory abnormality in those with mild disease.

• Prolonged PT or international normalized ratio (INR) is a key indicator of hepatic dysfunction and

Table 19.3 Laboratory abnormalities in liver disease.

Laboratory abnormality	Likely etiology
Isolated ↑ PT	FVII deficiency
	Vitamin K deficiency (cholestasis, dietary)
↑ PT + ↑ APTT	Coagulation factor deficiencies
↑ Thrombin time + ↑ reptilase time	Dysfibrinogenemia, hypofibringenemia
Thrombocytopenia	Hypersplenism, DIC
	Suppressed megakaryopoeisis
Abnormal platelet aggregometry	Acquired platelet function defect
↓ Euglobulin clot lysis time	Hyperfibrinolysis:
	↓ PAI
	↓ α_2-antiplasmin

APTT, Activated partial thromboplastin time; DIC, disseminated intravascular coagulation; PAI, plasminogen activator inhibitor; PT, prothrombin time.

commonly used as a trigger for liver transplantation; however, it is vitamin K-dependent.
• Factor V concentration is a sensitive indicator of hepatic disease as this protein is predominantly synthesized by hepatocytes and is not vitamin K-dependent.

Cholestasis

Patients with early vitamin K deficiency secondary to cholestasis have isolated prolongation of the PT, which is correctable by administration of intravenous vitamin K.

Factor VII has the shortest half-life of all the vitamin K-dependent factors and is therefore the first coagulation factor to decrease, hence isolated prolonged PT. With severe prolonged vitamin K deficiency there is reduction in factors II, IX and X with prolongation of both PT and APTT.

Advanced hepatocellular disease

These patients tend to have a more severe derangement of laboratory tests reflecting:
• high incidence of multiple coagulation factor deficiencies;
• hyperfibrinolysis; and
• DIC.

Fibrinogen level

Fibrinogen levels vary according to the type and severity of liver dysfunction. When measuring fibrinogen concentration, results may vary markedly depending upon the methods used. Assays based on the rate of clot formation (e.g. Clauss fibrinogen) result in low levels of fibrinogen more often than assays based on final clot weight. This is because dysfibrinogens and circulating proteins that impair fibrin clot formation may (e.g. fibrinogen degradation products; FDPs) influence rate-dependent assays.

Dysfibrinogenemia

This may prolong thrombin time and reptilase time but is not usually associated with bleeding.

Hyperfibrinolysis

This may lead to hypofibrinogenemia with prolongation of the PT, APTT, thrombin time and reptilase times. Other laboratory findings include a prolongation of the euglobulin clot lysis time, raised FDP levels and decreased plasminogen concentration.

Thromboelastography (TEG®) is an investigation measuring the dynamics of clot formation and has been shown to be a superior predictor of intraoperative bleeding in liver transplantation than standard coagulation tests.

Invasive procedures and liver disease

Liver biopsy

The risk of bleeding after liver biopsy is a small but significant one and has been estimated to occur in 0.4% of cases. In view of this risk, each case should be carefully reviewed to ensure that the procedure is only performed when absolutely necessary.

Percutaneous liver biopsy is relatively safe when the INR is below 1.5 and the platelet count is above 50×10^9/L. In subjects who do not fulfill these criteria, administration of vitamin K, plasma and platelets should be considered prior to the procedure. Subjects with prolonged bleeding time and history of bleeding may be given desmopressin (DDAVP). Alternative strategies include laparoscopic liver biopsy and biopsy via the transjugular approach.

A high mortality rate has been reported in patients with sickle cell disease undergoing percutaneous liver biopsy and extreme caution is recommended, particularly in the setting of acute liver failure.

Shunt insertion in liver disease

Portocaval and mesocaval shunts may be inserted to alleviate portal hypertension in decompensated liver disease. These procedures are frequently associated with increased fibrinolysis and DIC. Peritoneal–venous shunt insertion in patients with chronic ascites may trigger significant bleeding.

This is thought to be because of the flow of pro-coagulant and platelet-activating molecules from ascitic fluid into the systemic circulation triggering DIC. Clinically significant bleeding may be avoided by draining ascites prior to opening the shunt or by short-term occlusion of the shunt.

Liver transplantation

Liver transplantation is being increasingly offered to patients with end-stage decompensated liver disease. Marked hemostatic failure with substantial blood loss is frequently seen during liver transplant, with a strong association between blood loss and mortality rate. Research into the causes of liver transplant coagulopathy have led to improved intraoperative management strategies and decreased mortality rates.

The first operative (preimplantation) stage

There is mild deterioration in the baseline liver disease coagulopathy. This coincides with surgical dissection and mobilization of the diseased liver and is not usually associated with major blood loss.

The next three operative stages

The coagulation disturbance increases (Table 19.4) and is maximal during the anhepatic stage (because of loss of coagulation factor turnover) and early reimplantation (hyperfibrinolytic) stage.

Consumptive thrombocytopenia with DIC often occurs requiring massive blood product replacement.

This is followed by gradual resolution of hemostatic dysfunction in the third (reimplantation) stage and postoperative period.

Treatment of liver transplant coagulopathy

This varies according to stage of operation:
• Stage 1 is associated with mild surgical bleeding, not usually requiring aggressive hemostatic support.
• In the anhepatic and reperfusion stages, transfusion with blood, platelets, plasma and cryoprecipitate are required to correct profound coagulopathy and inevitable major blood losses.
• The reperfusion stage is associated with tPA and endogenous heparin-like substance release from the graft and antifibrinolytic therapy with aprotinin has been shown to be effective in reducing transfusion requirements in this setting.
• Stage 3 is usually associated with resolution of coagulopathy. However, if successful engraftment of the donor liver does not occur, tissue ischemia and necrosis may trigger DIC and further bleeding.

Treatment of liver disease coagulopathy

Treatment of coagulopathy in liver disease is required during episodes of bleeding or prior to invasive procedures. The type of treatment required will depend on the specific hemostatic abnormalities present and the nature of the bleeding event. It is important to remember that most patients with coagulopathy are stable and do not

Table 19.4 Coagulation abnormalities during liver transplantation.

Stage of transplant	Hemostatic abnormality
Stage 1: Preimplantation	Mild deterioration of baseline liver disease coagulopathy
Stage 2: Anhepatic	Loss of coagulation factor synthesis and clearance
	Accelerated fibrinolysis and DIC
	Consumptive thrombocytopenia
	tPA released from graft on reperfusion
Stage 3: Reimplantation	Restoration of coagulation factor synthesis and clearance
	Resolution of hyperfibrinolysis

DIC, Disseminated intravascular coagulation; tPA, tissue plasminogen activator.

require specific therapy. When bleeding does occur the associated triggers (e.g. oesophageal varices secondary to portal hypertension) need to be addressed in conjunction with strategies to correct coagulopathy.

Vitamin K

Deficiency of vitamin K may occur in liver disease resulting from poor diet or secondary to malabsorption. Administration of 10 mg vitamin K_1 will correct the PT, at least partially, in most patients within 48 h. The PT will not fully correct if there is a coexisting defect in hepatic synthetic function.

Plasma

Fresh frozen plasma (FFP) or solvent detergent plasma (SDP) contain all the coagulation factors synthesized by the healthy liver. It may be used to correct multiple coagulation factor deficiencies in bleeding patients or prior to invasive procedures. A significant problem with FFP is the large volume of transfusion required to correct the PT and APTT in severe liver disease, particularly in volume overloaded patients with ascites and peripheral edema. In addition, repeated transfusions are required to maintain circulating coagulation factor levels. Prothrombin complex concentrates should be used with caution in liver disease as their use has been associated with thromboembolism and DIC. Cryoprecipitate should be used to correct hypofibrinogenemia associated with hyperfibrinolysis or DIC.

Platelets

Platelet transfusions are indicated in bleeding patients with platelet counts of less than 10×10^9/L, or in patients undergoing invasive procedures. Platelet increments are generally poor in subjects with portal hypertension because of sequestration of transfused platelets in the spleen. DDAVP (0.3 μg/kg) may be of value in patients with acquired platelet dysfunction and prolonged bleeding time but its value in bleeding patients is uncertain.

Antifibrinolytics

Aprotinin, tranexamic acid and ε-aminocaproic acid have all been shown to reduce operative blood loss and transfusion requirements in liver transplantation. The use of these agents to reduce fibrinolysis associated with chronic liver disease is of uncertain value and their use in DIC is not recommended.

Other agents

Heparin and antithrombin

Their use in DIC has not led to significant improvements in blood loss or mortality and are therefore not recommended.

Estrogens

There are some reports on efficacy in bleeding related to chronic liver disease but further data from clinical trials is required before their use can be recommended.

Fibrin glue

Local endoscopic applications have been shown to be effective in the treatment of bleeding gastric varices.

Recombinant factor VIIa

Small studies have demonstrated reduced clotting times in chronic liver disease and a reduction in transfusion requirements in liver transplantation. The optimal role for recombinant factor VIIa in the treatment of liver coagulopathy has yet to be defined.

Further reading

Amirano L, Guardascione MA, Brancaccio V, Balzano A. Coagulation disorders in liver disease. *Semin Liver Dis* 2002;**22**:83–96.

Bernstein DE, Jeffers L, Erhardtsen E, *et al.* Recombinant factor VIIa corrects prothrombin time in cirrhotic patients: a preliminary study. *Gastroentrology* 1997;**113**:1930–7.

Datta D, Vlavianos P, Alisa A, Westaby D. Use of fibrin glue (beriplast) in the management of bleeding gastric varices. *Endoscopy* 2003;**35**(8):675–8.

DeLoughery TG. Management of bleeding with uremia and liver disease. *Thromb Haemost* 1999;**6**(5):329–33.

Narayanan KV, Shah V, Kamath PS. The Budd–Chiari syndrome. *N Eng J Med* 2004;**350**:578–85.

Porte RJ, Knot EA, Bontempo FA. Hemostasis in liver transplantation. *Gastroenterology* 1989;**97**:488–501.

Ratnoff OD. Hemostatic defects in liver and biliary tract disease. In: Ratoff OD, Forbes CD, eds. *Disorders of Hemostasis*. Philadelphia: WB Saunders, 1996:422.

Starzl TE, Demertris A, van Thiel DH. Liver transplantation. *N Engl J Med* 1989;**321**:1014–22, 1092–99.

Violi F, Ferro D, Basili S, *et al.* Hyperfibrinolysis resulting from clotting activation in patients with different degrees of cirrhosis. *Hepatology* 1993;**17**:78–83.

Chapter 20
Oncology

Anna Falanga and Marina Marchetti

Introduction

The association between cancer and thrombosis has been known for more than a century. The occurrence of venous thromboembolism as a common complication of cancer, which could often precede the onset of an occult neoplasia, was first reported by Armand Trousseau in 1865. Almost at the same time, the possibility that a relation between the clotting mechanisms and the development of metastasis might exist was postulated by Billroth in 1878.

In the last three decades remarkable progress has been made in this field, both by basic research and clinical studies. It is now clear that there is a two-way connection between coagulation and cancer:
• malignant disease results in a prothrombotic imbalance of the host hemostatic system; and
• prothrombotic mechanisms may promote tumor growth and dissemination.

Patients with cancer are exposed to a significant risk of thrombosis, particularly during chemotherapy and surgery. This situation is aggravated by the use of venous access catheters and antitumor drugs. Data derived from large randomized controlled trials have been used to determine the true incidence of this complication in cancer and its treatment; the incidence varies from 1% for limited stage patients with breast cancer treated with tamoxifen, to 60% for patients with any type of cancer who are subjected to orthopedic surgery and do not receive prophylactic therapy.

Very commonly, cancer patients present with abnormalities of laboratory tests of blood coagulation, even without clinical manifestations of thromboembolism and/or hemorrhage. These abnormalities reveal different degrees of blood clotting activation and characterize the so-called "hypercoagulable state" in these subjects. The results of laboratory tests in these patients demonstrate that a process of fibrin formation and removal is continuously ongoing during the development of malignancy.

The pathogenesis of thrombophilia in cancer is multifactorial; however, an important role is attributed to the tumor cell capacity to interact with and activate the host hemostatic system. Among other factors that contribute to the increased thrombotic diathesis in patients with cancer are the antitumor therapies.

Experimental studies show that fibrin and other coagulation proteins are involved in multiple steps of tumor growth and dissemination. Therefore, pharmacologic interventions to prevent thrombotic phenomena in malignancy may possibly contribute to the control of the malignant disease progression.

The aim of this chapter is to summarize the most recent advances in our knowledge on the thrombophilic state of cancer patients and the pathophysiologic mechanisms of blood clotting activation in this condition, giving also an overview of the current approaches to the prevention and treatment of venous thromboembolism (VTE) in cancer.

Clinical aspects

Although clinical manifest thrombosis in patients with cancer can involve both the venous and arterial systems (see Plate 8, facing p. 121), the thrombotic occlusions of the venous site have been more extensively studied (Fig. 20.1). VTE represents an important cause of morbidity in these patients;

Figure 20.1 Thrombotic disorders associated with cancer. Clinical manifestations of thrombosis in patients with cancer can vary from localized deep venous thrombosis, more frequent in solid tumors, to systemic syndrome, such as disseminated intravascular coagulation (DIC) with consumption of coagulation factors and platelets, which is generally associated with leukemias or widespread metastatic cancer.

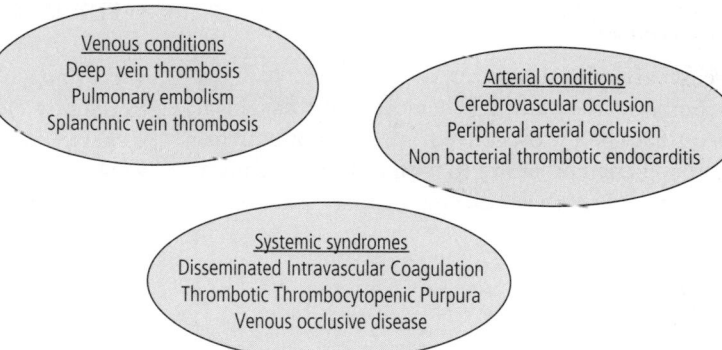

however, an exact quantification of the problem of VTE in cancer is not easy. Much of the early information comes from small series, retrospective analyses or autopsy studies.

Recently, our understanding of the epidemiology of VTE in cancer has started to become clearer with the advent of large, population-based studies, and data from prospective series describing outcome with regard to VTE. Deep vein thrombosis (DVT) of the lower limbs is the most common clinical manifestation in these patients. The next most common manifestations are DVT of upper limbs, pulmonary embolism, central sinus thrombosis and migratory superficial thrombophlebitis. Syndromes of more systemic involvement of the clotting system, such as disseminated intravascular coagulation (DIC) or thrombotic microangiopathy, have been described.

Occult malignancy

Thrombosis may be the earliest clinical manifestation of an occult malignancy. Initially, this observation was shown by anecdotal reports and retrospective clinical studies, but in more recent years this concept has become well documented. Particularly important is the clinical trial by Prandoni *et al.* (1992) which evaluated the occurrence of cancer after a first episode of VTE among 250 patients without cancer at diagnosis. This study clearly showed that patients with an "idiopathic" VTE episode have a four- to seven-fold increased risk of being diagnosed with cancer in the first year after thrombosis when compared with patients

with VTE secondary to known causes (e.g. surgery, congenital thrombophilia, oral contraceptives, pregnancy, immobilization). In the case of recurrent VTE, this risk is further raised by up to ten-fold.

In spite of this, the question as to whether aggressive diagnostic screening for cancer in patients with idiopathic DVT may lead to improved management of the malignant disease is so far unanswered.

In the prospective Italian multicenter study, "Screening for Occult Malignancy in patients with venous Thromboembolism" (SOMIT), extensive screening was found to be effective in identifying precociously an occult malignancy. Computerized tomography (CT) scanning of the abdomen and pelvis was the most effective diagnostic test, and CT scan and a gastrointestinal investigation (such as Hemoccult) was the best diagnostic combination. Larger clinical trials are needed to establish the impact of this finding on cancer survival.

Outcomes

Thrombotic events can influence the morbidity and mortality of the underlying disease. Epidemiologic data clearly show that patients with cancer have a significantly increased risk of having clinical overt thrombosis (secondary DVT) upon triggering conditions (e.g. long-term bed rest, trauma, surgery), compared with patients without malignancy. Medical treatments to cure cancer can worsen the patient's thrombophilic state and increase the thrombotic risk associated with this disease.

Breast cancer

Breast carcinoma is the only condition in which the thrombotic risk during chemotherapy has been quantified. In a prospective trial, 6.8% of patients receiving chemotherapy for stage II breast cancer developed thrombosis during the first 12 weeks of treatment.

Adenocarcinoma

Rectal cancer (particularly during radiotherapy), pancreatic cancer and advanced stage gastro-intestinal adenocarcinomas represent tumor categories likely to carry a high risk for VTE during pharmacologic treatment. However, in these conditions there are insufficient epidemiologic data to quantify this risk.

Drugs

There are insufficient data to identify drugs that can be directly incriminated, except for:
• L-Asparaginase in acute lymphoblastic leukemia (ALL); and
• tamoxifen, which has been shown to increase the thrombotic risk, independently from either tumor or chemotherapy.

Laboratory tests

Even without thrombosis and before any therapy, patients with cancer manifest multiple laboratory abnormalities of hemostasis that depict a hyper-coagulable state.

Routine laboratory tests

Coagulation profiles performed in the past have revealed that the most frequent routine abnormalities reported are:
• elevated plasma coagulation factor levels (i.e. fibrinogen, factors V, VIII, IX and X);
• increased levels of fibrin(ogen) degradation products (FDP or D-dimer); and
• thrombocytosis.

In two large prospective clinical trials evaluating routine coagulation tests on cancer patients:

• FDP levels and thrombin time were increased only in 8% and 14%, respectively.
• Fibrinogen and platelet count were found more frequently elevated (48% and 36% of the cases, respectively).
• The increase in the levels of these two markers over time directly correlated with the disease progression.
• Activation of the clotting system occurs in the absence of DIC or manifest thrombosis.

Specialized tests

Recently, the development of novel, more sensitive laboratory tests for the detection of the hyper-coagulable state or subclinical DIC (Table 20.1) has enabled the detection of markers of ongoing activation of blood coagulation *in vivo*.

These tests measure the final products of clotting reactions in plasma and include:
• Peptides released during the proteolytic activation of pro-enzymes into active clotting enzymes (i.e. prothrombin fragment 1 + 2 [F1 + 2], protein C activation fragment, factor IX and X activation fragments, fibrinopeptide A).
• Enzyme–inhibitor complexes produced during the activation of the coagulation and fibrinolytic systems (i.e. thrombin–antithrombin complexes [TAT], plasmin–antiplasmin complexes [PAP]).
• Cross-linked fibrin degradation product (i.e. D-dimer). Other markers are available to study the activation of cellular components of the hemostatic system, including platelets, leukocytes and endothelial cells.

Predictors of thrombosis

Studies on the plasma levels of these markers have provided a biochemical definition of the hypercoagulable state in humans. However, no studies of sound methodologic design have been performed to indicate if any of these tests of blood coagulation can serve as an adequate predictor of thrombosis in cancer patients. No studies have prospectively compared, in the same subjects, the levels of the plasma markers with the thrombotic events (confirmed by objective tests).

Recently, plasma markers of coagulation, fibrinolysis and activation of angiogenesis have

Table 20.1 Circulating markers of hemostatic system activation.

Coagulation
Activated factor VII (FVIIa)
Thrombin–antithrombin complex (TAT)
Prothrombin fragment 1 + 2 (F1 + 2)
Fibrinopeptide A and B

Fibrinolysis
Tissue plasminogen activator (tPA)
Plasminogen activator inhibitor type 1 (PAI-1)
Plasminogen
Plasmin–antiplasmin complex (PAP)
FDPs
Soluble fibrin
D-dimer

Platelets
β-Thromboglobulin
Platelet factor 4 (PF4)
TxA_2
Soluble P-selectin
Membrane CD62, CD63

Leukocytes
Monocytes
membrane Tissue Factor (mTF)
s-Tissue factor

Neutrophils
Membrane CD11b
Elastase
Myeloperoxidase

Endothelium
Thrombomodulin
Von Willebrand Factor (VWF)
tPA
PAI-1
s-E-selectin
s-VCAM-1 and s-ICAM 1
Tissue factor pathway inhibitor (TFPI)

been measured in cancer patients with acute VTE and compared with results from patients with VTE alone or cancer alone. While demonstrating enhanced coagulation activation in the setting of cancer patients with acute VTE, they do not give information on the clinical utility of measuring these markers in the single patient. Therefore, large studies are still required to answer the question as to whether the measurement of any of these laboratory markers may be useful in assessing the risk level in the individual.

Predictors of survival

Interestingly, a number of studies have been conducted with the aim of defining the predictive value of plasma markers for survival in different types of cancer. In a study of consecutive outpatients with different types of cancer, baseline TAT, fibrin monomer and D-dimer levels were predictive for survival at 1 and 3 years. Other small prospective studies have focused on specific types of cancer. Among these, a prognostic significance of TAT and PAP was found in the setting of lung cancer. However, other studies did not find any predictive value for plasma s-uPAR in breast cancer patients and for other fibrinolytic parameters in gastric cancer. Interestingly, plasma PAP levels were recognized to be useful in predicting fatal outcomes in the first 5 days after surgery for esophageal carcinoma.

Recently, an attempt has been made to establish whether the presence of a persistent biochemical hypercoagulabilty in clinically healthy men could predict for death from cancer. A study conducted on 3052 men from the UK National Health Service Central Registry found that subjects with hypercoagulability (defined as elevated F1 + 2 and FPA levels) have an increased risk of death from cancer.

Pathogenetic mechanisms

The activation of blood coagulation and thrombotic diathesis in patients with cancer is a complex and multifactorial phenomenon, which reflects the participation of different mechanisms. General mechanisms related to the host response to the tumor include the acute-phase reaction, paraprotein production, inflammation, necrosis and hemodynamic disorders, whereas tumor-specific clot promoting mechanisms include a series of prothrombotic properties expressed by tumor cells. In addition, an important part in cancer-related thrombosis is played by the procoagulant effects triggered by anticancer therapies (Fig. 20.2).

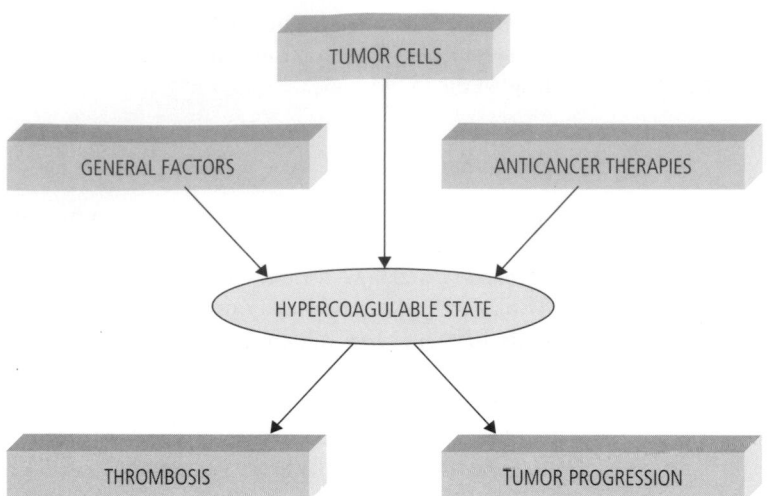

Figure 20.2 Mechanisms for activation of blood coagulation and thrombotic diathesis in patients with cancer. Even in the absence of overt clinical symptoms, almost all patients present with laboratory coagulation abnormalities, demonstrating a subclinical activation of blood coagulation, which characterizes a "hypercoagulable state." Multiple factors (i.e. general, tumor-specific and antitumor therapy-related) concur to the activation of blood coagulation and to thrombotic manifestation in cancer patients.

A. Tumor cell prothrombotic mechanisms

There are several ways in which tumor cells can interact with and activate the hemostatic system. The principal mechanisms can be summarized as follows:
- Production of tumor cell procoagulant activities, fibrinolytic proteins, and pro-inflammatory and pro-angiogenic cytokines.
- Direct interaction of tumor cell with host vascular and blood cells (i.e. endothelial cells, leukocytes and platelets) by means of adhesion molecules. All these properties are listed in Table 20.2.

A.1 Procoagulant activities

Tumor cells may express different types of procoagulants, the best characterized of which are:
- tissue factor (TF); and
- cancer procoagulant (CP).

Other tumor cell procoagulant activities described are:
- factor V receptor associated with vesicles shed from tumor cell plasma membranes, which facilitates the assembly of prothrombinase complex; and
- a factor XIII-like activity that promotes the cross-linking of fibrin.

TF is a transmembrane glycoprotein that forms a complex with factor VII (FVII)/FVIIa. The TF–FVII complex triggers blood coagulation by proteolytically activating factors IX and X. TF is the

Table 20.2 Tumor cell prothrombotic properties.

Expression of procoagulants that directly activate coagulation
Tissue factor
Cancer procoagulant

Release of pro-inflammatory and pro-angiogenic cytokines that stimulate the prothrombotic potential of endothelial cells
IL-1β, TNF-α, VEGF, FGF

Expression of fibrinolytic proteins
tPA, uPA, PAI-1 and PAI-2, uPAR

Expression of adhesion molecules for host vascular cells
Integrins, selectins, immunoglobulin family

procoagulant expressed by normal cells (including endothelial cells and monocyte–macrophages), which do not express TF in resting conditions, but expose this procoagulant in response to pro-inflammatory stimuli (i.e. interleukin-1β [IL-1β], tumor necrosis factor-α [TNF-α], bacterial endotoxin). Malignant cells are different in that they constitutively express TF in the absence of stimuli.

CP is a 68 kDa cysteine proteinase that activates FX independently of FVII. CP has been found in extracts of neoplastic cells or in amnion–chorion tissues but not in extracts of normally differentiated cells. CP antigen has been found to be elevated in 85% in the sera of cancer patients.

TF and CP have been identified in several human and animal tumor tissues. In recent years, a number of studies have characterized the procoagulant activities expressed by leukemic cells:

• Several authors have identified TF in leukemic cells.

• CP has been found in blasts of various acute myelogenous leukemia phenotypes, with the greatest expression in acute promyelocytic leukemia (APL) subtype.

• The differentiating treatment with all-*trans*-retinoic acid (ATRA) of APL blasts *in vitro* reduces the expression of both CP and TF.

• In patients with APL, the remission induction with ATRA treatment induces the rapid resolution of the severe coagulopathy of this disease and significantly affects the procoagulant activities expressed by the bone marrow cells *in vivo*.

• Similar observations have been reported for breast cancer.

Recent studies suggest a new role for TF in the tumor growth and metastasis, which is not entirely mediated via clotting activation, but may be dependent on signaling through the cytoplasmic domain, suggesting a "non-coagulation" role for TF in cancer disease.

A.2 Fibrinolytic activities

Tumor cells can express all the proteins of the fibrinolytic system, including the urokinase-type (uPA) and the tissue-type (tPA) plasminogen activators, and their inhibitors PAI-1 and PAI-2. Cancer cells also carry on their membranes the specific plasminogen activator receptor uPAR, which favors the assembly of all the fibrinolytic components, facilitating the activation of the fibrinolytic cascade. It has been suggested that in leukemia patients, the expression of these activities by blast cells may have a role in the pathogenesis of the bleeding symptoms.

An impaired plasma fibrinolytic activity has been found in patients with solid tumors, which represents *per se* another tumor-associated prothrombotic mechanism. Fibrinolysis is also a key component in tumor biology, as it is essential in releasing tumor cells from their primary site of origin, in neo-angiogenesis and in promoting cell mobility and motility. Fibrinolytic proteins are under evaluation as potentially valuable predictors

of disease-free interval and long-term survival in malignant disease. In breast cancer, patients with low levels of uPA and PAI-1 have a significantly better survival than patients with high levels of either factor, particularly in node-negative breast cancer.

A.3 Cytokine activity

Down-regulation of anticoagulant activity
Tumor cells synthesize and release a variety of cytokines and chemokines, which can act on the different hemostatic cells and affect their antithrombotic status:

• proinflammatory cytokines (i.e. TNF-α, IL-1β);
• proangiogenic cytokines (VEGF, bFGF).

These can induce the expression of TF procoagulant activity by endothelial cells. These cytokines also down-regulate the expression of thrombomodulin (TM), a potent anticoagulant, expressed by endothelial cell. TF up-regulation and TM down-regulation lead to a prothrombotic condition of the vascular wall.

Decreased fibrinolysis
The same cytokines stimulate endothelial cells to increase the production of the fibrinolysis inhibitor PAI-1, resulting in a subsequent inhibition of fibrinolysis, which further contributes to the prothrombotic potential of endothelial cells. Cytokines also contribute to enhance the adhesion potential of the vascular wall, through changes in the adhesion molecules of endothelial cells, which become more able to attract tumor cells of and support their extravasation.

Procoagulant properties
Further, tumor cells and/or tumor cell cytokines can induce the expression of monocyte TF. Mononuclear cell activation may occur *in vitro* and *in vivo*. Indeed, tumor-associated macrophages harvested from experimental and human tumors express significantly more TF than control cells. In addition, circulating monocytes from patients with different types of cancer have been shown to express increased TF activity. The generation of procoagulant activity by monocyte–macrophages *in vivo* is conceivably one mechanism for clotting activation in malignancy.

The cytokines and chemokines produced by malignant cells are also mitogenic and/or chemo-attractants for polymorphonuclear leukocytes. These cells, upon activation, secrete proteolytic enzymes, which can damage the endothelial monolayer, and produce additional cytokines and chemokines, which support tumor growth, stimulate angiogenesis and enable metastatic spread via engagement with either venous or lymphatic networks, but also produce VEGF which is chemotactic for macrophages and can induce TF procoagulant activity by monocyte and endothelial cell.

A.4 Cell adhesion molecules

During the hematogenous spread, tumor cells directly interact with endothelial cells, platelets and leukocytes. These interactions occur through surface cell-adhesion molecules (i.e. integrins, selectins and immunoglobulin superfamily). Particularly, the integrin family of cell-adhesion proteins promotes the attachment and migration of cells to the surrounding extracellular matrix (ECM). Through signals transduced upon integrin ligation by ECM proteins or immunoglobulin superfamily molecules, this family of proteins have key roles in regulating tumor growth and metastasis as well as tumor angiogenesis. Selectins are multifunctional cell-adhesion molecules that mediate the initial interactions between circulating leukocytes and activated endothelium as well as the adhesion reaction of tumors during malignancy.

The tumor cell capacity to adhere to the endothelium and the underlying matrix is well described and adhesion molecule pathways specific to different tumor cell types have been identified. The relevance of the tight interaction of tumor cell with endothelial cells in the pathogenesis of thrombosis in cancer is related to the localized promotion of clotting activation and thrombus formation. The tumor cell attached to endothelium releases its cytokine content into a protect milieu that favors their prothrombotic and proangiogenic activities. In addition, the adhesion of tumor cells to leukocytes or vascular cells represents the first step for cell migration and extravasation.

Experimental and *in vitro* studies have shown that polymorphonuclear leukocytes may function to promote tumor growth and metastasis. Tumor cell-derived factors can activate polymorphonuclear leukocyte function by up-regulating the expression of various adhesion molecules (i.e. the β_2-integrin CD11b/CD18) on leukocytes, which in turn attach to tumor cells and facilitate tumor cell migration through the endothelium. Similarly to leukocytes, clinical and experimental evidence suggests the importance of platelets in tumor cell dissemination via the bloodstream. Platelets can facilitate tumor cell adhesion and migration through the vessel wall by a variety of mechanisms, including bridging between tumor cell and endothelial cells, and by allowing migration of tumor cell through the endothelial cell matrix by heparanase activity.

Tumor cells can activate platelets directly or through the release of proaggregatory mediators including ADP, thrombin and a cathepsin-like cysteine proteinase. Upon activation, platelets aggregate and release their granule contents, as shown by the detection of elevated plasma levels of β-thromboglobulin and PF4, and increased platelet membrane antigens CD62P and CD63, in patients with malignancy.

In addition, activated platelets release VEGF and PDGF, which play an important part in the tumor neo-angiogenesis process.

B. Antitumour therapy prothrombotic mechanisms

The pathogenesis of thrombosis during antitumor therapies is not entirely understood, but a number of mechanisms have been identified (Table 20.3).

The first mechanism is caused by the release of procoagulants and cytokines by tumor cells damaged by chemotherapy (Fig. 20.3). The possible role of cytokine release in response to chemotherapy in increasing the thrombotic risk was suggested by experiments showing that plasma samples collected from women with breast cancer after

Table 20.3 Antitumor therapy prothrombotic mechanisms.

Release of procoagulants and cytokines from damaged cells
Direct drug toxicity on vascular endothelium
Induction of monocyte tissue factor
Decrease of physiological anticoagulants
Apoptosis

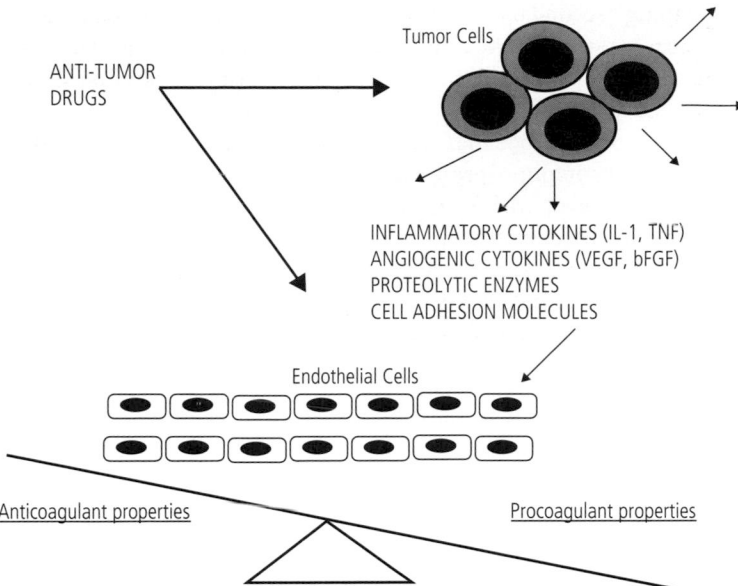

Figure 20.3 Antitumor therapy prothrombotic mechanisms. Tumor cells perturbed by antitumor drugs release a series of soluble mediators (i.e. proinflammatory and proangiogenic cytokines, proteolytic enzymes), which can act on endothelial cells by altering their normal antithrombotic and antiadhesive status or by damaging the endothelial monolayer, with the subsequent exposure of the highly procoagulant endothelial cell matrix. The same antitumor drugs can up-regulate the expression of adhesion molecules by tumor cells which become more adhesive towards the endothelium.

chemotherapy contained higher levels of mediators (likely cytokines) able to increase the reactivity of endothelial cells to platelets.

The direct damage exerted by chemo-radiotherapy on vascular endothelium represents another mechanism of drug-induced thrombosis.

Radiation therapy can cause endothelial injury, as demonstrated by the release of von Willebrand protein from endothelial cells irradiated with doses up to 40 Gy. In animal studies, bleomycin has been demonstrated to determine morphologic damage to the vascular endothelium of the lung, resulting in pulmonary thrombosis and fibrosis. In some experimental models, adriamycin can directly affect glomerular cells, impairing their permeability and leading to a nephrotic syndrome, accompanied by hypercoagulation and increased thrombotic tendency. Anti-angiogenetic drugs, such as thalidomide and SU5416, an anti-VEGF receptor, represent a new class of substances with endothelial toxic activity. In myeloma patients, an increased rate of VTE is associated with thalidomide therapy, especially when given in combination with chemotherapy.

The pathogenetic mechanisms underlying this prothrombotic effect are under evaluation. A significant increase in circulating markers of endothelial cell activation has been observed in cancer patients during anti-angiogenic therapy with SU5416, particularly in those patients experiencing a thromboembolic event. Profound changes in plasma markers of endothelial damage have been reported in patients receiving different types of chemotherapy. Some chemotherapeutic agents can directly stimulate the expression of TF procoagulant activity by macrophages and monocytes, thus inducing a procoagulant response from host cells.

The final mechanism observed involves the reduction in the plasma levels of natural anticoagulant proteins (antithrombin, protein C and protein S), which is a well-known risk factor for thrombosis, and is likely to be a consequence of a direct hepatotoxicity by radio- and chemotherapy.

Prevention and treatment of thrombosis in cancer

Prophylaxis of venous thromboembolism

Patients with diagnosed malignant disease are at an increased risk of developing "secondary" VTE in specific conditions (e.g. surgery, immobilization). These patients have been stratified by the Consensus Conference of the American College of Chest Physicians (ACCP) in their highest risk category for developing "secondary" VTE. In addition, the risk of recurrences is significantly increased in cancer compared with non-cancer patients, even during treatments for VTE.

There is no evidence that there is a benefit from giving antithrombotic prophylaxis to all cancer patients; however, there are indications to give prophylaxis in selected conditions carrying additional risk factors, such as surgical interventions; central venous catheters (CVC); administration of antitumor therapies and prolonged bed rest.

Cancer surgery

Cancer surgery carries a two- to three-fold increase in thrombotic risk compared with non-cancer surgery of equal intensity. Perioperative prophylaxis with low doses of unfractionated heparin (UFH) or with fixed dose low molecular weight heparin (LMWH) is effective in significantly reducing the incidence of postoperative VTE. LMWH has a good safety profile also in this condition. Further, a higher dose of LMWH has been shown to be more effective than a lower dose in surgical cancer patients, without increasing the hemorrhagic risk. A prolonged duration of postoperative prophylaxis up to 1 month after surgery for cancer carries an additional and significant benefit in reducing the incidence of "secondary" postoperative VTE.

Medical conditions

The advantages of thromboprophylaxis in non-surgical conditions, such as in patients with CVC or during chemotherapy, is still under evaluation. The true incidence of CVC-related thrombotic complications in cancer patients is not definitively established and it varies significantly on the basis of the diagnostic criteria utilized (i.e. from 0.02 to 0.92 symptomatic venous thromboses/1000 catheter days). The rate of thrombosis is much higher in those prospective studies in which asymptomatic thromboses are detected. The calculated rate of asymptomatic thromboses (i.e. venographically proven) is 30–62% compared with 4–19% of symptomatic clinically manifest thromboses.

The efficacy of prophylaxis with 1 mg/day fixed dose warfarin or with LMWH in reducing the CVC-

associated thrombosis (venographically assessed) was demonstrated some years ago, but more recent studies have failed to confirm these data. The decrease in incidence of CVC-related thrombosis in recent studies is believed to result from the use of newer catheters made from less thrombogenic materials.

The role of thromboprophylaxis in patients receiving chemo- and/or hormone therapy is still undefined because of the insufficient available information. Breast carcinoma is the only condition in which the thrombotic risk during chemotherapy has been accurately quantified. The analysis of randomized clinical trials to evaluate the efficacy of various treatments in this tumor type has provided useful information:

• The incidence of thrombotic complications in breast cancer is low (0.2–0.9%) in the absence of any treatment.

• The start of chemotherapy increases this incidence up to 5–13%, with the higher rate in the postmenopausal group (age > 50 years).

• The advanced stage of the disease further increases the thrombotic risk up to 17.5% in patients given chemotherapy for treatment of metastatic disease.

• The addition of tamoxifen to chemotherapy increments the thrombotic risk in comparison with chemotherapy alone and with tamoxifen alone.

In all of the above trials, the thrombotic events occurred during the administration of polychemotherapy courses (particularly within 7–9 months). However, it is not possible to identify the responsibility of a single drug over the others.

A randomized controlled trial of thromboprophylaxis demonstrated that low-dose warfarin (international normalized ratio [INR] range 1.3–1.9) is effective and safe in reducing the incidence of thrombosis in women with stage IV metastatic breast cancer receiving chemotherapy. In other tumor types and the respective treatments, there is not the same evidence available, although some useful information is deducible for ovarian carcinoma, cerebral glioblastomas and non-Hodgkin lymphomas.

The problems encountered using warfarin prophyaxis have prevented its use on a large scale. At present, indications for this type of prophylaxis are

Table 20.4 Advantages of low molecular weight heparin (LMWH) over oral anticoagulants.

Body weight adjusted dose without need for laboratory monitoring

Induction of a uniform anticoagulant response, as they are not sensitive to interference by other drugs or diet

Rapid onset of action and predictable clearance, which facilitate their management in case of interruptions/restorations of anticoagulation, when required (i.e. for thrombocytopenia or invasive procedures)

Rarely associated with heparin-induced thrombocytopenia

limited to cases considered at very high risk. The advent of LMWH has raised interest in this area because there is no need for laboratory monitoring and there is lower toxicity in terms of heparin-induced thrombocytopenia and osteoporosis (Table 20.4).

Treatment of venous thromboembolism

In general, treatment of newly diagnosed VTE in cancer patients follows the same lines as in patients without cancer. LMWH or UFH are administered for 5–7 days concomitantly with warfarin and thereafter vitamin K antagonists are continued for at least 3 months.

Complication rates

Oral anticoagulant therapy remains troublesome in cancer patients with VTE, and is associated with a higher number of failures (high rate of thrombotic relapses during anticoagulant treatment) and a higher rate of hemorrhagic complications compared with non-cancer patients.

Furthermore, the hemorrhagic risk can be aggravated by concomitant thrombocytopenias, secondary to the myelosuppressive effect of chemotherapeutic agents. Other problems during oral anticoagulant therapy in these patients may result from the invasive procedures (e.g. endoscopies, biopsies), which can require temporary discontinuation of treatment. Interruptions in anticoagulation coverage make the dose adjustment more difficult and, because of the narrow therapeutic window of these agents, unpredictable variations in the INR can lead to excessive bleeding or recurrent thrombosis.

In addition, infections, medications, malnutrition, gastrointestinal absorption and hepatic dysfunction may alter the dose–response to anticoagulants with important fluctuation of INR values with a consequent need for more frequent blood testing.

Clinical trials

New trials in these patients are addressing the issues of the duration and intensity of oral anticoagulation or are focusing on new modalities to treat thrombosis.

LMWHs have been the first antithrombotic agents to be evaluated for the long-term therapy of VTE in malignancy as they offer a number of potential advantages (Table 20.4). Furthermore, preliminary data from meta-analyses suggest a favorable role of these drugs on cancer survival.

The international randomized multicenter CLOT trial comparing long-term therapy with the LMWH dalteparin versus warfarin for a first episode of VTE in cancer patients has been recently published. The results show a 50% risk reduction of recurrence in the arm receiving LMWH, with no significant difference in bleeding complications. Therefore, long-term VTE treatment with LMWH can represent valuable choice for patients with cancer and venous thrombosis.

A number of studies are currently ongoing evaluating LMWH survival as a primary endpoint in patients with cancer. Preliminary results give some interesting suggestions in this direction, but no definite conclusions can be drawn from the data available so far.

Further reading

Barbui T, Finazzi G, Falanga A. The impact of all-*trans*-retinoic acid on the coagulopathy of acute promyelocytic leukemia. *Blood* 1998;**91**:3093–102.

Bertomeu MC, Gallo S, Lauri D, Levine MN, Orr FW, Buchanan MR. Chemotherapy enhances endothelial cell reactivity to platelets. *Clin Exp Metastasis* 1990;**8**:511–18.

Falanga A. Thrombosis and malignancy: an underestimated problem. *Haematologica* 2003;**88**:607–10.

Falanga A, Rickles FR. Pathophysiology of the thrombophilic state in the cancer patients. *Semin Thromb Haemost* 1999;**25**:173–82.

Falanga A, Marchetti M, Vignoli A, Balducci D. Clotting mechanisms and cancer: implications in thrombus formation and tumor progression. *Clin Adv Hematol Oncol* 2003;**1**:673–8.

Kuenen BC, Levi M, Meijers JCM, *et al.* Analysis of coagulation cascade and endothelial cell activation during inhibition of vascular endothelial growth factor/vascular endothelial growth factor receptor pathway in cancer patients. *Arterioscler Thromb Vasc Biol* 2002;**22**:1500–5.

Lee AYY, Levine MN, Baker RI, Bowden C, *et al.* for the CLOT Investigators. Low molecular weight heparin versus a coumarin for the prevention of recurrent venous thromboembolism in patients with cancer. *N Engl J Med* 2003;**349**:146–53.

Prandoni P, Lensing AWA, Buller HR, *et al.* Deep-vein thrombosis and the incidence of subsequent symptomatic cancer. *N Engl J Med* 1992;**327**:1128–33.

Rickles FR, Levine MN. Epidemiology of thrombosis in cancer. *Acta Haematol* 2001;**106**:6–12.

Verso M, Agnelli G. Venous thromboembolism associated with long-term use of central venous catheters in cancer patients. *J Clin Oncol* 2003;**19**:3665–75.

Zacharski LR, Ornstein DL. Heparin and cancer. *Thromb Haemost* 1998;**80**:10–23.

Chapter 21
Transfusion

Adrian Copplestone

Introduction

The most common request to hematologists for help in the emergency management of patients in the hospital setting, relates to the control of hemorrhage and the use of blood products. Whereas most treatment involves the use of purified drugs, blood and blood products are derived from human blood donors. They are rarely pure, they are subject to biologic variation and carry the risk of infection. This chapter discusses some of these issues and describes their use in specialized clinical settings.

Blood transfusion as a form of transplantation

Transfusion with red cells and other blood products is a form of tissue transplantation, which is made easier because the cells lack some or all of the HLA antigens. Because cells lack progenitor capacity, the benefit is temporary but allows time for the body's homeostatic processes to recover.

Table 21.1 Common red cell blood group systems.

Blood group	Gene location
ABO	9q34.1-q34.2
Rhesus	1p36.11
Lewis	19p13.3
Kell	7q33
Duffy	1q22-23
Kidd	18q11-q12
MN	4q28-31
Ss	4q28-31

However, the transfused cells contain surface proteins that are foreign to the host and give rise to an immune reaction. The common red cell blood grouping systems are listed in Table 21.1. The most important is the ABO group because individuals have naturally occurring circulating immunoglobulin M (IgM) antibodies to the A and B groups they lack, and these antibodies have the capacity to cause intravascular hemolysis and can lead to disseminated intravascular coagulation (DIC).

Red cell cross-matching

Just 100 years ago, Landsteiner discovered blood groups. Transfusion from donor to patient became feasible when it was possible to determine blood groups and store the blood in an anticoagulated form. In recent years, the speed of matching suitable blood for a patient has been enabled by:
• Monoclonal antibodies to achieve more consistent blood grouping results (phenotype).
• Knowledge of genetic basis of blood group to determine the genotype where relevant.
• Use of cell panels with wide representation of antigens to enable the exclusion of allo-antibodies (antibody screening).
• Use of new technologies to enhance the antibody–antigen reaction (low ionic strength saline, gel tubes, microtiter plate capture).

Confidence in the blood group results and the detection of clinically relevant allo-antibodies has led to increasing acceptance of electronic cross-matching, where the donor cells and patient serum is not actually tested against each other but a negative result is predicted.

These advances have dramatically reduced the time needed to supply suitable blood, enabling many operations to go ahead on a "blood grouped and screen basis." It also enables blood to be used in a more efficient manner and reduces waste because of expiry. However, the speed of the process may lead clinicians to forget that when antibodies are present or develop, more steps are necessary to provide suitable blood and this takes longer. In many circumstances (but not all) group O, Rh D-negative blood products may be required.

Risks of transfusion

Donor screening and testing have reduced the risks of transfusion but it should always be remembered that this process can never be "100% safe". New infections emerge and sometimes the steps taken to improve blood safety adversely affect other blood products.

Infective risks

Infections can be transmitted by transfusion by a wide variety of organism. Examples are listed in Table 21.2. Donor screening is designed to select out potential donors who are at higher risk of infection because of lifestyle or travel. All donor blood is tested for HBsAg, and antibodies to HIV1 and HIV2, syphilis, hepatitis C virus (HCV), human T cell leukaemia virus (HTLV) and some donors for cytomegalovirus (CMV). Despite these tests, there exist a small number of donors who are infected but lack antibody – this will be reduced further by nucleic acid testing (NAT) using polymerase chain reaction (PCR) technology to look for viral genome.

New agents (e.g. West Nile virus) continue to emerge as pathogens. Steps taken to reduce these risks include donor lifestyle screening, antibody testing, leukodepletion and DNA/RNA testing. For plasma products it is also possible to heat treat, nanofilter or disrupt lipid membranes with solvents, methylene blue and using psoralens with ultraviolet light.

Widespread leukodepletion was introduced in the UK in 1998 to reduce the risk of transmission

Table 21.2 Examples of transfusion transmitted infections.

Viruses	Hepatitis A
	Hepatitis B
	Hepatitis C
	HIV
	HTLV 1 & 2
	CMV
	EBV
	Parvovirus
Bacteria	*Treponema pallidum* (syphilis)
	Borrelia burgdorferi (Lyme disease)
	Staphylococcus spp.
	Diphtheroids
	Salmonella spp.
	Pseudomonas spp.
	Yersinia spp.
Protozoa	*Plasmodium* spp. (malaria)
	Toxoplasma gondii (toxoplasmosis)

CMV, cytomegalovirus; EBV, Epstein–Barr virus; human T cell leukaemia virus (HTLV).

of variant Creutzfeldt–Jakob Disease (vCJD). In addition, there was a major shift of procurement of plasma for plasma products from areas without bovine spongiform encephalopathy (BSE) – primarily the USA. No test is currently available to detect the abnormal prion. BSE has been transmitted in sheep by transfusion and in the UK, by 2004, there have been two cases of vCJD transmission by blood transfusion.

Transfusion reactions

Immediate hemolytic reactions

These are likely to be associated with shock, renal failure and DIC. The most common cause is patients receiving the wrong blood, 70% because of the labeling or checking errors at the bedside or in the laboratory. These errors are preventable by the adherence to clear transfusion protocols.

Delayed hemolytic reactions

These are usually caused by extravascular hemolysis and the boosting of allo-antibody levels.

Febrile transfusion reactions

Less common now that universal leukodepletion is in place, these are caused by the presence of cytokines and HLA antibodies. Urticarial and allergic reactions can still occur.

Transfusion-related acute lung injury

Transfusion-related acute lung injury (TRALI) is caused by donor leukocyte antibodies which cause adult respiratory distress syndrome. The patient becomes acutely short of breath and often requires artificial ventilation and circulatory support. TRALI needs to be distinguished from circulatory fluid overload which can occur following the transfusion of large volumes, especially in older patients.

Immunization

Alloimmunization can affect the efficacy of transfusion, especially platelets. It may also affect the subsequent choice of donors for organ transplantation. Immunomodulation can follow transfusion with an increase in infections and increase in relapse of carcinoma following surgery to patients who were transfused.

Post-transfusion purpura

Post-transfusion purpura (PTP) (Fig. 21.1) is a rare complication where severe thrombocytopenia occurs approximately 1 week after transfusion. The recipient is usually HPA1a-negative and HLA DR3*1010 and has anti-HPA1a antibodies, although on rare occasions other platelet groups are implicated. Treatment is high-dose intravenous immunoglobulin (IVIg).

Blood products available

Red cells

Whole blood

Donor blood is anticoagulated in 10% citrate anticoagulant and during storage the labile coagulant

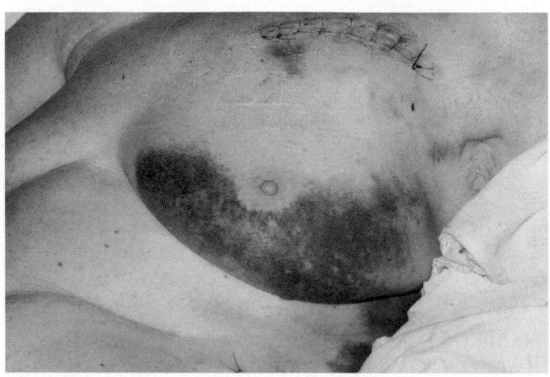

Figure 21.1 Post-transfusion purpura presenting with ecchymosis in a female patient with a platelet count of 10×10^9/L, subsequently shown to be HPA-1a negative with anti-HPA-1a antibodies. Transfusion had been given preoperatively. Reprinted from *Blood in Systematic Disease*, Greaves, 1997, with permission from Elsevier.

factors V and VIII and platelets are lost within a few days. Little whole blood is used in the UK because transfusion practice has adopted a component approach.

Leukodepleted red cells in additive solution

These donor cells collected in citrate anticoagulant, the white cells are removed by filtration and the red cells are stored in saline, adenine, mannitol and glucose (SAG-M). With storage at 4°C, the red cells have a 35-day shelf-life.

Washed red cells

For patients who have severe reactions to leukodepleted blood, or who have IgA deficiency, red cells washed in saline can remove plasma proteins that cause the reactions.

Frozen red cells

These are used for patients with rare blood groups. The red cells are frozen in glycerol as cryoprotectant and washed before use.

Platelets

Platelet concentrates are prepared from either:
• plateletpheresis of donors using a cell separator machine; or
• combining platelet-rich plasma from buffy coats and packed in four-donor pools.

At present, the shelf-life of platelet concentrates is only 5 days (with testing taking up the first 24–48 h), but the use of additive solution may extend this to 7 days.

Platelets are used to correct bleeding resulting from thrombocytopenia or abnormal platelet function, with the exception of immune thromocytopenia purpura (ITP), thrombotic thrombocytopenia (TTP) and heparin-induced thrombocytopenia (HIT). The latter two conditions are associated with thrombosis and platelet transfusions can exacerbate the disease.

Fresh frozen plasma

Fresh frozen plasma (FFP) is used to correct coagulation deficiencies and there has been considerable debate on the relative merits of different products.

In the ideal world, FFP would provide high concentrations of the relevant factor, be from a low number of screened regular donors, have a viral inactivation step in the production that does not adversely affect the coagulation factors, be procured in a country where BSE is not endemic, come from male donors (to reduce the risk of TRALI) and have appropriate ABO group.

The following are available:
• Single donor FFP.
• Methylene blue treated FFP for pediatric use is a single-donor product, procured in the USA. In the UK, it is used primarily for children born after January 1, 1996 when the risk of vCJD from meat was minimized, but its use will extend to other age groups as it becomes more available.
• Solvent detergent FFP (Octaplas®) is a pooled product that is solvent treated to reduce the infective risks. It is used in large quantities in TTP because it is low in high molecular weight multimers of von Willebrand factor (VWF), but it has been associated with thrombosis because of protein S deficiency.

British Committee for Standards in Haematology (BCSH) guidelines suggest that:
• FFP should only be used to replace single inherited clotting factor deficiencies for which no virus-safe fractionated product is available. Currently, this applies mainly to factor V.
• FFP is indicated when there are demonstrable multifactor deficiencies associated with severe bleeding and/or DIC. However, FFP is not indicated in DIC with no evidence of bleeding.
• FFP should not be used to reverse warfarin effect in the absence of bleeding as it has an incomplete effect and is not an ideal product as large quantities are required.

Cryoprecipitate

Cryoprecipitate forms when FFP is thawed slowly and the product, which is refrozen, is rich in fibrinogen, factors VIII and XIII. It is commonly used in the treatment of DIC to replace fibrinogen.

The complementary product **cryosupernatant** has been used in conjunction with plasmapheresis in TTP as it lacks high molecular weight multimers of VWF.

Human albumin solution

The final product of the plasma fractionation process, human albumin solution (HAS), comes in two strengths: 4.5 g/dl and 20 g/dl (salt-poor albumin). It is an important colloid for maintaining the oncotic pressure in the intravascular compartment, and its main indication relates to replacing albumin in severe edematous states. Its use as plasma expander has largely been superseded by crystalloids and gelatin solutions.

Intravenous immunoglobulin

IVIg solutions are pooled normal human donor immunoglobulins. In the coagulation disorders they are used as an immunomodulator for the treatment of ITP and PTP.

Coagulation factor concentrates

Concentrates are prepared from large pools of

donor plasma. They all have steps to reduce viral contamination and most have steps to remove impure proteins. Increasing use of recombinant coagulation factors as these become available is being encouraged:

- Factor VIII for hemophilia A. Some of the intermediate purity products contain useful amounts of VWF as well.
- Factor IX for hemophilia B.
- VWF concentrates are now available for von Willebrand disease (VWD).
- Prothrombin complex concentrate (combined factors II, VII, IX and X concentrate) is primarily used in the correction of life-threatening hemorrhage in patients on oral anticoagulants.
- Individual concentrates for factors VII, X, XIII and fibrinogen are available for patients with hereditary deficiencies.

Fibrin sealants

Mixing thrombin and fibrinogen forms "fibrin glue" which is applied to the site of bleeding and is a popular treatment in neurosurgery.

Autologous blood

In many situations it is possible to use the patient's own blood and thereby avoid exposure to the risks of donor blood. However, there are still risks with using autologous blood, mainly related to bacterial infection and the blood being transfused to the wrong patient. A number of approaches are possible.

Predeposit donation

Blood is venesected prior to elective surgery and retained for up to 4 weeks. By retransfusing older blood during the collection process, up to 4 units of blood can be stored. Surgery must take place on the planned date or the blood may expire.

Cell salvage

Blood can be aspirated during an operation and washed red cells returned to the patient. This is useful in vascular surgery and is also finding a place in cardiac surgery and trauma patients.

Intraoperative hemodilution

Blood is venesected at the time of anesthesia and crystalloid is used as fluid replacement. If bleeding occurs, less red cells are lost because of the lower hematocrit. At the end of the operation the blood, which also contains coagulation factors and platelets, is retransfused.

Cell salvage from wound drains

Blood is drawn into a sterile container by suction and transfused. This application has been used extensively in orthopedic surgery and has reduced the need for blood in joint replacement operations.

Drugs that reduce the need for transfusion

A number of drugs are used to either boost the hemostatic system or reduce fibrinolysis. Drugs that can increase the red cells mass are also important.

Desmopressin (DDAVP)

This analogue of antidiuretic hormone is used in mild hemophilia, VWD and some platelet disorders. Endothelial stores of VWF are released. Repeated administration is subject to tachyphylaxis.

Tranexamic acid and other fibrinolytic inhibitors

These are useful in major surgery but use needs to be balanced against the risk of venous thromboembolism (VTE). They are also useful in patients with marrow failure with mucosal bleeding from chronic thrombocytopenia in patients who are refractory to platelet transfusions.

Aprotinin is a bovine protease inhibitor which inactivates plasmin and kallikrein. It is used in cardiac surgery in patients on cardiopulmonary bypass.

Iron

There are many patients who have low iron stores or frank deficiency as a consequence of chronic hemorrhage, either through the disease process or the result of treatment (e.g. non-steroidal anti-inflammatory drugs). Correction with small doses of iron to improve compliance can avoid the need for transfusion. Where anemia has developed slowly, patients can tolerate quite low hemoglobin levels. Treatment with iron and patience are much safer than "top-up transfusions."

Vitamins

Other vitamins (such as folic acid) may also be required in anemic patients with poor intake (elderly or malabsorption) or increased turnover (pregnancy).

Erythropoietin

Erythropoietin (rhEPO) can be useful to boost the erythron. Concomitant iron therapy may also be needed to achieve a rapid response. Its cost has restricted its use in clinical practice, but many patients with renal failure no longer require regular transfusion.

Recombinant activated factor VII

This recombinant protein (rFVIIa) was originally used in hemophiliacs with inhibitors, but it is now increasingly being used in patients with severe bleeding from multiple trauma or major bleeding in a critical care situation.

Use of blood products

How much to give?

The decision of when to transfuse and how much to give can be difficult. In general, the rule should be to try to avoid transfusion if possible, but if it is necessary, to use sufficient quantities of the right product to achieve the desired effect (usually hemostasis).

Guidelines on the use of red cells have previously advised transfusion based of the reduction of red cell mass, but this can be difficult to estimate in clinical practice. As a result, "Hb triggers," have increasingly been used in the management of patients, particularly in the postoperative setting. In a landmark study, Hébert *et al.* showed that in patients in a critical care unit, a restrictive transfusion policy (Hb trigger 7.0 g/dL, aim Hb 7–9 g/dL) had a lower mortality than a more liberal policy (Hb trigger 10 g/dL, aim Hb 10–12 g/dL), with the possible exception of patients with acute myocardial infarction and unstable angina.

Although Hb trigger levels are easy for clinical teams to use, other factors also affect the Hb level and the Hb trigger level may need to be adjusted for individual patients based on comorbidities. Other measures may usefully aid the decision as to whether to transfuse, such as the rate of post-operative bleeding. Where this has been measured for a cohort of patients (e.g. postcardiac bypass surgery), deviations from the usual course can be spotted more rapidly and appropriate action taken. Similarly, if more attention was paid to improving anemia preoperatively, there would be less need for transfusion.

Assessment of hemorrhage

In situations where patients are bleeding, the first question is to determine whether this is surgically correctable. Simultaneously, blood should be sent for blood count and coagulation studies. The prothrombin time (PT) and activated partial thromboplastin time (APPT), combined with supplementary tests – fibrinogen level, thrombin time, equal volume mix with normal plasma – usually give an indication as to the type of hemostatic defect. Confirmation with specific factor levels can follow if necessary.

Blood sampling is important as these patients often have multiple cannulas and it is important that the sample is not taken through a line contaminated with heparin. The drug chart should be examined especially for anticoagulants, anti-fibrinolytics and antiplatelet drugs.

Near patient testing

Because coagulation tests take at least 20 min to complete (and usually longer, taking sample transport into account), there has been a move to use near patient testing (NPT) with a number of different devices.

• *Whole blood clotting time:* ACT – this is used in cardiac surgery to monitor heparin effect.

- *PT and APTT devices* (e.g. Coaguchek): these are designed mainly for testing patients on oral anticoagulants.
- *Thromboelastogram:* the TEG® is described in more detail in Chapter 18, and is used in liver and cardiac units. It gives information relating to platelet function, clot strength and fibrinolysis within approximately 15 min.
- Platelet function analyses (PFA-100®): an *in vitro* bleeding time test whose current role is determining mild VWD and platelet defects.

Although many hematologists dislike NPT equipment as being "uncontrolled" and lacking some of the strict supervision of laboratory procedures, the immediacy of results will lead to their increased use and both laboratory and clinical teams should work together to define their role in decision making.

Importance of good communication

When dealing with complex patients there needs to be good communication between the clinical team and the transfusion, hematology and coagulation laboratories. The hematologist is ideally suited to advise on suitable blood products, facilitate testing to minimize delays, ensure that blood products are dispatched rapidly and anticipate future requirements especially if the source of supply is offsite.

Special situations

Disseminated intravascular coagulation

DIC often requires transfusion of coagulation factors and platelets (see Chapter 10). Consumption of products may be dramatic and regular coagulation tests are required to guide therapy, although treatment is based on the degree of bleeding and organ failure rather than abnormalities in the tests. To reverse the process, the underlying cause must be treated.

Massive transfusion

The replacement of the blood volume with stored blood lacking platelets and factors VIII and V leads to mucosal bleeding and generalized ooze at operative sites. Recognition of the condition and correction with platelet and FFP transfusion, based on laboratory clotting studies, is usually all that is required. Antifibrinolytic drugs can help but their use can increase the risk of VTE.

Cardiac surgery

Cardiac surgery uses approximately 10% of the blood supply and is a major user of FFP, second only to critical care units (FFP) and oncology (platelets). This is discussed in detail in Chapter 18.

Obstetrics

Major hemorrhage in obstetrics is an emergency. It can occur for a number of reasons (Table 21.3). It can be dramatic and in rare cases of maternal mortality, the severity of the situation has often not been recognized. It requires immediate resuscitation, using the group O Rhesus D negative emergency blood if necessary, and ABO matched blood, FFP and platelets dispatched without delay. Further hematological support will depend on coagulation studies. DIC may be present.

Every obstetric unit should have a **major hemorrhage protocol**, agreed with the hematology laboratory. Good communication with the clinical team, laboratory and hematologist is essential.

Pediatrics

Neonates and young children have a number of considerations with respect to hemostasis and transfusion:

- Their size means that much smaller volumes are used.
- Donor exposure should be kept to a minimum.

Table 21.3 Causes of hemorrhage associated with pregnancy.

Ectopic gestation
Abortion
Placental abruption
Placenta praevia
Postpartum: atonic uterus, trauma due to childbirth, coagulation disorders

- Their relatively immature immune systems means that they may not make some antibodies (e.g. anti-A and anti-B) so that blood grouping will be different to adults (i.e. no reverse grouping available).
- Often group O red cells are used, but the plasma should not contain high-titer anti-A or anti-B antibodies. Similarly, note should be taken when using large volumes of FFP or platelets as red cell hemolysis resulting from ABO incompatibility has been reported.
- Their blood may contain maternal IgG antibodies (e.g. hemolytic disease of the newborn).
- Neonates who have received transfusion *in utero*, and children with immunodeficiency require irradiated blood products (to reduce the risk of transfusion-associated graft-versus-host disease).
- Severe coagulation disorders may present in the neonatal period. Coagulation studies can be difficult to perform and repeated tests will lead to institutional anemia.
- Neonatal thrombocytopenia may have an infective or immune basis. Treatment depends on the cause.

Jehovah's Witnesses

Jehovah's Witnesses belong to the Watch Tower Bible and Tract Society. They believe that transfusing blood is equivalent to eating it and this is prohibited by scripture. Although they refuse transfusion, they accept modern medical care and technology. As mentally competent adults, they have a right to refuse treatment. The situation is more complex in unconscious adults and children. Exactly which blood product is refused is an individual decision, although often guided by church elders (Table 21.4).

Surgery should be planned to minimize blood loss, with good consultation between patient, surgeon, anesthetist and hematologist. The patient should sign an Advance Directive.

Conclusions

Good transfusion practice in treating coagulation disorders is a combination of thinking ahead to reduce the need for transfusion and using the appropriate product in the right quantity. Clear

Table 21.4 Acceptance of blood products by Jehovah's Witnesses.

Refused	Accepted	Variable
Red cells	Crystalloids	Albumin
White cells	Synthetic colloids	Immunoglobulin
Platelets	EPO	Vaccines
Plasma	GCSF	Coagulation factors
	rFVIIa	Cell salvage
		Organ transplant

EPO, erythropoietin; GCSF, granulocyte colony-stimulating factor; rFVIIa, recombinant factor VIIa.

documentation of the reasons for transfusion and good institutional protocols also help.

Further reading

British Committee for Standards in Hematology

Guidelines for the use of platelet transfusions. *Br J Haematol* 2003;**122**:10–23.

Clinical use of red cell transfusion. *Br J Haematol* 2001;**113**:24–31.

Guidelines for the administration of blood and blood components and the management of transfused patients. *Transfus Med* 1999;**9**:227–39.

Guidelines for the use of fresh Frozen Plasma, Cryoprecipitate and Cryosupernatant. *Br J Haematology* 2004;**126**:11–28.

Hébert PC, Wells G, Blajchman MA, *et al.* A multicenter, randomized, controlled clinical trial of transfusion requirements in critical care. *N Engl J Med* 1999;**340**:409–17.

McClelland DBL. *Handbook of Transfusion Medicine*. Norwich: HMSO, 2001.

Murphy MF, Pamphilon DH. *Practical Transfusion Medicine*. Oxford: Blackwell Science, 2001.

Websites of interest

BCSH guidelines: www.BCSHguidelines.com
www.dh.gov.uk/PolicyandGuidance(BloodSafety)
www.transfusionguidelines.com
Guide to perioperative transfusion from Scottish Intercollegiate Guidelines Network: www.sign.ac.uk/guidelines/fulltext/54/index.html
National Blood Service: www.blood.co.uk/hospitals/guidelines/index.htm
Serious Hazards of Transfusion: http://www.shotuk.org

Normal ranges

Steve Kitchen and Michael Makris

Adult reference range

Interpretation of any laboratory result requires its comparison with a reference range based on the performance of the test in healthy normal individuals. The reference range is more commonly referred to as the normal range. The selection of individuals for testing and construction of reference ranges is important. Health is not well defined and results of some coagulation tests are influenced by age, sex, hormone replacement therapy, some oral contraceptive pills and blood group, which would suggest that matched normal ranges should be available. Effects of this type include increasing concentrations of factors VII, VIII:C, IX and fibrinogen with age. In the case of FVIII:C and von Willebrand factor (VWF) there are highly significant differences according to the blood group of the subject, with levels approximately 25% lower in group O individuals compared with non-O blood groups. However, many centers do not take this latter effect into account when screening for von Willebrand disease (VWD) because the clinical management will normally depend on the levels of FVIII and VWF in relation to the clinical needs of the patient irrespective of blood group.

The lower levels of protein S activity in women compared with men are probably sufficiently great (approximately 20% different at age under 45 years) that this should be taken into account when interpreting results obtained by some methods. In general, establishing these types of group-specific reference ranges may not always be practical and clinically it is of debatable value for many hemostatic parameters.

When constructing normal ranges the samples from normal subjects should be collected, processed and analyzed locally using identical techniques to those used for the analysis of the patient samples. The literature and reagent manufacturer's information should only be used as a guide. In the case of some activated partial thromboplastin time (APTT) reagents, there is sufficient variation between different production lots or batches of the reagent to affect the results obtained. In this case it is necessary to reassess the normal range before introducing a new lot number. This should also be the case for other screening tests including the prothrombin time (PT).

The reference or normal range is usually constructed from individual results in such a way that it contains 95% of the reference distribution. When the results are normally distributed, the normal range is conventionally calculated to be the mean plus or minus 2 standard deviations, which include 95% of the population. If the results are not normally distributed, other statistical tests such as log transformation should be used first to obtain a normally distributed population. In some cases non-parametric methods may be used to identify the central 95% of values.

The number of normal subjects required for analysis and construction of a normal range depends on a number of issues. From a statistical validity aspect, the number of subjects required is considered to be at least 40 and preferably at least 120. However, for many tests of hemostasis, the effect of increasing numbers of subjects from 25–30 up to more than 40 leads to entirely minor and clinically irrelevant differences in the calculated ranges and in these cases 25–30 is adequate. Results of normal subjects can be inspected graphically to identify skewedness or particularly to identify outliers amongst the group. Any outliers (i.e. any result that lies unexpectedly far from the majority of others) should then be excluded from calculations. This can be done statistically but visual inspection is normally sufficient.

Reference intervals may be required for patient groups other than healthy normal subjects to take account of particular physiological or pathological states. Because of considerable variations in the concentration of clotting factors during pregnancy and development, specific normal ranges for neonatal, pediatric and pregnant subjects should be available. This is a particular problem where, because of ethical and practical reasons, it is virtually impossible for each laboratory to establish their own neonatal normal ranges, so many laboratories use the same published ranges in newborns. Data on the expected results of clotting tests in older children have also been published. For these studies it is important to note that ranges for screening tests are only appropriate for the particular technique used in the study, whereas the results of clotting factor assays are normally influenced much less by the method employed and may therefore be a useful guide to centers employing other techniques.

In some cases, the effects of drugs on coagulation tests should be taken into account. For example, if attempting to diagnose protein C (PC) or protein S (PS) deficiency during oral anticoagulant therapy a reference range constructed from subjects receiving oral anticoagulant prophylaxis is necessary to take account of the reductions in PC and PS induced by the therapy.

In general, the normal range should be used only as a guide and an aid to clinical interpretation in conjunction with all other available relevant clinical information. The most appropriate normal reference range is one that has been established locally using the same system as for patient samples. It is important to use a technique for which such a local range is in broad agreement with the published literature.

The following are the reference ranges used at the Royal Hallamshire Hospital in Sheffield, UK at the time of publication of this book.

General tests

Prothrombin time	10–12 s
APTT	24–36 s
Thrombin time	24–32 s
Fibrinogen	1.7–3.3 g/L
FDP	< 8 µg/mL
D-Dimer	< 0.25 µg/mL
Platelet count	$150–400 \times 10^9$/L
Reptilase time	Control time ± 2 s

Lupus tests

DRVVT ratio	0.9–1.09
DRVVT 50/50 ratio	0.9–1.09
Exner KCT 80/20 ratio	< 1.2
Anticardiolipin IgG	< 8.0 IU
Anticardiolipin IgM	< 5.0 IU
Anti-beta II glycoprotein	< 8.8

Bleeding disorders

Bleeding time (simplate)	< 8.0 min
FVIII:c	0.52–1.40 IU/mL
FVIII:VWFAg	0.46–1.46 IU/mL
FVIII:Rcof	0.50–1.72 IU/mL
Platelet FVIII:VWFAg	$0.144–0.367$ IU/10^9 platelets
Platelet FVIII:Rcof	$0.126–0.420$ IU/10^9 platelets
FIX	0.62–1.44 IU/mL
FII:C	0.66–1.06 IU/mL
FV	0.73–1.37 u/mL
FVII	0.60–1.56 IU/mL
FX	0.79–1.31 IU/mL
FXI	0.60–1.39 u/mL
FXII	0.51–1.47 u/mL
FXIII screen	Negative
FXIII	0.75–1.55 u/mL
PIVKAII	< 0.8 ng/ml
α_2-Antiplasmin	0.67–1.03 u/mL

Thrombotic disorders

Antithrombin activity	0.84–1.17 IU/mL
Antithrombin antigen	0.83–1.24 IU/mL
Ratio of AT act/ag	0.93–1.08
Plasminogen activity	0.75–1.31 u/mL

Plasminogen antigen	0.76–1.36 u/mL
Protein C activity	0.71–1.42 IU/mL
Protein C antigen	0.75–1.31 IU/mL
Ratio of PC act/ag	0.59–1.47
FII:Ag	0.72–1.20 IU/mL
Ratio of PC/FII Ag	0.62–1.54
FVII:Ag	0.58–1.60 IU/mL
Ratio of PC/FVII Ag	0.67–1.73
FX:Ag	0.60–1.34 IU/mL
Ratio of PC/FX Ag	0.80–1.58
Protein S Total	0.71–1.36 IU/mL
Protein S Free	0.64–1.31 IU/mL
C4BP Ag	0.43–1.45 u/mL
Patio of PS Act/Ag	0.70–1.26
Fragment F 1 + 2	0.10–1.06 nmol/L
Protein S antigen Total on warfarin	0.49–0.87 IU/mL
Protein S antigen Free on warfarin	0.27–0.79 IU/mL
APC resistance ratio	2.77–4.31
APC resistance ratio (V-corr)	1.96–2.45

Platelet aggregation

ADP threshold	1–3 µmol
Adrenaline threshold	< 3 µmol
Collagen threshold	< 2 µg/mL
Ristocetin threshold	0.7–1.0 mg/mL

Platelet parameters

Beta thromboglobulin	< 58 ng/mL
Platelet TXB2 to 4 µg collagen	6.9–27.5 pmol/ 10^7 platelets
Platelet TBX2 to 1.5 mmol arachidonic acid	87.3–172.2 pmol/ 10^7 platelets
Platelet ATP release to 4 µg collagen	0.7–2.25 nmol/ 10^8 platelets
Platelet ATP release to 1.5 mmol arachidonic acid	1.0–5.14 nmol/ 10^8 platelets
Platelet nucleotide ATP	2.66–8.40 nmol/ 10^8 platelets
Platelet nucleotide ADP	1.07–6.45 nmol/ 10^8 platelets
Platelet nucleotide AMP	0.07–1.32 nmol/ 10^8 platelets
Platelet ATP/ADP	0.93–1.83
5-HT uptake at 30 min	35–92%
5-HT uptake at 60 min	44–97%
5-HT uptake at 90 min	45–92%
5-HT leakage	< 8%
5-HT release to 4 µg collagen	12–61%
5-HT release to thrombin	69–92%
Spontaneous platelet aggregation	Nil

Pregnancy normal ranges

Few laboratories have specific normal ranges for pregnant subjects. It is rarely necessary to have a precise range, but it is important for clinicians to be aware of the range and type of changes that occur during this period. The following table from a published study indicates some of the hemostatic variables that change during pregnancy. Shown are the mean values and the calculated normal ranges from the mean ± 2 standard deviations (Adapted from Kjellberg *et al. Thrombosis and Haemostasis* 1999;**81**:527–31.)

Variable (non-pregnant normal range)	Pregnancy (weeks gestation)				Postpartum	
	10–15	*23–25*	*32–34*	*38–40*	*1*	*8*
Classic APCR (> 2.3)						
Mean	2.89	2.74	2.64	2.66	2.87	3.16
Normal range	2.33–3.45	2.18–3.30	2.16–3.12	2.02–3.30	2.09–3.65	2.34–4.00
Modified APCR (V depleted) (> 2.0)						
Mean	2.63	2.59	2.57	2.62	2.68	2.71
Normal range	2.39–2.87	2.35–2.83	2.35–2.79	2.36–2.88	2.40–2.96	2.43–2.99
FVIII:C IU/mL (0.50–2.0)						
Mean	1.41	1.69	2.06	2.31	2.24	1.25
Normal range	0.51–2.31	0.81–2.49	1.02–3.10	1.43–3.19	0.86–3.62	0.49–2.01
Fibrinogen g/dL (2.0–4.0)						
Mean	3.3	3.5	4.1	4.5	4.6	2.6
Normal range	2.1–4.5	2.3–4.7	2.9–5.3	3.5–5.5	3.2–6.0	1.8–3.4
Protein C IU/mL (0.70–1.25)						
Mean	0.95	1.04	1.02	1.00	1.16	1.02
Normal range	0.65–1.25	0.68–1.40	0.64–1.40	0.62–1.38	0.76–1.56	0.68–1.36
Free protein S IU/mL (0.63–1.12)						
Mean	0.62	0.53	0.51	0.51	0.59	0.74
Normal range	0.36–0.88	0.35–0.71	0.33–0.69	0.31–0.71	0.27–0.91	0.52–0.96
D-dimer ng/mL (< 120)						
Mean	35	81	130	193	251	11
Normal range	0–93	0–175	0–286	0–417	0–867	0–22

Neonatal normal range

Reference values for coagulation tests in the healthy full term infant during the first 6 months of life. Values shown are mean with the normal range based on mean ± 2 standard deviations. (Adapted from Andrew M, Paes B, Johnston M. Development of the hemostatic system in the neonate and young infant. *Am J Pediatr Hematol Oncol* 1990;**12**:95–104.) *Values are indistinguishable from those of the adult.

Tests	Day 1	Day 5	Day 30	Day 90	Day 180	Adult
PT (s)	13.0 (10.1–15.9)*	12.4 (10.0–15.3)*	11.8 (10.0–14.2)*	11.9 (10.0–14.2)*	12.3 (10.7–13.9)*	12.4 (10.8–13.9)
INR	1.00 (0.53–1.62)	0.89 (0.53–1.48)	0.79 (0.53–1.26)	0.81 (0.53–1.26)	0.88 (0.61–1.17)	0.89 (0.64–1.17)
APTT (s)	42.9 (31.3–54.5)	42.6 (25.4–59.8)	40.4 (32.0–55.2)	37.1 (29.0–50.1)*	35.5 (28.1–42.9)*	33.5 (26.6–40.3)
TCT (s)	23.5 (19.0–28.3)*	23.1 (18.0–29.2)	24.3 (19.4–29.2)*	25.1 (20.5–29.7)*	25.5 (19.8–31.2)*	25.0 (19.7–30.3)
Fibrinogen (g/L)	2.83 (1.67–3.99)*	3.12 (1.62–4.62)*	2.70 (1.62–3.78)*	2.43 (1.50–3.79)*	2.51 (1.50–3.87)*	2.78 (1.56–4.00)
FII (u/mL)	0.48 (0.26–0.70)	0.63 (0.33–0.93)	0.68 (0.34–1.02)	0.75 (0.45–1.05)	0.88 (0.60–1.16)	1.08 (0.70–1.46)
FV (u/mL)	0.72 (0.34–1.08)	0.95 (0.45–1.45)	0.98 (0.62–1.34)	0.90 (0.48–1.32)	0.91 (0.55–1.27)	1.06 (0.62–1.50)
FVII (u/mL)	0.66 (0.28–1.04)	0.89 (0.35–1.43)	0.90 (0.42–1.38)	0.91 (0.39–1.43)	0.87 (0.47–1.27)	1.05 (0.67–1.43)
FVIII (u/mL)	1.00 (0.50–1.78)*	0.88 (0.50–1.54)*	0.91 (0.50–1.57)*	0.79 (0.50–1.25)*	0.73 (0.50–1.09)	0.99 (0.50–1.49)
VWF (u/mL)	1.53 (0.50–2.87)	1.40 (0.50–2.54)	1.28 (0.50–2.46)	1.18 (0.50–2.06)	1.07 (0.50–1.97)	0.92 (0.50–1.58)
FIX (u/mL)	0.53 (0.15–0.91)	0.53 (0.15–0.91)	0.51 (0.21–0.81)	0.67 (0.21–1.13)	0.86 (0.36–1.36)	1.09 (0.55–1.63)
FX (u/mL)	0.40 (0.21–0.68)	0.49 (0.19–0.79)	0.59 (0.31–0.87)	0.71 (0.35–1.07)	0.78 (0.38–1.18)	1.06 (0.70–1.52)
FXI (u/mL)	0.38 (0.10–0.66)	0.55 (0.23–0.87)	0.53 (0.27–0.79)	0.69 (0.41–0.97)	0.86 (0.49–1.34)	0.97 (0.67–1.27)
FXII (u/mL)	0.53 (0.13–0.93)	0.47 (0.11–0.83)	0.49 (0.17–0.81)	0.67 (0.25–1.09)	0.77 (0.39–1.15)	1.08 (0.52–1.64)

Test	Day 1	Day 5	Day 30	Day 90	Day 180	Adult
Antithrombin (u/mL)	0.63 (0.39–0.87)	0.67 (0.41–0.93)	0.78 (0.48–1.08)	0.97 (0.73–1.21)*	1.04 (0.84–1.24)*	1.05 (0.79–1.31)
Protein C (u/mL)	0.35 (0.17–0.53)	0.42 (0.20–0.64)	0.43 (0.21–0.65)	0.54 (0.28–0.80)	0.59 (0.37–0.81)	0.96 (0.64–1.28)
Protein S (u/mL)	0.36 (0.12–0.60)	0.50 (0.22–0.78)	0.63 (0.33–0.93)	0.86 (0.54–1.18)*	0.87 (0.55–1.19)*	0.92 (0.60–1.24)

Further reading

Andrew M, Paes B, Milner R, *et al.* Development of the human coagulation system in the full-term infant. *Blood* 1987;**70**:165–72.

Andrew M, Vegh P, Johnston, Bowker J, Ofosu F, Mitchell L. Maturation of the hemostastic system during childhood. *Blood* 1992;**80**:1998–2005.

Gill JC, Endres-Brooks J, Bauer PJ, Marks WJ, Montgomery RR. The effect of ABO blood group on the diagnosis of von Willebrand's disease. *Blood* 1987;**69**:1691–5.

International Federation of Clinical Chemistry (IFCC) and International Committee for Standardization in Hematology (ICSH). Approved recommendation on the theory of reference values, 1987. *J Clin Chem Clin Biochem* 1987;**25**;645–56.

Kjellberg U, Andsersson NE, Rosen S, Tengborn L, Hellgren M. APC resistance and other haemostatic variables during pregnancy and puerperium. *Thromb Haemost* 1999;**81**:527–31.

Lowe GDO, Rumley A, Woodward M, *et al.* Epidemiology of coagulation factors, inhibitors and activation markers: the third Glasgow MONICA survey I. Illustrative reference ranges by age, sex and hormone use. *Br J Haematol* 1997;**97**:775–84.

Appendix 2
Useful websites

Michael Makris

For all websites you will need to add the prefix http://
Although most websites start with www after the prefix this is not always the case.

Guidelines

British Committee for Standards in Haematology: www.bcshguidelines.org
The Thrombosis Interest Group of Canada: www.tigc.org
Seventh ACCP Consensus Conference on Antithrombotic Therapy:
www.chestjournal.org/content/vol126/3_suppl/index.shtml
Scottish Intercollegiate Guidelines Network (SIGN): www.sign.ac.uk/
SIGN Antithrombotic therapy guideline: www.sign.ac.uk/guidelines/fulltext/36/
Royal College of Obstetricians and Gynaecologists: www.rcog.org.uk/guidelines.asp?PageID=106

Societies and organizations

International Society for Haemostasis and Thrombosis: www.med.unc.edu/isth
American Society for Haematology: www.hematology.org
European Haematology Association: www.ehaweb.org/
College of American Pathologists: www.cap.org
British Society for Haematology: www.b-s-h.org.uk
British Society for Haemostasis and Thrombosis: med6.bham.ac.uk/bsht
Australian Society for Thrombosis and Haemostasis: www.asth.org.au/
Mediterranean League against thromboembolic diseases: www.medleague-thrombosis.org
World Federation of Haemophilia: www.wfh.org
The Haemophilia Society: www.haemophilia.org.uk
National Hemophilia Foundation: www.hemophilia.org

Journals

Internal medicine

New England Journal of Medicine: www.nejm.org
Annals of Internal Medicine: www.annals.org
Archives of Internal Medicine: archinte.ama-assn.org/
The Lancet: www.thelancet.com
British Medical Journal: www.bmj.org

Hematology

Blood: www.bloodjournal.org
British Journal of Haematology: www.blackwell-science.com/bjh
The Hematology Journal: www.nature.com/thj/
European Journal of Haematology: www.blackwellpublishing.com/ejh
Blood Reviews: www.harcourt-international.com/journals/blre/
Haematologica: www.haematologica.org
Haematology: www.tandf.co.uk/journals/titles/10245332.html
Clinical and Laboratory Haematology: www.blackwellpublishing.com/clh
Best Practise & Research Clinical Haematology: www.harcourt-international.com/journals/beha/
Current Opinion in Hematology: www.co-hematology.com/

Hemostasis

Journal of Thrombosis and Haemostasis: www.journalth.com
Thrombosis and Haemostasis: www.schattauer.de/zs/startz.asp
Circulation: circ.ahajournals.org/
Atherosclerosis Thrombosis and Vascular Biology: atvb.ahajournals.org/
Blood Coagulation and Fibrinolysis: www.bloodcoagulation.com/
Pathophysiology of Haemostasis and Thrombosis:
 content.karger.com/ProdukteDB/produkte.asp?Aktion=JournalHome&ProduktNr=224034
Thrombosis Research: www.elsevier.com/locate/thromres
Platelets: www.tandf.co.uk/journals/titles/09537104.html
Seminars in Thrombosis and Hemostasis: www.thieme.de/sth/
Haemophilia: www.blackwellpublishing.com/journal.asp?ref=1351-8216&site=1
Vascular Medicine: www.vascularmedjournal.com/

Mutation databases

Hemophilia A: europium.csc.mrc.ac.uk/WebPages/Main/main.htm
Hemophilia B: www.kcl.ac.uk/ip/petergreen/haemBdatabase.html
Factor XIII: www.med.unc.edu/isth/mutations-databases/Factor_XIIIA.htm
Factor XI: www.med.unc.edu/isth/mutations-databases/Factor_XI.htm
Factor X: www.med.unc.edu/isth/mutations-databases/Factor_X.htm
Factor VII: 193.60.222.13/index.htm
Factor V: www.med.unc.edu/isth/mutations-databases/Factor_V.htm
Factor V + VIII: www.med.unc.edu/isth/mutations-databases/combined_FV_&_VIII.htm
Fibrinogen: www.geht.org/databaseang/fibrinogen/
Prothrombin: www.med.unc.edu/isth/mutations-databases/prothrombin.htm
Von Willebrand disease: www.sheffield.ac.uk/vwf/
Glanzmann thrombasthenia: sinaicentral.mssm.edu/intranet/research/glanzmann/menu
Antithrombin: www1.imperial.ac.uk/medicine/about/divisions/is/haemo/coag/antithrombin/default.htm
Protein C: www.xs4all.nl/%7Ereitsma/Prot_C_home.htm

Index